Headache

HEADACHE
Through the Centuries

Mervyn J. Eadie MD, PhD

Emeritus Professor of Clinical Neurology and Neuropharmacology
Honorary Research Consultant
University of Queensland
Brisbane, Australia

OXFORD
UNIVERSITY PRESS

OXFORD
UNIVERSITY PRESS

Oxford University Press, Inc., publishes works that further Oxford University's objective of excellence in research, scholarship, and education.

Oxford   New York
Auckland   Cape Town   Dar es Salaam   Hong Kong   Karachi   Kuala Lumpur   Madrid   Melbourne
Mexico City   Nairobi   New Delhi   Shanghai   Taipei   Toronto

With offices in
Argentina   Austria   Brazil   Chile   Czech Republic   France   Greece   Guatemala   Hungary   Italy
Japan   Poland   Portugal   Singapore   South Korea   Switzerland   Thailand   Turkey   Ukraine
Vietnam

Published by Oxford University Press, Inc.
198 Madison Avenue, New York, New York 10016
www.oup.com

Oxford is a registered trademark of Oxford University Press

Library of Congress Cataloging-in-Publication Data
Eadie, Mervyn J.
  Headache : through the centuries / Mervyn J. Eadie.
    p.; cm.
  Includes bibliographical references and index.
  ISBN 978-0-19-986097-5 (hardcover : alk. paper)
  I. Title.
  [DNLM: 1. Headache—history. 2. Headache Disorders—history. WL 11.1]
  616.8'4914—dc23
                                        2011039086

9 8 7 6 5 4 3 2 1
Printed in the United States of America
on acid-free paper

CONTENTS

PREFACE

At least in modern times, there would probably be relatively few people who could truthfully assert that they had never experienced headache (or "headach" in its earlier spelling) at any stage in their lives, so long as they had reached at least their middle years. So frequently indeed is headache encountered in medical practice that, a century ago, the London physician Samuel Gee (1908) seems to have thought it worth mentioning, as the 188th in his list of *Aphorisms*: "Some people seem incapable of headache, even when they suffer from disease which is usually accompanied by this symptom, i.e. typhoid fever" (p. 285). More than two centuries earlier, Thomas Willis (1621–1675), Sedlian Professor of Natural Philosophy in the University of Oxford (Hughes 1991; Isler 1968), had similarly acknowledged the high prevalence of headache in the community. He wrote, at the outset of his chapter on *De Cephalalgia*, which appeared at the beginning of the second part of his *De Anima Brutorum* (1672), a work "English'd" by Samuel Pordage in 1683 as *Two Discourses Concerning the Sole of Brutes*:

> The pain of the Head is wont to be accounted the chiefest of the Diseases of the Head, and as it were to lead the troops of the other Affections of that part; for that it is the most common and most frequent symptom, to which indeed there is none but is sometimes obnoxious, so that it has become a Proverb, as a sign of a more rare and admirable thing, *that his Head did never ake.* (p. 105)

The beginnings of the human experience of headache are now lost, probably irretrievably, in the impenetrable obscurity of prehistory. However, the story of the symptom can be traced back through some six millennia of existing records. Over that long period of time a great deal has been written about the disorder, and undoubtedly a great deal more spoken but not committed to more durable form. Yet, until little more than half a century ago, scientific work concerning headache, when any was done, was mainly observational and interpretative, and the experimental approach was hardly utilized. Before comparatively recent times, the situation tended to be, as the Guy's Hospital, London, physician William Moxon in 1875 somewhat pungently put it:

> Now these headaches, which are not pains in the special organs of the head itself, have been a good deal written about in a semi-popular sort of way; opinions about them in plenty have been given, opinions which express not the knowledge of the opiner, but his sense of saying something advantageous, whereof his conscience is almost the only check.... Every old woman, or nearly every old woman, is an authority on headache in this general way. Indeed it is not easy to find any other good authorities on them. (p. 749)

That situation has changed rapidly in the past few decades, with a flowering in published scientific work on headache, but also with a considerable growth in "popular" writing on the topic, some of it of rather variable, if not of dubious, scientific quality.

In this time of growing interest in the disorder, a number of short- and medium-length accounts of the history of headache have been published. Some of this historical writing seems more concerned with recording the historical material itself than with systematically interpreting how headache has been understood at different times. It therefore seems that there might be a place for a longer account of the history of knowledge of human headache, especially its more scientific aspects, that takes a particular interest in the ways the symptom has been understood and that translates the understanding into attempts to benefit headache sufferers.

This book has resulted from the perception of Craig Panner, of Oxford University Press, that there might be a place for such a work at the present time. I am very grateful to him for the suggestion that I might attempt to write it, and for all his help, and that of his Oxford University Press colleagues, particularly Kathryn Winder and Emily Perry. I am also grateful to Smitha Raj and Veena Deepak, of Glyph International, who saw the book through its production stages, and to Mary Anne Shahidi, for her meticulous copyediting and unfailing tact when drawing attention to the embarrassingly numerous errors and infelicities that she detected in the text.

It would have been difficult to have practiced clinical neurology over much of a professional lifetime without having acquired at least some interest in headache, that most common of all presenting neurological symptoms. I do appreciate the knowledge and insights that I have gained from listening to the accounts of headache sufferers over the years, and for the understandings that an increased acquaintance with the earlier headache literature has brought me during the writing of this book.

Until quite recent years, gaining access to much of the earlier medical literature was often rather difficult, tedious, and protracted for someone working in a relatively newly settled country such as Australia, distant from the centers of European civilization, and where library collections rarely contain material more than two centuries old. This situation has been transformed by the almost instant access to such early material that is now possible by virtue of electronic communications and the activities of numerous unnamed librarians and their staffs throughout the world who have ensured that material from their collections has increasingly been made available in electronically transmissible form. To them, and in particular to those responsible for the invaluable resources at the BIUM (Bibliothèque Interuniversitaire de Médicine) and EEBO (Early English Books Online) websites, I offer most grateful thanks. I suspect that the resources that they have made available may have shortened the time of writing of this book by as much as a year. What they have already done has provided an enormous blessing to those interested in the earlier medical literature.

I would also like to express my gratitude to those who have provided illustrations, or permission to use illustrations, for this book, especially the staff of the Wellcome Library, London, of the Royal College of Physicians of London, Sage Publications, and Oxford University Press, and also to Professor Ann Scott for making available a photograph of her great grandfather, Sir William Gowers.

Last, I would express my gratitude to Margaret, who has shared life with me over these many years and who, without vocal protest, has endured my repeated withdrawals from her presence to sit in front of a computer or in an armchair, pen in hand, paper on lap, with the surrounding floor and nearby table submerged in books and photocopies. Whether she will regard the completion of this book with unalloyed pleasure or merely with relief is, like some aspects of the understanding of headache, a matter still to be settled.

Mervyn Eadie
Brisbane
August 2011

INTRODUCTION

Before taking up the actual topic of this book—namely, the history of the human encounter with headache and the development of the understanding of the disorder—there are several matters that may seem largely of a technical nature but may be advantageous to mention.

First, it should be appreciated that in what follows, the history of headache has been approached predominantly from a medical standpoint and with a particular interest in the ways in which the disorder has been understood from time to time, trying to relate the understandings to the patterns of thought through which Western medicine has evolved. To have traced the history of the understanding of headache in non-Western cultures would have required talents and knowledge that I lack. Further, a superficial attempt to look at the matter even in relation to a modern account of Chinese medicine (Liu and Liu 2009) led to a realization that the understanding of the disorder in that tradition is so different to the Western one that it seems almost impossible to equate the major types of headache in the two traditions in any manageable way.

In this book, approaches to the understanding of headache from other than a medical standpoint—for example, from the sociological, the psychological, or perhaps the religious—would have been possible. However, it can be argued that the medical one has, so far, yielded greater benefits for headache sufferers than the others, and therefore is the one best pursued. This course of action raises the question of whether events in the past should be related primarily to medical knowledge as it existed in the times when the events occurred, or to present-day medical understandings. From a purely historical perspective, the former approach may have been more appropriate. However, over much of its history headache has been classified and thought about in ways that do not readily interdigitate with present-day medical thinking. It therefore seems that it may be more useful to the prospective contemporary reader to try to interpret the past in relation to modern concepts, while also trying to maintain sympathy with earlier ideas and events as they were understood in their own day.

There is also the issue of the point in time when the account ceases to deal with what is historical and begins to abut on the present, when the present itself is merely an ever-changing moment between past and future. This is a matter of some importance at a time when the scientific understanding of headache and its mechanisms is growing apace. On purely arbitrary grounds, the year 2000 A.D. has been taken as the later limit of headache history for the purposes of this book, though that limit has then been treated as somewhat flexible. Material that became available after 2000 and that throws important light on earlier material has not been ignored, but other post-2000 material has not been used, important though it may prove to be in the future.

A further issue is the range of headache types whose histories are to be pursued. The present-day internationally agreed classification of headache types includes an extensive array of entities. Should each be dealt with individually? It is generally believed that headache is a symptom and not a disease in its own right, but it is also realized that in the majority of headache sufferers no causal disease can yet be identified, so that their headaches are regarded as primary ones. To have attempted to deal with the histories of all the symptomatic (i.e., secondary) varieties of headache and the diseases that may cause them would have been an almost prohibitive task, and perhaps would not have been of great value when headache is often only an occasional and relatively unimportant manifestation of the recognized underlying pathologies. Therefore the topic of this book has been limited to that of the history of the primary headaches. Of course, in the past, when the diagnostic capacity of medicine was much more limited than it now is, headache that would now be considered symptomatic would sometimes have been regarded as a disorder in its own right, in other words, as falling into a primary headache category. Historical material concerning such headache has been regarded as dealing with primary headache for the purposes of the present account, unless it is completely clear that, in the light of latter-day knowledge, such material must have been dealing with a specific manifestation of now recognizable disease.

Writing on the history of headache depends heavily on access to relevant documents from the past. Many such documents were written in languages other than English. One must then rely on the adequacy of the translations made by others, or on one's own decidedly limited efforts to convert other languages into English. There is always the possibility that a translator who lacks medical knowledge will fail to perceive the medical import of a particular wording in an original; there is also the converse danger that a translator with modern medical knowledge may tend to read this knowledge into material where the originator did not intend it. Further, the material translated may not be the original version of a text, but a transcript into which inadvertent errors or transcribers' interpretations have already found their way. From some of the early surviving material, it is clear that authors have sometimes borrowed from other even earlier writings that have subsequently been lost. There is in addition a tendency, pervasive in medical writing in earlier times, to include material without formal acknowledgment of its sources. As a result, later attributions of priority and of information sources may prove to be incorrect. The material quoted in various parts of this book, almost always originally written in English or subsequently translated into English, has been left with its spelling unmodernized, in the expectation that this will probably not unduly trouble the reader.

When the classificational criteria for the major types of contemporary primary headaches are applied to pre-19th-century materials dealing with the symptom, it soon becomes apparent that there often is not sufficient detail available to permit headache type categorization. As will be explained in more detail later, over the years a number of authors have taken the view that, because the word *migraine* is derived from the Latin *hemicrania*, the two words are essentially interchangeable in relation to identifying this particular contemporary type of headache. Undoubtedly this will often be the case, simply on probability grounds in that migraine is such a frequent type of headache in the community.

However, some authors in more recent centuries have acknowledged that the earlier category of *hemicrania* also included entities such as unilateral frontal sinusitis and supraorbital and trigeminal neuralgia. Moreover, accounts of what probably was migraine, but where the headache was not unilateral in its distribution, may be found in earlier writings on *cephalalgia* and *cephalaea*. The present account has taken the stance that *hemicrania* and migraine in the literature do not necessarily refer to the same entity, and has treated the earlier literature conservatively in this regard. The idea of migraine as a distinct headache entity began to emerge in the medical, as distinct from the lay, literature in the later decades of the 18th Century. At about the same time, the centuries-old main headache categories of *cephalalgia, cephalaea,* and *hemicrania* began to disappear in the wake of the attempt to classify all disorders on the basis of their underlying structural pathologies.

Up to the end of the 18th century, the history of headache can be dealt with as a whole, largely regardless of headache category, in view of the rather poor correlation between the old and the modern headache types. Thereafter, partly as a result of the growing bulk of the available material, there are advantages in taking up the histories of the major modern-day headache categories individually. Admittedly, this arrangement results in a disadvantage in that some clearly identifiable material relating to members of these modern headache categories can be found in the pre-1800 literature, and therefore needs to be mentioned twice over, to ensure that particular topics can be followed from their beginnings.

As the outcome of these considerations, this book has been organized into chapters dealing seriatim with the history of the headache as follows:

Chapter 1	Headache and Its Classification
Chapter 2	The "Seat" of Headache
Chapter 3	Headache before 1800
Chapter 4	Migraine: Clinical Phenomena
Chapter 5	Migraine: Pathophysiology
Chapter 6	The Treatment of Migraine
Chapter 7	The Trigeminal Autonomic Cephalalgias
Chapter 8	Tension-Type Headache
Chapter 9	Cranial Neuralgias
Chapter 10	Some Thoughts from the History of Headache

Hopefully, mentioning these various matters at the outset may help explain the approach that has been adopted in the present book to the history and understanding of headache.

Headache

CHAPTER 1
Headache and Its Classification

Those who often speak with headache sufferers soon learn that not all headaches are identical, even those occurring in the same individual at different times. As descriptions of headache accumulated over the passage of time, it seems almost inevitable that we would realize that different varieties of the disorder must exist, and that they could be identified by the presence or absence of particular phenomena. As James's *Medical Dictionary* put it:

> Pains of the Head are widely different from each other, according to the Parts in which they are seated, as also according to their Degrees: for this Reason Authors have assign'd different Names to different Species of Head-achs. (Anonymous 1745, p. 207)

Over the long course of the recorded history of headache knowledge, a number of classifications of the disorder have appeared. These have been based on various criteria and have survived for various periods of time, some short, though one lasted for many centuries.

There is mention of the occurrence of headache in ancient cuneiform texts from Mesopotamia dating from perhaps as long ago as 4000 B.C., in accounts in Egyptian papyri of around 1500 B.C., and in the Old Testament Second Book of Kings (ca. 700 B.C.). Headache is described at several places in the *Genuine Works of Hippocrates* (ca. 400 B.C.; Adams 1849), in the later Hippocratic corpus of writings, and in the works of the Latin authors Celsus (early first century A.D.—Spencer 1938) and Pliny the Elder (later first century A.D.). In none of these accounts is there any indication of a formal attempt being made to discern characteristic patterns in features of the headaches mentioned, and thereby to designate different varieties of the disorder. However, Celsus did suggest different treatments for acute and for long-standing headache, raising the possibility that he may have seen some usefulness in recognizing the existence of different types of headache.

The first known account of the recognition of different varieties of headache appears in the surviving writings of Aretaeus the Cappadocian, which probably date from early in the second century A.D. Aretaeus and, as judged from the wording of Adams's (1856) translation of his writings, his contemporaries used the term *cephalalgia* for a sudden head pain that was attributed to a temporary cause, even if the pain lasted for several days. If the pain was protracted or recurred frequently over a long period, or if it was more severe and if more intractable symptoms developed in conjunction with it, the disorder instead was termed *cephalea*. Aretaeus indicated that there were infinite varieties of such *cephalea*. In these, the pain could be present continuously or be intermittent; it could involve the whole head, one or other side of the head, the forehead or the top of the head, and from time to time its site might vary between these different locations. When such *cephalea* was confined strictly to one side of the head, Aretaeus applied the term *heterocrania* to it. Thus, for Aretaeus, the distinction between *cephalalgia* and *cephalea* appears to have been based mainly on a combination of the time course of the head pain and the severity of its effects on the sufferer. In his account, *heterocrania* seems to have been regarded simply as a particular variety of *cephalea* determined by its site of occurrence rather than its being a more independent headache entity in its own right.

Galen (131–200 A.D.), probably writing later than Aretaeus and in the latter half of the second century, preserved the *cephalalgia–cephalea* distinction, but replaced the term *heterocrania* with *hemicrania*. In so doing, he created a terminology of headache types that continued in use for some 1700 years. However, not every author over that long period employed the terms or used them in exactly their initial senses. According to the author of the section on *Cephalalgia* in Robert James's *Medical Dictionary*, Galen "beautifully described" *cephalea*:

> A Cephalea is a lasting Pain of the whole Head, which is with Difficulty remov'd, and which, by the slightest Accidents, is so increased, that the Patient can neither endure any Noise, any loud Voice, the Splendor of the Light, or any Motion, but seeks Retirement from Noise, and a dark Chamber, on account of the intense Pain: For some imagine, that they are beaten with a Mallet, others that their Heads left contus'd and distended, and in some few the Pain reaches to the Roots of the Eyes, so that, in this Species of Pain, we have no Reason to doubt but the whole Membrane of the Head is severely affected. (Anonymous 1745, p. 207)

In terms of present-day diagnostic criteria, such a description would very probably be taken to represent migraine without aura. There is another

English-language version of the same set of ideas available in the earlier account provided by Philip Barrough (1610; see chapter 3 in this volume).

For Galen, as for Aretaeus, *hemicrania* was a variety of *cephalea* and not a separate type of headache. Such *hemicrania* embraced a more limited type of headache than present-day migraine, instances of which would have also fallen within the ambit of (non-*hemicranial*) *cephalea*, as in the description cited immediately above. Caelius Aurelianus (fifth century A.D.), whose account was based on now lost writings of Soranus of Ephesus (90–138 A.D.), restricted the idea of *cephalalgia* to acute headache accompanying fever, and employed *cephalea* for chronic nonfebrile episodic headache, the latter a usage more or less similar to that of Galen. The terminology of Caelius, of course, would seem to leave other types of headache without a designation. Paul of Aegina (635–690 A.D.), in his *Seven Books* (Adams 1844), wrote of *cephalalgia* and, separately, of *cephalea* and *hemicrania* (which he considered together). He added little to what was already available in the writings of his predecessors. His position seems to have been largely that of Galen several centuries earlier.

Beginning with the account of Alexander of Tralles (515–ca. 600 A.D.; translated into German by Puschmann, 1878), in the late ancient world the entity of *hemicrania* seems to have been increasingly accepted as a full member of a triad of headache types rather than merely a subset within the category of *cephalea* (De Villiers 1819; Allory 1859). However, in one part of his writings, Galen had dealt with the treatment of *hemicrania* as if it were a separate type of headache, and one that possessed a status similar to that accorded to *cephalea* and *cephalalgia* (Kühn 1821–1833). This full triad of headache types continued to feature in medieval Arabic medical writing, for example that of Avicenna (980–1037), though different names were applied to each of its members. Simple nonrecurrent headache was *soda*, recurrent bilateral headache was *bayzeh*, and recurrent unilateral headache *shaqhiqheh* (Karenberg and Leitz 2001).

In early modern times Jean Fernel (1497–1558), in his *Medicina* (1544), translated into French as *La Pathologie ou Discourse des Maladies* (1655), retained the triad *la céphalalgie, la céphalée, la migraine* in his account of headache. Lazarus Riverius (1589–1655) stated that the word *cephalalgia* was used as a general term for all head pain, while *cephalaea* signified an old headache (Culpeper 1658). For him, *hemicrania* had its then usual meaning. Riverius began to employ a new classificational principle, rather than using the older classificational basis of the time course and the severity of the pain. He subdivided headache into types in which the pain originated internally or externally in relation to the skull. A little later than Riverius, according to Koehler (1997), the Dutch physician Johan van Beverwijck (1594–1647), writing in 1641 in a little known and relatively inaccessible work, also used the presumed site of pain origin as his headache classification basis. He considered that *hemicrania* originated within the skull.

A little afterward, in the period of the 17th-century scientific revolution, Thomas Willis (figure 1-1), in England, also departed from the long standing phenomenologically based headache triad in his *De Anima Brutorum* (1672, and 1683 when it was translated as *Two Discourses Concerning the Soul of Brutes*; figure 1-2). Willis based his approach on first defining those parts of the contents of the head from which, in theory, pain could arise (the latter-day "pain-sensitive structures of the head"). He then settled on those from which he thought headache actually seemed to originate, in other words, he developed further the line of approach that Riverius had adopted. In the words of Pordage's translation (Willis 1672/1683, p. 106), "As to the differences of the Headache, the common distinction is, That the pain of the head is either without the skull, or within its cavity." In *De Anima Brutorum*, in relation to *cephalalgia* (translated by Pordage as "headach,"

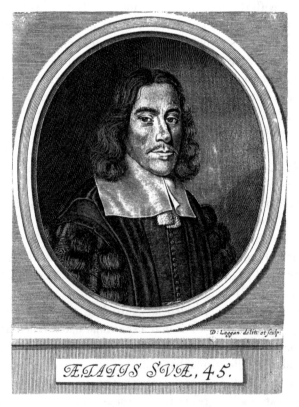

Figure 1-1 Thomas Willis (1621–1675). The frontispiece from *The Remaining Medical Works of That Famous and Renowned Physician Dr Thomas Willis*, edited and translated by Samuel Pordage (Willis 1684).

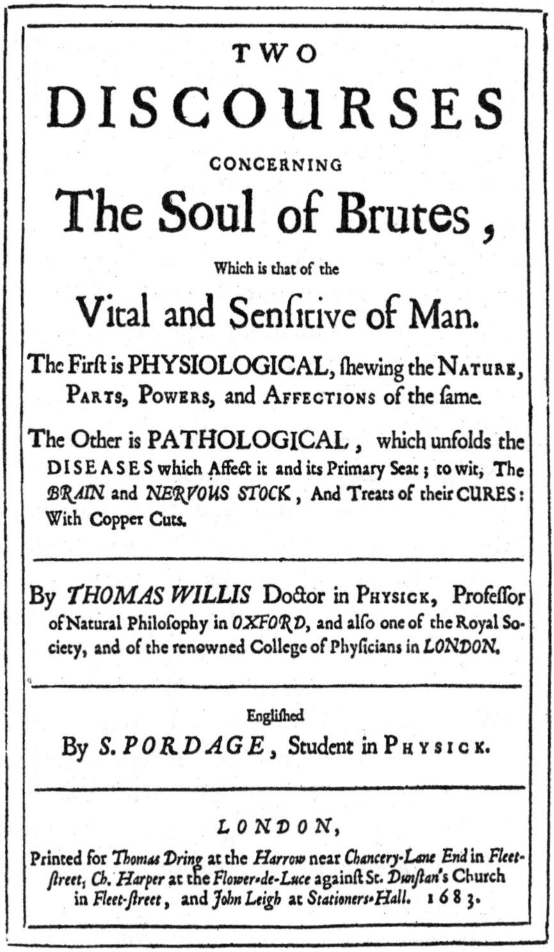

TWO

DISCOURSES

CONCERNING

The Soul of Brutes,

Which is that of the

Vital and Senſitive of Man.

The Firſt is PHYSIOLOGICAL, ſhewing the Nature, Parts, Powers, and Affections of the ſame.

The Other is PATHOLOGICAL, which unfolds the DISEASES which Affect it and its Primary Seat; to wit, The *BRAIN* and *NERVOUS STOCK*, And Treats of their CURES: With Copper Cuts.

By *THOMAS WILLIS* Doctor in Physick, Profeſſor of Natural Philoſophy in *OXFORD*, and alſo one of the Royal Society, and of the renowned College of Phyſicians in *LONDON*.

Engliſhed

By *S. PORDAGE*, Student in Physick.

LONDON,

Printed for *Thomas Dring* at the *Harrow* near *Chancery-Lane End* in *Fleet-ſtreet*, *Ch. Harper* at the *Flower-de-Luce* againſt St. *Dunſtan's* Church in *Fleet-ſtreet*, and *John Leigh* at *Stationers-Hall*. 1683.

Figure 1-2 The title page of Samuel Portage's translation of Willis's *De Anima Brutorum*. This translation is the source of the quotations from Willis in the present book.

with the word being used to embrace all forms of headache), Willis (1672/1683, p. 105) admitted that "it seems most difficult to deliver an exact Theorie of its appearance." Having apparently settled on a classification of headache based more on functional anatomy than on phenomenology, Willis did not proceed to apply the approach consistently in the remainder of his account of "headach." He explored the causes and mechanisms of head pain, for which he used as a general term *cephalalgia*. He made no mention at all of *cephalea*. At one point in his text he did touch on *hemicrania*, a word rendered by Pordage as "meagrim." This particular type of pain, Willis indicated, could be experienced in the front or the rear half of the head, and not necessarily only in one side half (as is now usually expected to be the intention when the word *hemicrania* was used). Willis's was a logical interpretation, but one that that subsequent authors did seem to not take up, though Petroz (1817) did mention it a century and a half later.

For some time after his death, Willis's English-language successors did not follow his approach in attempting to depart from the conventional tripartite headache classificational basis. When they began to do so, many years later, they were probably unaware of the precedent he had set, because his ideas, with his speculative iatrochemistry, were rather lost on succeeding generations. For the most part Willis's achievements have come to be appreciated mainly within living memory. One of Willis's contemporaries, the great Thomas Sydenham (1624–1689), did not deal with headache as a formal topic in his writings, but in discussing "the affection called hysteria in women; and hypochondriasis in men," he mentioned an entity called *clavus hystericus* (Sydenham 1848, p. 231), describing it as "a racking pain in the head, so limited as to be covered by your thumb, accompanied by the vomiting-up of green matter like rancid bile." The term *clavus* continued to be used for such very localized headache for some considerable time. Campbell (1894), for instance, devoted a chapter to the subject in his monograph on headache. There he traced the probable origin of the recognition of this headache variety, under terms such as *ovum* and *passio galeata*, back to the Arabian Haly Abbas in the Middle Ages. The head pain that had earlier been included in the *clavus*-type concept was more extensive in its extent than was indicated by Sydenham, whose account Campbell thought probably simply represented migraine. It seems possible that the entity of *clavus* has resurfaced in the first decade of the 21st century under the designation of *nummular headache*.

Very occasionally some authors (e.g., Anonymous 1745) resurrected the word *crotaphos*, which first appeared in the writing of Caelius Aurelianus, and was applied to a *hemicrania* in which the pain was limited to one temple.

The venerable *cephalalgia, cephalaea, hemicrania* triad, with *clavus* sometimes added as a fourth component, remained the usual basis of headache classification until around the end of the 18th century. However, as already mentioned, the traditional headache terms were not always applied to exactly the same patterns of headache as they originally had been. Thus Hoffman (Lewis 1783) seemed to use *cephalaea* for generalized headache, *cephalalgia* for a pain in some particular part of the head, and *hemicrania* for one-sided head pain. Tentative indications began to appear that the categories were not proving entirely satisfactory in their customary patterns of usage. In James' *Medical Dictionary* of 1745 the three traditional headache varieties were dealt with under the overarching designation of *cephalalgia*

(Anonymous 1745), suggesting that this word was beginning to be employed as the Latin equivalent of the English-language "headache." This attitude to the word *cephalalgia* seemed to be increasingly adopted in the writings of some later 19th-century authors (e.g., Colin 1873). As early as 1830, Jolly had stated that *céphalalgie* was the generic term for headache, though some writers still used the term *céphalée* for chronic continuous or intermittent *céphalalgie* (Jolly 1830).

As well, some 17th- and 18th-century authors began to make more explicit the range of the headache patterns that they included in the category of *hemicrania*, which in the then contemporary medical literature was increasingly considered more or less equivalent to the vernacular term *migraine*, in one or other of its variant spellings (Anonymous 1745). According to Riley (1932), over the years the word *hemicrania* had become corrupted in low Latin into *hemigranea*, thence to *emigranea*, *migranea*, and *migrana*. In English *hemicrania* became *mygrame* (1398), *meygrym* (1460), *migrim* (1579), and *megrim* (1713), before, in 1777, becoming *migraine*.

As an example of the range of the disorders that had come to be included under the designation of *hemicrania* in the late 16th and 17th centuries, Willis's contemporary Johan Jakob Wepfer (1727), in his posthumously published *Observationes Medico-practicae de Affectibus Capitis*, included probable trigeminal neuralgia. Boissier de Sauvages (1706–1767) in his *Nosologie Méthodique* (1772), an attempt to produce a comprehensive classification of disease along the lines in which Linnaeus had classified the plant kingdom, included instances of sinusitis, eye disease, and dental disease within the *hemicrania* category. Such inclusions could certainly be regarded as etymologically justifiable in relation to the original meaning of *hemicrania*. Sauvages continued to employ the terminology of the classical three types of headache in his comprehensive classification. He equated *cephalalgia* with acute headache or a "heavy pain of the head" (Vaughan 1825), *cephalea* with chronic periodic headache, and *hemicrania* with pain on either side of the forehead, in other words, a partial or local headache. He then subdivided each of the three major categories on a basis of their assumed causal mechanisms or circumstances of occurrence. As well, Sauvages included *ophthalmia*, *otalgia*, and *odontalgia* within his category of headache. His attempt to be consistently logical produced an outcome that appeared contrary to some aspects of customary medical and lay thought. Interestingly, in his explanatory commentary, Sauvages seemed to suggest that the difference between *cephalea* and *cephalalgia* was more a matter of degree than of kind. Every *cephalaea*, of course, would have begun as an episode of *cephalalgia*, and no one had set a sharp and generally agreed boundary line beyond which the latter was considered to have become the former. William Heberden, in his posthumously published *Commentaries*, also was conscious of uncertainty in his mind as to the fundamental difference between *hemicrania* and other headaches:

> the hemicrania, or pain of one half of the head, was very early distinguished by medical writers from the other species of head-achs: but we have not yet advanced much in how this differs from other pains of the head, except in the circumstance which the name denotes. (1802, p. 75)

In addition, by the end of the 18th century, some authors were prepared to allow *hemicrania* to transgress the midline of the head (Pelletan de Kinkelin 1832; Labarraque 1837).

Near the end of the 18th century, in 1789, William Cullen avoided all consideration of the topic of headache in his influential and long surviving *First Lines of the Practice of Physic* (1789/1805), and in his nosology. A contemporary, the Swiss author Samuel Tissot (figure 1-3), the so-called (medical) educator of Europe, in his *Traité des nerfs* (1778–1780), when writing specifically on *De la Migraine*, first stated that there were four, rather than three, varieties of head pain. These were the usual triad plus *le clou* or *l'oeuf,* a very localized form of headache that was more or less equivalent to *clavus.* To Tissot, *cephalalgia* was the ordinary headache to which everyone was vulnerable, and which could be recurrent, whereas *cephalea* was a very severe and almost continuous headache that was usually due to organic disease that involved the head. For him, the category of *cephalea* did not therefore include migraine and was obviously very much more limited in range of headache types than earlier authors had indicated. In a few lines of text, Tissot proceeded to dismiss all varieties of headache apart from migraine. He then wrote at considerable length on the latter disorder, reflecting its importance in his eyes. Frank (1819) recognized the existence of Tissot's four headache categories but then subdivided them further, on the basis of their assumed etiologies.

It would seem that, by the latter part of the 18th century, the traditional tripartite phenomenologically based categorization of headache was increasingly being considered not entirely satisfactory as a consequence of growing medical and pathological knowledge, new interpretations of disease mechanisms, and a continuing inconsistent use of the ancient headache type terminology. Data were accumulating on correlations between anatomical pathology appearances and disease manifestations, and were consolidated in Morgagni's *De Sedibus* (1779). The time of the final eclipse of the long-standing humoral basis of the pathogenesis of disease had arrived, and migraine emerged in the writings of Tissot as a major type of headache in its own right. The circumstances seem to have brought about a

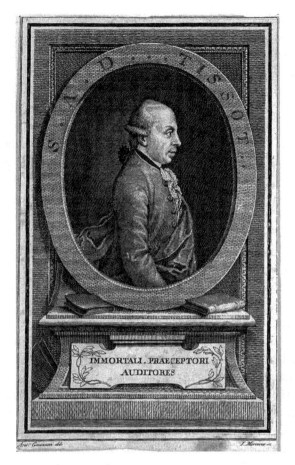

Figure 1-3 Samuel Tissot (1728–1797). Courtesy of Wellcome Library, London.

situation in which attempts to reclassify headache on a basis of its underlying structural or pathogenic mechanism must have seemed desirable. For the better part of a century, in parallel with dwindling use of the old phenomenologically based headache type triad terminology, attempts at new classifications based on etiology and underlying structural pathology went on. They took various forms until their individual shortcomings finally led to the necessity of modifying the philosophical basis of the classificational approach itself.

The early part of the 19th century saw the appearance of monographs devoted to the topic of migraine written mainly by French authors (e.g., Piorry 1831; Labarraque 1837). There seems to have been a general surge of medical interest in France in relation to this specific type of headache during the 19th century, with a number of doctoral theses being based on the topic, including one by the Englishwoman Elizabeth Garrett Anderson

(1870; translated by Wilkinson and Isler, 1999). Near the end of the century, Thomas (1887) designated the existence of two types of migraine: that with, and that without, an aura. This subdivision has continued in general use ever since. The French 19th-century headache literature seems to show some disenchantment as to the reality of any fundamental distinction between *céphalalgie* and *céphalée*. Georget and Calmeil (1834) and Martineau (1867) wrote on the combined topic of *céphalalgie, céphalée* in French dictionaries of medicine, dealing with the two traditional headache types as if they comprised a single entity for which they preferred the designation *céphalalgie*. On the whole, types of headache apart from migraine seem to have been largely ignored by the French authors of the 19th century.

At much the same time, English-language authors dealing with headache tended to discreetly drop the traditional triad classification, though Vaughan (1825), who was heavily dependent on Sauvages, retained it. In its stead, a variety of relatively simple, though perhaps not totally comprehensive, headache classifications appeared. Some were based predominantly on clinical characteristics, some on the underlying pathological process or interpretations of the disordered physiology, and others on mixtures of these. Weatherhead (1835) used a rather simple classification based on a pragmatic mix of mechanism and pathology, namely (i) dyspeptic or sick headache, (ii) nervous headache, (iii) headache from cranial arterial or venous plethora, (iv) rheumatic headache, and (v) headache from organic brain disease. Weatherhead's monograph was followed by a flurry of publications in the 1850s that employed various categorizations of headache types.

Murphy (1854) provided a correlation between the classification he proposed and the familiar terms of the old triad of headache types (table 1-1). To Murphy, whose classification was based mainly on presumed headache mechanism, migraine did not equate with *hemicrania*, and his *cephalalgia* and *cephalea* would appear not have had the exact meanings that Aretaeus,

Table 1-1 MURPHY'S (1854) CLASSIFICATION OF HEADACHE

Common Type of Headache	Site of Headache Origin	Equivalent Older Term
Anemic	Intracranial	*Cephalea* or migraine
Congestive	Intracranial	*Cephalalgia* if congestion passive; sick headache if congestion active
Neuralgic	Extracranial	*Hemicrania* or *clavus hystericus*
Rheumatic	Extracranial	
Periosteal	Extracranial	

for instance, had originally given them. Edward Sieveking (1854) took a pathophysiological approach, subdividing headaches into those due to too much, to too little, or to vitiated (i.e., qualitatively abnormal) blood within the cranial cavity. He then further divided the causes of these cranial intravascular abnormalities into those that involved the cerebral cortex (e.g., psychological factors and his *cephalalgia epileptica*, to be discussed in chapter 5), the organs of nutrition, or the sexual apparatus (see table 1-2). John Russell Reynolds (1855), with his customary clarity of thought, simply designated two major varieties of headache, *cephalalgia* and *hemicrania*, in addition to the focal cranial neuralgias. However, he then proceeded to subdivide his *cephalalgia*. He regarded *hemicrania* as a disease due to excessive experience of sensation and did not subdivide it further but cited its alternative names of *neuralgia cerebralis* and *la migraine*.

Copland (1858), in his *Dictionary of Practical Medicine*, classified headache as: (i) nervous, from depression or exhaustion, (ii) congestive, (iii) plethoric and inflammatory, (iv) dyspeptic and bilious, (v) cerebral, (vi) pericranial, (vii) hemicranial or neuralgic, (viii) rheumatic or arthritic, (ix) periodic, (x) hypochondriacal, or (xi) sympathetic (from the uterus and urinary organs). This classification seems based on a mix of principles: the assumed causative mechanisms, the site of headache origin, and the time course of headache occurrence. In that same year, Symonds (1858) proposed what appeared to be a reasonably simple scheme of headache classification: that headaches were (i) primary (idiopathic) or (ii) secondary to (a) local intracranial changes, (b) morbid changes in the blood, and (c) disorders of distant organs (i.e., they were sympathetic headaches). After so doing, he then proceeded to discuss the topic of headache on a somewhat different basis under the designations of (i) structural headache, (ii) hyperemia headache, (iii) nervous and neuralgic headache (including migraine), and (iv) toxemic headache.

Table 1-2 SIEVEKING'S (1854) SUBDIVISION OF TYPES OF *CEPHALALGIA*

1. *Cephalalgias* of extrinsic origin
   a. Those from acute specific diseases
   b. Rheumatic cephalalgias
   c. Symptomatic headache, related to disease of other organs
2. *Cephalalgias* of intrinsic origin
   a. Congestive
   b. Inflammatory
   c. Due to organic disease
   d. Neuralgic

Other English-language writers later in the 19th century devised somewhat different and rather complex personal classificational approaches, mainly based on presumed headache pathogenesis rather than diseased anatomy (e.g., Wright 1867; Day 1875; Shuldham 1876; Ross 1885; Campbell 1894; Copeman 1901). Corning (1888), in the United States, classified headaches into those of intracranial and those of extracranial origin, there being six subsets of the first type and two of the second. Most of these classificational schemes seemed to involve the designation of around 10 main subtypes of headache. It is rather noticeable that migraine received relatively little prominence in most of these 19th-century English-language approaches to headache classification.

In France, Martin (1829) had simply divided headaches into migraine and *cephalalgia*, applying the latter term to headache in general, and Labarraque (1837), who embraced all headache within the term *cephalalgia*, split this entity into symptomatic and idiopathic (essential) varieties, the latter including migraine. Martineau (1867) listed several different classifications of *cephalalgia* drawn from the literature, again taking *cephalalgia* to be a synonym for headache. He employed his own classification, which split headaches into primary and symptomatic types, and then split each of these main types into headaches originating in intracranial structures: ones originating in extracranial structures and those mediated by sympathy (and therefore originating outside of the head). Dheur (1900) later employed Martin's (1829) primary *cephalalgia* and migraine headache categories before subdividing the former into neurasthenic, hysterical, uremic, syphilitic, adolescent, alimentary disturbance related, and other types.

The plethora of 19th-century headache classifications contained a good deal of content in common, but the overall variety of headache entities that were proposed must have seemed rather overwhelming. No single classification appears to have achieved anything like widespread acceptance. Criticism of pathogenesis-based classifications of headache began to appear in print quite early, probably mainly because the evidence for the assumed etiologies was perceived to be inadequate. Thus Vaughan wrote the following:

> As for the division of Headachs into bilious, nervous, spasmodic, gouty, rheumatic, &c., as every one of these epithets contains a hypothesis, which I do not understand, and which I am persuaded, nobody else does, I shall not enter into any formal refutation of it. (1825, p. 93)

Although the clinical features of the various headache types had nearly always been described by those who specified their existences, diagnosis based on the features as described must have often been difficult to achieve in practice. Despite these deficiencies, and the number of existing and not readily compatible schemes that existed, the headache classification situation did not seem to change significantly in the early part of the 20th century. Possibly World War I and its aftermath had seriously disrupted intellectual endeavors in the countries where there had been most interest in headache and its problems. In Germany, Oppenheim (1904) and, on the eve of the war, Auerbach (1913) had clung to the old terms *cephalalgia* and *cephalea*, the latter author indicating that the former term referred to mild headaches and the latter term to more severe ones. Auerbach's preferred subdivision of headache was into (i) more independent forms of headache (migraine, neurasthenic headache, and nodular or rheumatic headache), (ii) headache associated with disease of particular organs (brain disease, disorders of the organs of special sense, of the digestive tract and of the kidneys), (iii) headache associated with general disease (infection, acute intoxication, constitutional disorders), and (iv) headache representing various combinations of the above types. Almost a century after headache classifications based on pathogenesis had begun to appear, Spriggs (1935), after excluding cranial neuralgias from consideration, divided the topic of headache into (i) organic headache, (ii) vascular headache, (iii) toxic headache, (iv) reflex headache, (v) functional headache, which included migraine, and (vi) headache due to causes such as asthenia and mental disturbance.

By the mid-20th century, the old *cephalalgia, cephalea, hemicrania* classification of headache had completely disappeared from use. The multiple idiosyncratic classifications that had attempted to replace it had all proved to have unacceptable drawbacks. However, migraine had increasingly emerged in medical thinking as both a distinctive and a very major headache entity that needed clear recognition in any adequate headache classification. Further, it was increasingly accepted that the headache of migraine need not be confined to one side of the head (Gowers 1907), though certain authors had also held this view at least seven decades earlier (Pelletan de Kinkelin 1832; Labarraque 1837), and Allory (1859) not long afterward. Indeed, Willis had adopted a similar position in the 17th century, as mentioned earlier in this chapter, though in his case it was on grounds of logic rather than of general word usage. In the wake of the relative suspension of advance in medical knowledge of headache during and immediately after World War II, recognition of the need to tidy the existing rather chaotic headache classificational situation led to action in the United States. An Ad Hoc Committee on the Classification of Headache (1962), under the aegis of the American Neurological Association, produced a new classification of headache. This classification was based on contemporary understandings of headache pathogenic mechanisms. It was highly dependent on

Table 1-3 THE AMERICAN NEUROLOGICAL ASSOCIATION'S (1962) CLASSIFICATION OF HEADACHE

1. Vascular headache of migraine type
2. Muscle contraction headache
3. Combined headache (migraine plus contraction headache)
4. Nasal vasomotor headache
5. Headache of delusional, conversion, or hypochondriacal states
6. Nonmigrainous vascular headache
7. Traction headache
8. Headache from overt cranial inflammation
9. Headache from eye, ear, nose, nasal sinus, dental, other cranial structure, and neck disease
10. Cranial neuritides
11. Cranial neuralgias

the work and ideas of Harold Wolff, who had contributed so greatly to knowledge of headache mechanisms over the previous decades. The 1962 classification itself was moderately extensive, but not so bulky as to be unmanageable for use in clinical practice. Its main categories are listed in table 1-3.

This 1962 headache classification progressively gained reasonably wide acceptance and supplanted nearly all the others then extant. For several decades it provided a helpful framework for terminology and research into headache. However, it became increasingly inadequate as knowledge of headache phenomenology and mechanism advanced with the great blossoming and increasing internationalization of headache research in the later decades of the 20th century.

In 1988 the International Headache Society produced a new and much more exhaustive headache classification (Headache Classification Committee 1988). This, by 2004, required some modification and further amplification as new clinical patterns of headache phenomena were recognized and headache mechanisms sometimes became clearer (International Headache Society 2004). The details of this most recent classification, running to 160 pages of text, are much too extensive to reproduce in full here. Its major primary headache categories are listed in table 1-4. The initial classificational criterion has tended to revert to a mix of etiology and clinical phenomenology, with a subsidiary classificational level based on clinical phenomenology; however, in the state of contemporary knowledge, the phenomenology often can be correlated with what is known of headache mechanisms.

Table 1-4 MAJOR CATEGORIES IN THE INTERNATIONAL HEADACHE SOCIETY'S (2004) CLASSIFICATION OF HEADACHE

1. Primary headache, not causally associated with structural pathology
   - Migraine
   - Cluster headache and other trigeminal autonomic cephalalgias
   - Tension-type headache
   - Other primary headaches
2. Secondary headache, related to structural, biochemical, traumatic or psychiatric causes
3. Cranial neuralgias (some idiopathic, others due to structural disease) and primary facial pain and other headaches

Even though the present book's cutoff time was set arbitrarily at the year 2000 (see the introduction), it has seemed likely that using the 2004 Headache Classification, rather than earlier versions, as a point of reference will better serve the intellectual comfort of much of its prospective readership, which is expected to be mainly those with medical backgrounds.

CHAPTER 2
The "Seat" of Headache

I n the English language literature of the past, the word *seat*, when used in relation to headache, was intended to refer to the anatomical site in the head from which the pain was thought to originate. Unlike what happened in relation to the development of the classification of headache, in which over the centuries major changes were found desirable to cope with a growing understanding of the situation, ideas concerning the seat of headache have tended to remain relatively static since they first appeared in the written record. However, some important additional material became available in relatively recent times.

THE ANCIENT WORLD

It seems very likely that primitive man would not only have experienced headache but might have begun to think about where in the head the pain arose. This might have been particularly the case if the pain was experienced only in a restricted location, or at or near the site of an injury, or where there was a recognizable local abnormality of the shape of the head. Nonetheless, in the surviving writings until the early centuries of the Christian era, there appears to be little documented evidence that such considerations led to any systematic thought about the site of headache origin. The available writings of the Hippocratic school contain no indication that the intellects of its members were exercised by the issue. Nor were those of the Latin authors of the first century A.D., Celsus and Pliny the Elder.

In the surviving writings of Aretaeus the Cappadocian, dating probably from the early second century A.D. (Adams 1856), with one possible exception there was no consideration of the anatomical seats of the types of headache that he discussed. When Aretaeus mentioned the treatment of *cephalea*, he stated that measures similar to those used for this type of headache could also be applied to the side of the head affected by his entity of *heterocrania*. This statement might be interpreted as suggesting that he believed that the site of origin of localized headache might be close to the place where the pain was experienced.

Galen, probably a little later than Aretaeus in the second century A.D., dealt with the topic of headache at various places scattered through his voluminous surviving writings (Kuhn's edition 1821–1833). Galen seems to have been the first to specify sites within the head where he believed headache originated. For him, the main sources of headache were the meninges and the pericranium, but he was aware that the cerebral arteries and veins were sensitive to stimulation. He cited an observation that apparently originated in the now long lost writings of one Archigenes (ca. 100 A.D.), which suggested that the scalp blood vessels played a role in headache production. In the words of Siegel's (1976, p. 52) translation of Galen's *De locis affectis*,

> If blood vessels which are not inflamed are strongly compressed, the headaches [Kephalgias] are stopped as if the influx [of humors] is prevented. This is usually achieved by the foreign bandage. Gangrenous pain on one side of the head can be confined by cutting [these blood vessels], especially by arteriotomy. (Kühn 1821–1833, vol. 6, p. 91)

Henry Campbell, a late 19th-century London physician, provided a translation of part of the *Sepulchretum* of Theophile Bonet (1700) in which Galen's views on the site of origin of head pain were set down:

> The pain may be spread throughout the entire head or affect only some one part of it, and it may be internal or external. By internal pain I mean pain in the membrane or the substance of the brain or the veins, arteries and nerves, of which some are more, others less, sensitive. (1893, p. 185)

The differentiation between internal and external headache was made possible by Galen's belief that the pain of the former, but not that of the latter, extended into the roots of the eyes, in other words, the back of the eyeballs. He had some anatomical grounds for this idea because he knew that the dura mater, one of his major sites of origin of head pain, was continuous with the sheath of the optic nerve and the tunic of the orbit. A further point of distinction was that in headache of external origin, there was local tenderness of extracranial structures.

The evidence on which Galen based his nomination of the cranial sites of headache origin is often not readily apparent. It must have been more than merely a matter of his having knowledge of anatomy and then thinking of parts of the head that he might invoke on anatomical grounds as pain sources. If he had done that, it is unlikely that he would have excluded the brain itself from the list of sites, and he did this. By Galen's time, it seems possible that transmitted knowledge obtained from centuries of observing the effects of head injury may have already shown which cranial structures, when injured in various ways, appeared to cause pain. Galen also believed that the pain of *hemicrania* could originate in the temporal muscle of the side where the headache was experienced (Kuhn, vol. xii, p. 591).

Galen's views regarding the seats of headache origin were reiterated, though with some variation, by subsequent Byzantine authors in the late ancient world, for example Paul of Aegina. In expressing basically similar views regarding headache origin sites, Caelius Aurelianus wrote the following:

> Some hold that the membrane of the brain is affected, others the membrane surrounding the skull, others the entire skin of the head and still others the muscles of the temples and jaws. But our view is that in some cases some of these parts are affected, while in other cases all these parts are affected. (Drabkin 1950, p. 445)

Thus Caelius's list of headache sources, like that of Galen centuries earlier, came to include the majority of the major anatomical structures that are present in the part of the body where headache was experienced. Neither Caelius nor Galen mentioned the bones of the skull or the air-filled sinuses within the skull bones, or the brain itself, as possible sites of head pain origin.

THE MEDIEVAL WORLD

The early medieval Arabian physicians added no significant insights to the situation, in general merely repeating Galen's views concerning the seat of headache.

In the later medieval world, Jean Fernel (1497–1558) in Paris criticized Galen's grounds for believing that his headache of internal origin extended into the eye sockets while his headache of external origin did not. Fernel (1655) pointed out that the dura and the pericranium formed a continuous membrane within the orbits. Therefore, purely on anatomical grounds, he contended that there was as much justification for asserting that extracranial headache extended into the back of the orbit as for claiming that headache of internal origin did. Fernel's own view was that the main types of headache originated in the membranes of the head, by which he meant the meninges and the pericranium.

Up to that time, in the available writings, there still was little evidence as to the grounds on which the sites of headache origin were designated, apart from the obvious anatomical considerations and, one assumes, knowledge of the effects of local disease and head injury. There does not seem to have been any attempt made to identify any pain-producing site by means of any experimental procedure.

EARLY MODERN TIMES

Early in 17th century, Charles Le Pois (1563–1633; figure 2-1), foundation professor of medicine at the University of Pont-à-Mousson in northeastern France, stated, as it were ex cathedra, that headache arose from the membranes of the head when they were distended by vapors or humors (Le Pois 1618). He thus simply repeated Fernel's view as to the site of headache origin, though he also added to the situation a hypothetical pain-producing mechanism. Half a century after Le Pois, Thomas Willis in England at least provided a rationale when he nominated the sites from which he thought headache

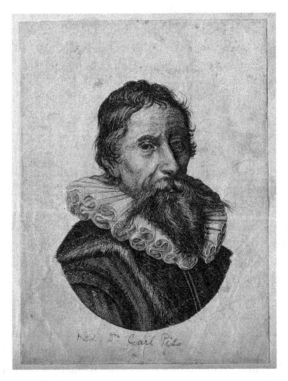

Figure 2-1 Charles Le Pois (Carolus Piso; 1563–1633). Courtesy of Wellcome Library, London.

might arise. When he attempted to do this, he based his views on the richness of the innervation of the tissues concerned, in combination with an implicit belief that the experience of pain was mediated through sensory nerves:

All pain is a violated Action, or a troublesome tension or feeling, depending on a Convulsion, or a Congestion of the Nerves, the Subject of the Headachs are the most nervous parts of the Head, that is, the Nerves themselves, as also the Fibres and Membranes, and such as are more and most sensible, seated both without and within the skull. But the parts of this kind, which are affected with pain, are first the Meninges, and their various processes, the Coats of the Nerves, the Pericranium (or skin compassing the Skull) and other thin skinny Membranes, the fleshy Panicle of the Muscle, and lastly the skin its self. As to the Brain and Cerebel, and their Medullary dependencies, we affirm, that these bodies are free from pain is, because they want sensible Fibres, apt to be unskilled and distended: the same, for the like reason, may be said of the Skull. (Willis 1672/1683, pp. 105–106)

Later in his chapters on headache in *De Anima Brutorum*, Willis (1672) added to his list of structures that could produce head pain the nervous fibers that belong to the tendons. Thus he extended the spectrum of headache-producing structures as compared with those described by his forerunners.

Although he lived at much the same time as Willis, the publication in which the Swiss physician and pathologist Johann Jacob Wepfer (1620–1695; figure 2-2) discussed headache, his *Observationes*, did not appear in print until 1727, some years after his death and then only by virtue of his grandsons' efforts (Fischer 1931). In it, Wepfer argued that pain did not originate in the pericranium in at least one patient with headache because, in the words of Campbell's translation,

the pain is not increased by external contact, but the dura mater, because it becomes more severe after coughing, screamings &c, and because it is diminished by mental exercise. It is not in the pia mater, because there is no vertigo or sleepiness . . .; nor is a pain superficially situated or in the interior of the brain, because the sharper pain is felt chiefly in the forehead. (1893, p. 186)

A few of the points made in Wepfer's argument for the location of the origin of head pain in this particular instance—for example, the effects of external contact—seem valid in the light of modern knowledge. Others are more doubtful, depending as they do on ideas of nervous system function that are no longer held.

Overall, by the end of the 17th century, the list of sites of headache production remained much as Galen had suggested a millennium and a

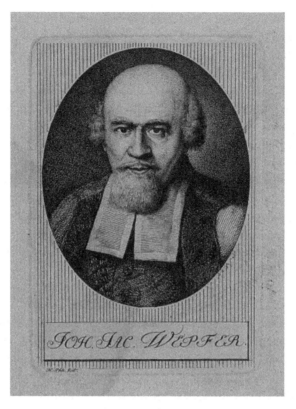

Figure 2-2 Johann Jakob Wepfer (1620–1696). Courtesy of Wellcome Library, London.

half earlier. Willis, at least, had provided some rationale for his identification of the structures he considered responsible for head pain production. Further, it is a rationale that remains plausible today. If he possessed evidence either from experience of the effects of disease or from experimentation that supported his views, Willis did not provide it as part of his neurological legacy.

THE 18TH CENTURY

More medical literature dealing with headache is available from the 18th century, particularly from its latter half, than from any earlier era. On the whole, authors in this period were less dogmatic about the seats of origin of head pain and some evidence from experimentation began to become available. Haller (1755) published his experimental animal studies on sensibility and irritability. He considered that irritability was present if voluntary and involuntary muscles in living creatures contracted after they were stimulated, and if no other disturbance in the experimental animal was obvious. The presence of such "irritability" would not necessarily warrant the interpretation that pain was being experienced as result of the stimulation. On the other hand, Haller's "sensitivity" involved witnessing the animals react to stimulation in ways that might be expected if they were experiencing pain. The matter was explained in the words of Tissot's English-language translation of Haller's text:

> I call that a sensible part of the human body, which on being touched transmits the impression of it to the soul; and in brutes, in whom the existence of a soul is not so clear, I call those parts sensible, the Irritation of which occasions evident signs of pain and disquiet in the animal. (1752, p. 4)

Haller's experimental observations enabled him to state that the pericranium was sensitive because nerves were present in it. He noted that trephining of the human skull did not cause pain. He could burn the dura with oil of vitriol (sulfuric acid), butter of antimony (antimony trichloride), or spirits of niter (nitric acid), cut it with a knife, or tear it with pincers without his conscious animals appearing to suffer pain. Despite such observations, he then proceeded to state that the dura was the seat of headache. The pia mater was not sensitive to butter of antimony. The skin was sensitive, and "the nerves, which are the source of all sensibility, are themselves of course extremely sensible." Haller's overall conclusion pointed in the direction of a tissue's sensibility being proportionate to the richness of its innervation, in conformity with Willis's earlier reasoning.

On the whole, Frederick Hoffman (1660–1742), in the words of his translator Lewis, tended to agree with Haller:

> The seat of pain in the head is most frequently the pericranium or its membrane which immediately covers the skull; sometimes the cutis itself, particularly its interior surface contiguous to the pericranium; sometimes also the dura mater, which communicates with the pericranium through the sutures; and sometimes the production of the pituitary tunic which lines the sinuses of the frontal bone. The other membranes immediately, investing the brain, as the pia mater and arachnoides, seem little adapted to be the seat of pain, as no elastic fibres or nervous branches are distinguished in them. (1783, pp. 459–460)

Hoffman held that the brain itself was incapable of feeling, as the cerebral cortex could be severely injured without any pain being felt. Thus he identified a slightly wider range of anatomical structures than Haller as sites of headache origin, but provided no evidence to support his identification of these seats of pain.

Lorry (1760) had noted that pressure applied to the cerebral hemispheres of dogs, cats, rabbits, and pigeons produced behavior suggesting that the animals were experiencing pain. Because he believed that the brain itself was insensitive to stimulation, he assumed that the pressure that had been exerted had been transmitted to affect the origins of the emerging cranial nerves (Neuberger 1897/1981).

At about the same time that Haller, Hoffman, and Lorry had recorded their views in print, Robert Whytt (1714–1766), professor of the theory of medicine at Edinburgh and a considerable experimentalist, put forward the view that the membranes of the brain in health possessed relatively little capacity for feeling (Whytt 1764/1768). However, elsewhere in his writings he stated that the membranes and the pericranium could be the site of origin of violent head pain. John Fordyce (1758), in his *De hemicrania*, seemed to suggest that hemicranial pain could originate in the temporal muscles and the falx cerebri, the latter a part of the dura not specifically mentioned previously in relation to the site of head pain origin.

Boissier de Sauvages (1772), in his attempted classification of all disease, located the site of origin of *cephalalgia* to the meninges (which he thought possessed the ability to contract), that of *cephalea* to the membranes outside the skull, and that of *hemicrania* to the internal membranes of the frontal sinus on the side of the pain, or to the parts of the head that are innervated by sympathetic nerves. (He probably used the term *sympathetic* here to convey the idea that such nerves were involved in the experience of pain occurring at a distance from its true site of origin, rather than in the latter-day sense of nerves that are part of the sympathetic nervous system.) Sauvages did not reject the possibility that headache could originate in the brain. Soon afterward, at the close of the 18th century, the English physician William Heberden (1802), in his posthumously published *Commentaries*, went further and openly stated that he regarded the brain itself as the seat of headache, without providing any evidence to support this view.

THE 19TH CENTURY

The 19th century saw the cranial vasculature being increasingly recognized as a major source of headache. This happened at least partly because of increasing interest in migraine and its pathogenesis. The disorder emerged not only as a distinct but as a very frequent type of headache (see chapter 4). However, some authors, particularly English-language ones, still tended to adhere to the old *cephalalgia, cephalaea, hemicrania* approach and deal with the topic of headache as a whole, not considering migraine as a major entity until well into the century.

There was some diversity of opinion among authors concerning where in the brain headache might have its origin. Seller (1848), Handfield-Jones (1867), and J. A. Symonds (1858) considered that the nerves that accompany the cerebral blood vessels were a source of headache. They also thought that the brain itself could be a site of headache origin. Colin (1873) took a quite different view. He believed that nearly all headache was of extracranial origin and arose in the muscles in the back of the neck and in the epicranial aponeurosis. Samuel Wilks (1878; figure 2-3) rejected the possibility that headache could arise in the normal brain. David Ferrier (1879) based his opinion on data obtained in the course of his experimental animal studies on the localization of representation of function in the cerebral cortex. From his work, he concluded that the dura was definitely sensitive, the arachnoid not sensitive, and the pia-arachnoid capable of producing a burning pain when it was infected or inflamed. Ferrier also noted that posterior fossa disease consistently produced pain experienced at the back of the head but that there was not such a close correlation between where headache was experienced and disease that was present in the anterior cranial fossa.

Despite all the foregoing material emanating from his contemporaries, William Gowers (1845–1915; figure 2-4), in the first edition of his

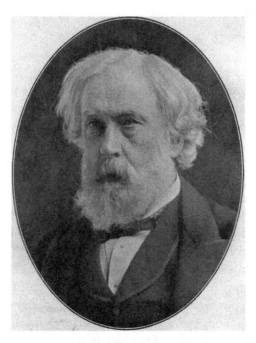

Figure 2-3 Sir Samuel Wilks (1824–1911) when aged about 60 years. The frontispiece from his *Biographical Reminiscences* (1911), now in the public domain.

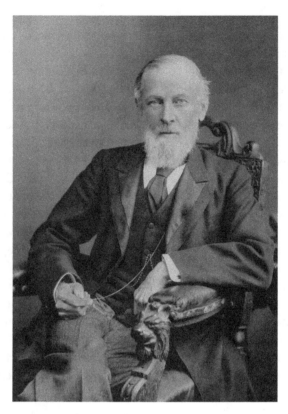

Figure 2-4 Sir William Gowers (1845–1915). Courtesy of Gowers's great-granddaughter, Professor Ann Scott.

Manual of Diseases of the Nervous System (1888, vol. 2), was prepared to state that "we know almost nothing of the structures in which the pain of headache is felt or the mechanism of its production." Gowers thought that the site of pain origin might well be different in different types of headache. He considered that neuralgia could arise in scalp nerves, in which case the pain would follow the line of the nerve involved, that apparently deep-seated pain might arise from sites in the brain membranes, and that diffuse headache might originate in the higher cerebral centers. He thought that vasodilatation per se could probably produce pain and the headache that preceded the onset of hemiplegia due to syphilitic endarteritis originated in the affected artery itself (Gowers 1888).

Henry Campbell (1893), who seemed to take a particular interest in the history of attempts to locate the sites of the structures from which head pain originated, put forward his own view on the matter somewhat tentatively. In his opinion, the extracranial structures involved in headache production were the muscles of the back of the neck and the temple, possibly the aponeurosis of the temporal muscle, the epicranial aponeurosis, the pericranium, the skin of the scalp, the scalp nerves, the scalp arteries (in particular, the superficial temporal arteries), and the lymph glands that drained the scalp (if the latter became infected). Intracranially, the dura was certainly a source of headache, but the possible roles of the pia-arachnoid and brain itself were more doubtful. However, Campbell thought that events that occurred in them probably contributed to the pain associated with intracranial structural disease.

In all, from the days of Galen over a millennium and a half earlier, up to the end of the 19th century, there was relatively little expansion of the list of cranial structures identified as responsible for the production of headache. There had been a few additions—for example, the neck muscles, the epicranial aponeurosis, the mucous membrane of the frontal sinuses—but the pericranium and the dura mater remained the sites most commonly mentioned. The role of the brain itself in pain production continued to be contentious, opinions about the matter differing among authors. Relatively little experimental work relevant to the matter had been carried out, either in animals or in humans. While an experimental animal may behave as if it is in pain, it does not possess the capacity to communicate in any other way whether or not it actually experiences headache at the relevant time. One can hardly escape the suspicion that until this time, much of what was written about the sites of headache origin simply reproduced the statements of earlier writers without further personal attempts at verification of the claims. Too much seems to have been written without its evidence base being made explicit.

THE 20TH CENTURY

Shortly before the outbreak of World War I, Auerbach (1913) raised what seems to have been the then novel possibility that the dura might not possess a uniform degree of pain sensitivity over its whole extent. He suggested that the dura at the base of the brain appeared to be more sensitive than that overlying the cerebral cortex. He also mentioned that the existence of the phenomenon of thalamic pain implied that there might be a possible role for the brain itself as a seat of headache production. Thalamic pain, a persistent pain experienced in the opposite side of the body as result of damage to the posterior part of one thalamus and the neighboring posterior limb of the internal capsule, comprises one component of the so-called thalamic syndrome. If such pain could arise within the human brain itself from a strategically sited abnormality, even though the brain contains no sensory nerves and appears to be insensitive to stimulation applied from outside its surface, could not headache also originate in the brain? There was a further relevant observation: that pain in the contralateral trigeminal nerve territory of supply could occur as an occasional residue of Wallenberg's lateral medullary syndrome, usually due to ischemic damage to one side of the medulla oblongata. This was additional evidence that head pain may arise, albeit rarely, from within the central nervous system itself.

Wolff

In the mid-20th century, under the leadership of Harold Wolff in New York, a very important series of planned but essentially opportunistic studies on the sites of head pain origin in conscious humans undergoing neurosurgery was carried out. The outcomes of the individual studies were consolidated in the detailed account that appeared in the second edition of Wolff's book *Headache and Other Head Pain* (1963; figure 2-5). Wolff completed the text of this edition of his book shortly before his own death and did not live long enough to read the proofs. For the first time, extensive systematically collected data from conscious humans became available, enabling the sites of stimulation of individual cranial structures to be correlated with the location and character of any induced headache (figure 2-6). In essence, the conclusions that emerged from these studies were as follows:

- The periosteum of the skull is not particularly sensitive, and is not sensitive at all at the brow.
- The cranial bones and diploic veins are not sensitive.
- The dural arteries are sensitive, irritation of the middle meningeal artery usually producing localized aching pain behind the eye on the same side. However, pain can be experienced at the back of the head if the more posterior branches of the middle meningeal artery are stimulated. Stimulation of the distal middle meningeal artery branches does not produce pain.
- The supratentorial dura is not sensitive unless it is stimulated close to middle meningeal artery branches, but faradic stimulation of the dura of the floor of the anterior cranial fossa produced pain experienced in the eye on the same side. The falx cerebri is not sensitive.
- Similarly, the dura over the convexity of the cerebellum is insensitive to stimulation but the dura of the floor of the posterior cranial fossa is sensitive, with pain being felt at the back of the head and behind the ear on the same side.
- Pain from stimulation of the upper surface of the tentorium cerebelli is felt in the forehead on the same side; that from stimulation of the lower surface can be experienced behind the ear, in the forehead, or in both of these sites.

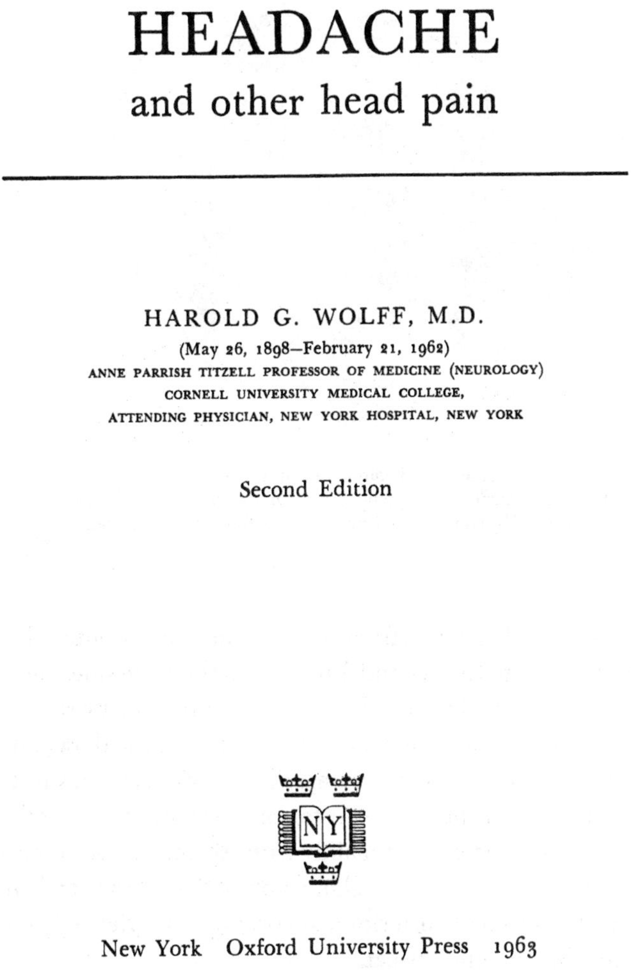

HEADACHE
and other head pain

HAROLD G. WOLFF, M.D.

(May 26, 1898–February 21, 1962)

ANNE PARRISH TITZELL PROFESSOR OF MEDICINE (NEUROLOGY)
CORNELL UNIVERSITY MEDICAL COLLEGE,
ATTENDING PHYSICIAN, NEW YORK HOSPITAL, NEW YORK

Second Edition

New York   Oxford University Press   1963

Figure 2-5 Title page of the second edition (1963) of Harold Wolff's *Headache and Other Head Pain*, the last edition for which Wolff was responsible. Courtesy of Oxford University Press.

- Stimulation of the superior sagittal sinus and nearby cerebral veins, the transverse and straight sinuses, causes pain.
- The pia-arachnoid is insensitive except near the great arteries at the base of the brain. The stimulation of these arteries, but not their more distal branches, produces deep dull aching and sometimes throbbing pain felt behind and above the eye on the same side. Stimulation of vertebral artery and certain of its accessible branches causes pain at the back of the head and neck.
- Stimulation of the cerebrum and cerebellum themselves does not elicit pain.

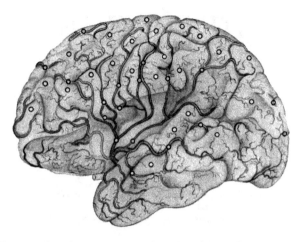

Figure 2-6 Illustration from the second edition of Harold Wolff's *Headache and Other Head Pain* (1963, p. 72) showing a result of his mapping of sites on the surface of the human brain from which headache could be evoked by stimulation. Courtesy of Oxford University Press.

Thus Wolff found that pain from stimulation of supratentorial structures tends to be referred to the eye and forehead on the same side. The supratentorial structures from which head pain can be produced by stimulation are mainly at the base of the brain where they comprise the dura and the large cerebral arterial and venous structures; the superior sagittal sinus region is also pain sensitive but the brain substance is not. As regards infratentorial structures, pain can be evoked mainly from structures on or close to the floor of the posterior fossa of the skull; stimulation of the cerebellum does not produce pain. Pain of posterior fossa origin is experienced in the region of the occiput and behind the ear.

Wolff also listed the extracranial structures whose stimulation could produce local head pain. These were the scalp, the epicranial aponeurosis, the temporal and occipital muscles and their overlying fascia, the scalp arteries and nerves, and, to a lesser extent, the veins in the scalp. Posterior neck muscle contraction produced pain in the back of the neck and the back of the head, and also caused pain around the circumference of the head.

Wolff's data demonstrated the existence of different degrees of pain sensitivity in different regions of the same intracranial structure. This finding helped explain some of the apparently conflicting identifications of pain-producing sites in the past. His series of studies in humans provided what was perceived as the definitive identification of the cranial structures from which headache could arise. It was not too different from the set of structures that Galen had identified nearly two millennia before. For a time it must have seemed that the story of the seats of headache was complete, but there lurked in the background Auerbach's hints that head pain might arise from local disturbances within the brain itself.

In the final quarter of the 20th century, there was a considerable expansion of laboratory and clinical investigations into headache mechanisms, particularly in relation to migraine, studied in both humans and experimental animals. Various highly sophisticated investigational tools were employed. These studies are discussed in some detail in later sections of the present book. Here it may suffice to indicate that they have provided reasonably persuasive evidence that altered functioning of quite localized areas in the dorsal pons and the hypothalamus appears capable of inducing, respectively, attacks of migraine headache and of cluster headache. Further, various investigations, some of them pharmacological, have been interpreted as suggesting that altered activity in central pain modulating mechanisms, mainly in the descending spinal nucleus of the trigeminal nerve (the nucleus caudalis), can augment the pain experienced during headaches, and indeed perhaps maintain it.

It now seems established that parts of the brain itself can be added to the list of cranial pain-producing structures, a list that comprises virtually every major structure above the line of the base of the skull. Time will tell whether the story of locating the seat of headache has now reached finality.

CHAPTER 3

Headache before 1800

U ntil around the end of the 18th century, most published accounts of headache dealt with the disorder as a single overall entity, or in terms of the individual members of the old *cephalalgia, cephalaea, hemicrania* triad of categories, or in such other ways that the appropriate present-day accepted headache type cannot be recognized with reasonable certainty. The present chapter is concerned with the history of such pre-1800 headache that cannot be assigned with a sufficient degree of confidence to a modern headache category. When a modern headache type can be recognized in a pre-1800 account with a reasonably high probability, that account will be dealt with subsequently in relation to the modern category of headache to which it belongs, though the existence of the account may also be mentioned here.

THE ANCIENT WORLD

Babylonia

There have been suggestions that human skulls may have been trephined for headache even earlier than 4000 B.C., and that the bone reaction around some of the trephine holes suggests that the procedure was not invariably fatal. However, there really is no unambiguous evidence as to why the trephining was carried out.

As already mentioned, the earliest known recorded descriptions of headache are believed to date from around 4000 B.C., and come from ancient Mesopotamia. Thompson (1903) published a translation of a set of Babylonian cuneiform tablets, dating from around the end of the eighth century B.C., in which headache was mentioned. In the introduction to his translation, Thompson expressed the view that the material recorded on the tablets originated in a much earlier era, some 6000 years before the time when he wrote. The contents of the tablets indicated that headache had been believed to emanate from malign, invisible, supernatural beings and influences (evil spirits, one named *Ti'i*, and demons). On tablet 3, a concept of headache origin was recorded:

> Headache hath come from the Underworld,
>> It hath come forth from the dwelling of Bel. (Thompson 1903, p. 45)

And on tablets 8 and 9, the unpredictability of its occurrence was reflected in these lines:

> Headache roameth in the desert, blowing like the wind
>> Flashing like lightning, it is loosed above and below;
>> It cutteth off him who fears not his god like a reed,
>> Like a stalk of henna it slitteth his thews. (p. 65)

The uncertainty as to the course and the outcome of headache, ranging in severity from simple self-limited instances to potentially lethal varieties, was appreciated by those ancient people:

> Headache whose course like the dread windstorm none knoweth,
>> None knoweth its full time or its bond. (p. 67)

Spells and other courses of action intended to drive away headache were recorded on the tablet. A treatment approach was described that involved an admixture of magical ritual and possible rational therapeutic actions. The latter involved binding the head, which may at times have reduced the pulsatile element of the pain in migraine or febrile headache. To expel the headache demon, one Marduk sought the advice of the great god Ea, who dwelt in water. Marduk was directed to take water from the junction of two streams and, after following a prescribed ritual described immediately below, was to sprinkle it over the headache sufferer:

> Take the hair of a virgin kid
>> Let a wise woman spin [it] on the right side
>> And double it on the left
>> Bind knots twice seven times
>> And perform the incantation of Eridu
>> And bind the head of the sick man
>> And bind the neck of the sick man

And bind up his limbs
And surround his couch
And cast the water of the Incantation over him,
  That the headache may ascend to heaven like the smoke from a peaceful homestead.
(Thompson 1903, p. xxxviii)

Zayas described the existence of a translation of other ancient texts from the Sumerian city of Nippur. These texts are believed to date from between 2113 and 2038 B.C. One incantation identified a demon, *Namtar*, as a source of headache:

In heaven the wind blows,
  on earth the mice proliferate,
  and Namtar inflicts headache. (2007, p. 46)

According to Zayas, the original translators of the tablets had available to them further material containing additional incantations against headache that they intended to publish.

These scanty fragments from ancient Mesopotamian civilization indicate that headache was being experienced by members of that population, perhaps with some frequency. The nature or natures of the headaches cannot be determined from the available translated wordings, but it appears that the suffering was attributed to the activities of demonic powers. Understandably, the remedial actions that were attempted were basically magical in nature. In the records that survive from those distant times, there seems to be no evidence that headache was understood in any other more physical way, or that natural or other nonmagical remedies were deliberately employed in its treatment. Bruyn (1989) collected from various sources other rather similar material from the ancient Near East that mentioned headache and that was interpreted it along similar lines.

Ancient Egypt

Headache is mentioned at various places in surviving Egyptian papyri from the period around 1500 B.C. to 1200 B.C. In these, the main interest lay in the treatment of headache rather than in its nature and mechanism. Karenberg and Leitz (2001) stated that the disorder was mentioned in the Papyrus Ebers, Papyrus Hearst, Papyrus Berlin, and Papyrus Edwin Smith, all of which were written around 1550 B.C. and are what can be regarded as medical in their orientations. There was additional material on headache in the so-called magical papyri of the New Kingdom (the Papyri Leiden,

Deir el-Medinch, and Beatty). In these, incantations, conjurations, and spells against the symptom were recorded. Karenberg and Leitz estimated that some 1.5 percent of the 900 prescriptions in the Papyrus Ebers were concerned with treating headache. The remedies recommended were of (i) animal origin—for example, synodontis (catfish) skull, lates (perch) fish bones, stag's head, ass's grease, cattle or goose fat (ii) vegetable origin— for example, castor oil plant roots, honey, frankincense, wax, grass, reed, coriander seed, carob tree fruit, cumin, myrtle, juniper fruit, lotus, dill seed, and (iii) mineral origin—for example, natron (mainly sodium carbonate and bicarbonate), malachite, clay, stibium, or yellow ochre. These substances were usually applied directly to the sufferer's head. For instance, Nunn mentions the following: "Another [remedy] for suffering (meret) in half the head (ges-top). The skull of a cat-fish (nor), fried with oil. Annoint the head therewith" (2002, p. 93).

Bryan (1930) had earlier described how in the Papyrus Ebers the goddess Tefrut attempted to treat the great sun-god Ra, but the treatment caused him to suffer headache. Isis cured Ra of this headache and also of "all sufferings and evils of any sort" by smearing a mixture on his head. This mixture was composed of the following: berry of the coriander, berry of the poppy plant, wormwood, berry of the sames plant, and berry of the juniper plant, all mixed with honey. One might wonder whether this mythical account grew out of a possible awareness that any opium in the poppy plant might be absorbed transdermally and then produce a degree of genuine analgesic effect.

Bryan also mentioned other head pain remedies described in the papyrus. All were applied to the head, and rubbed in: for example, a mix of "inner of onions, fruit of the am tree, natron, setself seeds, cooked bone of the swordfish, cooked redfish, cooked skull of the crayfish, honey and abra ointment." For more resistant headache, a poultice of crocodile earth broken up with ostrich egg could be used.

In the Papyrus Leiden, various spells were commended for use in relieving headache. At one place in the papyrus, the mythological deities Horus and Thoth were described as themselves being headache sufferers. The deity Ra called on the human headache sufferer to turn on the demon Apropis, who had caused the headache, and threaten the demon with the tmmt-loop of Ra. Following this action, the sufferer's head was to be rubbed with the tmmt-loop of a snake to effect a headache cure.

As far as can be judged from the available records, the ancient Egyptians, like the people of Mesopotamia centuries before, understood headache as a form of suffering imposed by external supernatural powers. As well as employing measures such as incantations, which were believed appropriate to counter the supernatural influences of these occult powers, the Egyptians used locally applied agents to which they presumably attributed some therapeutic efficacy. These agents may have had some soothing effects and, if rubbed in, some muscle relaxing ones. There did not seem to have been attempts to identify any headache varieties.

Ancient Israel

The Old Testament Second Book of Kings, chapter 4, records the story of the only son of a Sunammite woman who had been befriended by the prophet Elisha. One morning the boy went out to his father in the fields. There the boy cried out, "My head, my head!" He was carried back to his mother and sat on her knees till noon, when he died. The mother sent for Elisha who, when he came, found that the child had "neither voice nor hearing." Elisha then seems to have carried out what may have been a form of mouth-to-mouth resuscitation. The child became warm and then, after an interval, opened his eyes. From that point on, the boy disappeared from the Old Testament record, except for brief mention that he was alive at least seven years later (2 Kings 8:5). Whatever the religious importance of the story, the medical nature of the seemingly catastrophic event that occurred in relation to the boy's head is likely to forever remain uncertain, though it does invite speculation as to whether the headache may have been, for instance, an attack of childhood migraine that was followed by a period of deep sleep during which the pain subsided.

Ancient Greece and the Hippocratic Corpus

Ancient Greek mythology contains mention of a headache that affected Zeus before Athena emerged from his head as it split open (Trompoukis and Vadikolias 2007). The earlier ideas that the supernatural had a role in headache origin continued to persist in ancient Greek thought. For instance, in one of the Dialogues of Plato, dating from the same general period as the older Hippocratic writings, there is an account of how Socrates was asked by Critias to advise on the treatment of his cousin and ward, Charmides:

> And turning to the attendant, he [Critias] said, Call Charmides, and tell him that I want him to come and see a physician about the illness of which he spoke to me the day before yesterday. Then again addressing me [Socrates], he added: He has been complaining lately of having a headache when he rises in the morning; now why should you not make him believe that you know a cure for the headache? . . .
> He came as he was bidden, and sat down between Critias and me. . . .

When he asked me if I knew the cure of the headache, I answered, but with an effort, that I did know.

And what is it? He said.

I replied that it was a kind of leaf, which required to be accompanied by a charm, and if a person would repeat the charm at the same time that he used the cure, he would be made whole; but that without the charm the leaf would be of no avail. (Jowett 1892, pp. 11–12)

Socrates went on to explain to the youth:

For the charm will do more, Charmides, than only cure the headache. I dare say that you have heard eminent physicians say to a patient who comes to them with bad eyes, that they cannot cure his eyes by themselves, but that if his eyes are to be cured, his head must be treated; and again they say that to think of curing the head alone, and not the rest of the body also, is the height of folly. And arguing in this way they apply their methods to the whole body, and try to treat and heal the whole and the part together.

Whatever other motives underlie the events described in this story, it would seem that charms probably retained an accepted place in the Greek thought of the time, and that there was realization that problems and situations outside the head could contribute to headache causation.

There was also brief and simple factual mention of headache in Aristotle's *The History of Animals*, dating from around 350 B.C. The following appears in Thompson's (2007) translation:

After conception women are prone to a feeling of heaviness in all parts of their bodies, and for instance they experience a sensation of darkness in front of the eyes and suffer also from headaches. These symptoms appear sooner or later, sometimes as early as the tenth day, according as the patient be more or less burthened with superfluous humours.

The Hippocratic Corpus

Turning to what can be regarded as the surviving medical literature of the time, there is no part of the Hippocratic corpus of writings, much of it dating from around 400 B.C., that dealt specifically with the topic of headache. The symptom was mentioned, sometimes almost in passing, in a number of places, in some of which various infective processes were under consideration. Thus, in the writing on *Prognosis*, particularly in relation to fevers, one reads in the translation of Chadwick and Mann that "severe continuous headache accompanied by fever is a certain sign of death" (1978, p. 182).

The discussion on *Regimen in Acute Diseases*, records the observation that "sweet wine is less likely to produce headache than is heavy wine" (p. 199), and among the *Aphorisms*, "warmth . . . [applied] to the head, it relieves headache" (p. 223), "milk is not recommended for those who suffer from headaches" (p. 226), and "when there is pain at the back of the head, some help may be given by dividing the vessel which runs vertically in the forehead" (p. 227).

From such passages it may be deduced that members of the Hippocratic school knew that drinking wine might cause headache (perhaps migraine in the light of latter-day experience) and that local application of heat could ease the symptom (possibly when it was part of a tension-type headache). Why milk was not recommended, and how dividing a vein in the mid-forehead might relieve headache, do not seem particularly obvious to present-day understandings, so that one might wonder about the quality of the observations on which these recommendations presumably were based. The surviving Hippocratic texts contain no explicit interpretations of headache mechanisms, provide no consolidated account of the treatment of the disorder, and give no indication that particular varieties of headache were recognized within the overall clinical spectrum of the disorder. However, as was also the case in relation to epilepsy, there were no suggestions in the Hippocratic corpus that headaches were produced by the influences of supernatural powers such as devils or demons.

It should be mentioned that one of the later writings of the Hippocratic school, not usually regarded as part of the genuine works of Hippocrates himself, contains a reasonably convincing description of a migraine attack. This particular account is considered further in chapter 4, in relation to the history of the latter disorder.

Early Christian Era Greco-Roman Medicine

Celsus

In the early part of the first century A.D., Aulus Cornelius Celsus (ca. 25 B.C.–ca. 50 A.D.) dealt with aspects of headache at several places in the text of in his *De Medica*. He observed that winter and a costive bowel could provoke headache, as could "weakness of the stomach." In the latter situation, the headache occurred only when the stomach was empty. He mentioned the outlook for headache in a number of circumstances. In the words of Spencer's translation, "Pains in the head, accompanied by dimness of vision and redness of the eyes, along with an itching of the forehead, may be relieved by a haemorrhage, whether fortuitous or procured" (1938, pp. 139, 141).

Celsus stated that prolonged headache could be treated by rubbing the head, though not when the pain was at its height. Headache that accompanied fever could be relieved by pouring a mixture of rose oil and vinegar over the head, with strips of linen or unscoured wool soaked in the mixture then applied to the forehead. He mentioned the possible local use of other cooling applications in treating the symptom.

In Book IV of *De Medica*, Celsus gave a detailed description of an acute and dangerous disease of the head that he said the Greeks called *cephalaia*. Under this designation he appears to have included several types of headache: those from potentially lethal severe infective illnesses (which caused intolerable pain in the temples and back of the head, blurred vision, vomiting, alienation of the mind, and possibly nose bleeding), chronic lifelong headaches, and temporary severe headaches (caused by wine, indigestion, cold, heat, or the sun). The latter headaches might involve the entire head or only part of it, and might or might not be associated with fever. In addition, he wrote of another type of headache that he said the Greeks termed *hydrocephalus*. This might become chronic and was due to a humor that infiltrated the scalp so that it became swollen and could then be indented by pressing a finger into it. The meaning of the term *hydrocephalus* has since changed. If Spencer's interpretation of Celsus's Latin is correct, the term *cephalaia* seems to have taken in a spectrum of headache patterns that was more extensive than the one that later ancient writers included in the words *cephalalgia* and *cephalaea*.

When headache was of sudden onset but not of intolerable severity, Celsus advised immediate abstinence from food and drink, except for water. On the second day, clystering of the bowels was to be carried out, and sneezing induced. Such measures would often dispel headache due to wine or indigestion. If they failed, the sufferer's head was to be shaved. Then, if the cause of the headache was hot weather, cold water was to be poured over the head. It was then to be anointed with rose oil and vinegar, or a pad of unscoured wool that had been saturated with the same cooling mixture was to be applied to it. If, instead, a recalcitrant headache was thought due to cold exposure, the head was to be bathed with warm seawater and then rubbed briskly, warm oil poured on it, and the head then covered. If the cause of the headache could not be determined, the warming approach was to be tried in preference to the cooling one. For severe headache of acute onset, bloodletting was the primary remedy to be employed.

For chronic headache, Celsus recommended general measures such as provoking sneezing, rubbing the legs smartly, having the sufferer gargle to provoke salivation, cupping the temples and occiput, making the nostrils bleed, applying mustard to the headache site so that local ulceration developed, and even employing a cautery to produce an area of ulceration. For the type of headache that he had attributed to a humor that had inflated the scalp, mustard was applied to the scalp until ulceration occurred (presumably to allow the retained humor to escape). If the headache still persisted despite this, an incision was to be made into the scalp.

If the writings of Celsus reflected the overall situation, at the outset of the Christian era at least one stream of Greco-Roman thought, one later perceived as medical in its orientation, appears to have abandoned the notion that supernatural influences were the cause of headache. Rather, the causes were perceived to lie within the sufferer's own body, or in the impact of extraneous physical factors on the body. Though Celsus did not go into the natures of possible headache-producing mechanisms, it seems clear that he envisaged that a humor, or humors, played a significant role in it. Many of the treatments that he proposed might be expected to remove undesirable humors from the headache sufferer's body, through various routes of elimination. Logically enough, before applying such remedies, he proposed attempts to counter the effects of any causal factors that could be identified. As mentioned in chapter 1, Celsus seemed to appreciate that certain varieties of head pain were recognizable within the overall spectrum of headache. To some extent, he tailored his recommended treatments to what he regarded as the causes of these varieties, but he did not formally define these individual headache types as distinct entities, and hence did not provide any formal classification of headache.

Pliny the Elder

Later in the first century A.D., Gaius Plinius Secundus (23–79) touched briefly on headache in some of the volumes of his *Natural History*. He mentioned that the wine of Mesag may cause headache, and also remarked that headache could be relieved by applying to the head a number of apparently disparate substances: for example, the juice drawn from roses, locally applied flowers and tendrils of *Agnus Castus* (monks' pepper) dissolved in rose oil, a liniment made from the ashes of cloth stained in menstrual blood and tempered with oil of roses, the skin from the head of a hyena, a chaplet made of smilax, and white earth Eretria (a pigment). For the purposes of his writings, Pliny had simply collected information from any source he could find. He provided little indication that he had assessed its validity in any critical way before recording it. His material is therefore probably more of curiosity value than an indication of the evolution of the human understanding of headache and its management.

The *Herbal* of Pedianus Dioscorides (ca. 40–90 A.D.), of Anazarba in Cicilia, has been the prototype of most subsequent published works on *material medica*. There has been only one English-language translation of Dioscorides's manuscript, that of the botanist John Goodyer, completed in 1655. This version was never published at the time. The manuscript remained in an archive in Magdalene College, Oxford, until recognized by R. T. Gunther, who edited it and ensured its publication in book form (Gunther 1959). The published version contains black-and-white illustrations of the numerous plant drawings that an unknown Byzantine artist, around 512 A.D., prepared for Juliana Anicia, daughter of Anicius Olybrius, Emperor of the West. Gunther was very circumspect in providing a date for the text of the Greek version on which the English-language translation was based. Headache was mentioned in relation to at least 41 different plants, but in no instance was the Greek ever translated by Goodyer as *hemicrania* or migraine (or its equivalent). This would be consistent with the text antedating Aretaeus and Galen and originating in the first century A.D.

Gunther pointed out that there was uncertainty about the exact natures of some of the botanicals dealt with in Dioscorides. Several were stated to be capable of causing headaches: namely, Absinthium (wormwood), arbutus fruit (when ripe), date palm, hellebore, *Meum Athamanticum*, oil of Narcissus, *Peucedanum*, pickled olives, Polion, rosin wine, and styrax ointment. A greater number were described in various ways as being of benefit for headache, for example, for *Aloe vulgaris*: "It assuageth Scabritas and the itchings of ye eye corners, and ye headache being anointed with acetum [vinegar] and Rosaceum [rose oil], on ye forehead and the temples." In the great majority of instances, the plant materials, with or without extraction of components, were applied locally to the head in the forms of plasters, softened leaves or plant roots, or as liquid extracts. The only materials that were mentioned as being of benefit after oral intake were black poppy seed and *Myrtus silvestris*. The botanical sources of the materials applied locally to the scalp were almond oil, almond, anise, asaron, *Britanica*, *Chamaedaphne*, *Conzya*, flower of *Lawsonia alba* (henna), *Iris Germanica*, iuncus, *Melanthium*, melilot, *Mentha sativa*, mountain rue, *Peristereon*, Portulaca, psyllium, *Rhodia radix*, *Rosa lutea*, *Rosaceum* oil, *Scamonia*, *Serpyllum*, *Sisymbrium*, *Solanum hortense*, *Sphondylium*, and *Vitex* (chaste tree).

It seems unlikely that, perhaps apart from some opium in the poppy seed, these materials would have provided more than local soothing actions, but the extent of the list perhaps gives an indication both of the magnitude of the community headache problem in ancient times and of the dearth of effective therapies.

Aretaeus the Cappadocian

Relatively little is known of the life of Aretaeus. As judged from his writings, he was an approximate contemporary of Galen in the second century A.D. The majority of modern opinion seems to consider that his work dates from slightly earlier than that of Galen. It seems likely that Aretaeus wrote on short lived headache, his *cephalalgia*, in the parts of his works that have been lost. Therefore, except for differentiating *cephalalgia* from the more chronic headache of *cephalaea*, only Aretaeus's ideas about the latter are now accessible.

Aretaeus (Adams 1856) stated that *cephalaea*, which was due to coldness with dryness, occurred in an infinite range of varieties, from slight continuous head pain to periodic pain occurring at more or less regular, or at regular, intervals. The headache could be constant or variable in site, even within a single episode.

> And in certain cases the whole head is pained; and the pain is sometimes on the right and sometimes on the left side, or the forehead, or the bregma; and these may all occur the same day in a random manner. (Adams 1856, p. 294)

If the pain was strictly localized to one half of the head he termed it (*h*)*eterocrania*. Such pain was often intermittent and sometimes slight, but it could begin acutely with

> unseemly and dreadful symptoms; spasm and distortion of the countenance takes place; the eyes either fixed intently like horns, or they are rolled inwardly to this side or that; vertigo, deep-seated pain of the eyes as far as the meninges; irresistible sweat; sudden pain of the tendons, as of one striking with a club; nausea; vomiting of bilious matter; collapse of the patient; but, if the affection be protracted, the patient will die, or, if more slight and not deadly, it becomes chronic; there is much torpor, heaviness of the head, anxiety, and *ennui*. For they flee the light; the darkness soothes their disease; nor can they bear readily to look upon or hear anything agreeable. (Adams 1856, pp. 294–295)

Such a description of *heterocrania* in some instances could represent modern-day migraine but, in others, the presence of a structural disorder such as frontal sinusitis. Aretaeus's statements about the subsequent courses sometimes being followed by instances of *cephalaea* (see immediately below) suggest that more than present-day migraine was included within his category of *cephalaea*. Aretaeus proceeded to indicate that *cephalaea*, if it persisted and increased in severity, might develop into *vertigo*, which term he defined in the following way:

> If darkness possesses the eyes, and if the head be whirled around with dizziness, and the ears ring as from the sound of rivers rolling along with a great noise, or like the wind when it roars among the sails, or like the clang of pipes or reeds, or like the rattling of a carriage, we call the affections *Scotoma* (or *Vertigo*). It has a humid and cold cause. (Adams 1856, p. 295)

Aretaeus interpreted the mechanism of *cephalaea* in terms of humoral pathology. The headache syndrome was attributed to coldness with dryness, and the transition into vertigo resulted from the dryness being replaced by humidity. This vertigo was liable to develop into other disorders: mania if yellow bile was involved, melancholy if it was associated with black bile, and epilepsy if excess phlegm was present.

As to treatment, for progressing *cephalaea* Aretaeus recommended bleeding from an elbow vein followed by use of the purgative hiera (a material whose nature is now unclear). This treatment was believed to draw the pabulum of the disease from the head. Further bleeding from a vein in the forehead could be carried out, and the head could be shaved and then cupped at the vertex. There was an alternative cupping site between the shoulder blades. The scalp might need to be scarified to remove redundant fluid. If it became necessary, the great remedy for *cephalaea* could be resorted to, namely, excising portion of the superficial temporal or postauricular arteries. Purgatives or clysters (enemas) were also used to remove phlegm via the alimentary tract route, sternutatories were employed to remove it via the nostrils (by promoting sneezing), and sialogogues to achieve its removal via the mouth. The sternutatories that Aretaeus recommended for blowing into the nostrils were powdered pepper, root of the herb soapwort and beaver's testicle, these materials being used individually or in combination. Alternatively, an oily solution of *euphorbium* (a resin from a cactus-like plant) could be instilled into these orifices. Salivation was promoted by local use of pepper, mustard, *granum Cnidium*, or stavesacre (a species of larkspur).

Aretaeus also provided advice on general supportive and lifestyle measures for *cephalaea* sufferers. For instance, he indicated that milk and cheese could cause headache, but that white wine did not, and wrote that sexual intercourse was a self-inflicted evil. In a final therapeutic note, he stated that *heterocrania* was in general to be treated similarly to *cephalaea*, but that local remedies should be applied to the parts of the head where the headache was being experienced.

Thus Aretaeus proposed a range of therapeutic measures, ranging from the comparatively innocuous to the drastic, with the apparent intention of removing phlegm from the body of the headache sufferer through a variety of possible routes. This suggests that he regarded excess phlegm as the humoral medium primarily responsible for this type of headache. Although his account was more detailed than that of Celsus a century earlier, in many respects it was reasonably similar in content. The main conceptual advance between the two was that Aretaeus had formalized a simple subdivision of types of headache, ones that in retrospect were probably recognizable in his predecessor's account.

Galen

Galen lived between 121 and circa 200 A.D. No English-language translation of the full text of his complete works has yet become available. At the present time, his writings on headache are usually accessed in the Latin of Kühn's translation of Galen's *Opera Omnia* (1821–1833). Material concerned with headache is to be found at various places scattered through the twenty-two volumes of Kühn, most of it in volumes 8 and 12, with small sections in volumes 6, 16, and 19. *De locis affectis*, comprising a large part of Kühn's volume 8, has been translated into English as *Galen on the Affected Parts* (Siegel 1976). Parts of *De locis affectis* are in effect a commentary and criticism of the identically named but now lost work of Archigenes (late first and early second centuries A.D.). Book 2 of volume 12 of the Kühn edition, dealing at length with therapeutic matters, contains individual chapters on head pain (*dolor capitis*, seemingly equivalent to *cephalalgia*), on *cephalaea*, and on *hemicrania*. As mentioned in chapter 1, this suggests that Galen at some stage in his thinking accorded *hemicrania* the dignity of a status comparable with that of *cephalaea*, rather than considering it merely a subdivision of the latter. As also indicated in chapter 1 of the present book, Galen's *cephalaea* almost certainly contained instances of modern-day migraine without aura, and in the terms of his definition it could also have contained other types of primary headache and, as well, headache secondary to brain and systemic disease. His *hemicrania* (*heterocrania*) would probably have comprised mainly instances of one-sided migraine, but could have included other types of one-sided head pain, whatever their cause. The headache-related material in volume 19 involved little more than brief descriptive definitions of *cephalaea, dolor capitis* (noninveterate *cephalalgia*), and *heterocrania* (not *hemicrania*, though in most other places in Kühn's translation of the Greek the latter term was employed for the same entity).

The external causes of Galen's category of *dolor capitis* (i.e., *cephalalgia*) included heat and a hot brain (the latter bringing to mind the latter-day idea of a hotheaded temperament), cold, inebriation, blows to the head, and exertion. Causative factors intrinsic to the sufferer included fever, suppression of the menses, uterine irritation, sympathy (consent), bilious, acrid or complex humors, and stomach disturbances. Galen wrote of headache arising from bilious humors (yellow bile) being retained in the stomach. He commented that such headache resolved quickly once the bile was vomited: "How constantly do we see the head attacked with pain when yellow bile is contained in the stomach; as also the pain forthwith ceasing when the bile has been vomited" (Kühn, vol. 8, in Liveing's 1873 translation). If the headache persisted after the vomiting, Galen believed that the disorder originated in the head itself rather than in the stomach. He knew enough anatomy to have some idea of the functions of the vagus, and may have seen in its ramifications a mechanism that could mediate the sympathy believed to exist between stomach and brain, since he wrote, "For the brain transmits to the stomach, and the stomach to the head, its own affections, by reason of the abundance of nerves passing from the brain to the mouth of the stomach" (in Campbell's 1892 translation of Kühn, vol. 8, p. 934n). In some of his interpretations of headache pathogenesis, Galen envisaged a hot vaporous pneuma, rather than bile, accumulating in the stomach and rising to the head to cause the aching, but he also suggested that stomach disturbance could be responsible for headache via direct neural connections.

In volume 12 of Kühn, Galen dealt with the treatment of headache in general, and also that of headaches attributable to the various internal and external causes mentioned above. As well, he went into the treatment of *cephalaea* and *hemicrania*. He discussed his own choice of remedies and those recommended in earlier times by other authors, including Archigenes. The list of medications that he favored, as well as the numerous alternatives that he considered worth mentioning, was extensive, and it would add little to most readers' enlightenment to reproduce it in full. The categories of agent to be found in it included phlegm-removing apophlegmatics, which were to be taken by mouth or inserted into the nostrils, clysters, cataplasms (plasters or poultices), sternutatories, local applications, and even amulets. In headaches attributable to heat, he recommended that snow be applied to the sufferer's head; in bilious headaches, the bile should be evacuated from the body by means of various aperients.

It has sometimes been stated that the fifth century A.D. account of *Acute and Chronic Diseases*, authored by Caelius Auralianus (Drabkin 1950), is largely responsible for knowledge of the contents of a lost writing of the late first and early second centuries A.D. author Soranus of Ephesus (Patsioti and Rose 1995). If this is true, and if Caelius did not interpolate later ideas into the original material, the *cephalalgia, cephalaea, hemicrania* subdivision of types of headache may have been in use even prior to the time of Aretaeus. Neither Aretaeus nor Galen was mentioned in Caelius's text, though the first century A.D. physician Themison of Laodicea was. As mentioned in chapter 1, to Caelius *cephalalgia* was a temporary febrile headache; all other more chronic nonfebrile headaches, whether intermittent or continuous, were included in the category of *cephalaea; hemicrania* was a one-sided *cephalaea*, and headache localized to the temple was termed *crotaphoe*. According to Caelius, the common causes of *cephalaea* were severe cold or chill, the burning heat of the sun and prolonged lack of sleep. *Cephalaea* tended to be experienced more severely in women because they dressed the hair of their heads repeatedly. He stated that there was a variety of opinions about the part of the head that was affected in *cephalaea*. Different authorities mentioned the meninges, the pericranium, the whole scalp, the temples, and the jaws. As mentioned in chapter 2, Caelius thought that in some instances one or other of these structures was involved, and in other instances all of them.

The pain of *cephalaea* was situated deep to the eyes, in the back of the head and the neck, and could extend down the spine. Dizziness, dimmed vision, nausea and the vomiting of bile could occur if the *cephalaea* sufferer wanted to sit down. When the headache of *cephalaea* grew more severe there was also redness and prominence of the eyes and intolerance to light, dimness of vision, ringing in the ears, aversion to food, and insomnia, a range of manifestations that might suggest that present-day migraine was being described. Some of the description of Caelius resembles parts of the account of *cephalaea* in the surviving writings of Aretaeus.

Caelius indicated that it was advisable for the *cephalaea* sufferer to rest, lying on the side of the pain if *hemicrania* was present, or on the back if the headache was generalized. Olive oil was to be applied to the head, either alone or mixed with various astringent materials. Alternatively, plasters containing astringent substances—for example, knotgrass, plantain, endive, bramble, or pimpernel—were to be placed on head. If the pain grew worse, hot foments could be applied to the head. For even more severe pain, venesection might be required. Should the headache persist despite such measures, the scalp should be shaved, plasters applied to it, and the head then cupped and, during periods when the headache was easing, the scalp should be scarified. Leeches could be applied to the skull if that structure's configuration made it difficult to carry out cupping satisfactorily. While all this therapeutic activity was going on, if the sufferer was constipated clysters were to be used, since the motion of the feces and their rising emanations caused congestion of the head. It was therefore better in treating headache to ensure that the bowel was empty.

As well as describing the above treatment measures, Caelius mentioned others and devoted considerable space to general supportive measures for the sufferer. He provided quite detailed advice as to diet, physical activity, exercise, and bathing, particularly when the headache was subsiding, and also afterward, with the aim of preventing recurrences of the pain.

Caelius's account reveals little indication of his thinking (or perhaps that of his predecessor Soranus) concerning the mechanism of headache production, though it would seem that congestion of the head may have been regarded as a factor in the pain production. Some of the treatments that he recommended, and the rationales he provided for their use, suggest that he considered that humoral abnormalities (whose details were left unspecified) were involved in the pathogenesis of at least some types of headache. Caelius's account leaves the impression that he may have been considering a more limited spectrum of headache types (perhaps mainly migraine) than those that other ancient authors wrote about.

Oribasius

The collected works of Oribasius (ca. 320–400 A.D.) comprised a compilation of earlier writings that was prepared at the request of the Byzantine emperor Julian the Apostate. In book 5 of the French translation of the surviving writings (Bussemaker and Daremberg 1873), the arrangement of the material concerning headache was rather similar to that in the treatment-oriented book 12 of Kuhn's translation of Galen's *Omnia opera*. First, headache in general was dealt with, then chronic headache, followed by migraine. Later in book 5 of Oribasius, *cephalaea* and *hemicrania* were considered again. In the following account, the material in these two parts of the whole book has been brought together to minimize overlap.

According to Oribasius, the causes of headache were heat, cold, humors arising from the origin of the stomach, excesses of wine, and physical injury to the head. Severe headache indicated that there was a superabundance of humors. When headache was chronic and the pain was accompanied by a sense of heaviness, a state of plentitude was considered to be present.

(Elsewhere in the text it was indicated that "plentitude" referred to a large amount of humors spread throughout the meninges). If there were accompanying tinglings, the presence of vapors or sharp humors could be deduced. If there was pulsation, inflammation was believed to be present. If the headache was accompanied by a sense of tension in the head but not by pulsation or heaviness, the presence of a large quantity of warm, flatulent wind could be anticipated. If in the latter situation pulsation was present, inflammation of the meninges existed. If the pain had a gnawing character, there was acrimony of the involved vapors or humors. If headache with a sensation of tension was accompanied by a feeling of heaviness, the pain was due to excess humors being retained in the meninges. When the presence of excessive vapors or humors was diagnosed, the question arose as to whether this resulted from an intrinsic local weakness of the parts where the humors had accumulated, or whether it was a consequence of plentitude throughout the body. The distinction between the two was an important matter. It was necessary to treat plentitude by an evacuation of the whole body, whereas a local tissue weakness was managed differently.

The treatments recommended in the text of Oribasius were on the whole comparatively mild in nature and rarely were as drastic as bloodletting. They were directed against the presumed cause of the headache. In headache of recent onset and thought due to heat, agents intended to cool, for example oil of roses, were to be applied to the top of the head. These were followed by the local application of materials with a greater cooling capacity, for example oil of camomile. The cooling capacity of oil of roses might be enhanced by adding to it juice of joubarbe (houseleek), or of pourpier (purslane), or of lettuce or green grapes. It might even be necessary to add juice of pavot (poppy) or of magdragora (mandrake), though these substances could be damaging to the local tissues. Conversely, when headache was thought due to cold, warming materials were to be applied to the head.

If headache had become chronic, medications in the form of plasters or ointments were applied to the shaved head over more prolonged periods. Humors thought to emanate from the orifice of the stomach had to be dealt with by inducing vomiting. If that did not suffice to produce relief by emptying the stomach, the use of harsh purgatives was indicated. Headache following excess of wine required evacuation of the stomach and the use of cooling medicaments such as those already mentioned. Therapeutic bleeding might become necessary when headache followed blows to the head.

Oribasius stated that *hemicrania*, a pain that occupied half of the head, was caused by an afflux of humors or vapors. It might require treatment by purging or bleeding, though topically applied medications could also be employed. Before the anticipated onset of *hemicrania*, warming remedies might be applied to the forehead and this area rubbed with the hand or a linen rag. Once *hemicrania* was actually present, agents specific against this type of headache could be used. If in the attack the patient experienced great warmth, cooling agents and medicaments with styptic properties were to be applied to the head. If these failed to afford relief, or if there had been no feeling of heat in the first place, agents that possessed a degree of warming capacity, for example euphorbe (euphorbia), were employed. Lukewarm oil injected into the ear might provide some headache relief.

Oribasius acknowledged that the treatment of the inveterate head pain of *cephalaea* (which would have included instances of present-day migraine), was difficult.

Thus Oribasius was another ancient authority who interpreted the pathogenesis of headache in terms of the effects of humors and vapors, or of the local actions of physical factors, for example blows to the head. At least to the modern mind, he had sidestepped the issue of explaining how humors or vapors could affect one side of the head only and thus produce *hemicrania*. Perhaps if imagined properties were conferred on existing bodily substances, or the effects of nonexistent substances were invoked, it was allowable to bypass other limitations of physical reality in considering how they behaved. On the whole, Oribasius treated the matter of headache in a rather perfunctory manner. The treatments he recommended for what seem to have been regarded as different types of headache were rather similar to one another, though in general, they were relatively innocuous. His account did not contain nearly as much information on pharmaceutical agents as was present in Galen's writings. In the surviving material from Oribasius, there was no identifiable conceptual advance over Galen's position regarding headache.

Alexander of Tralles

Alexander of Tralles (525–ca. 605 A.D.) dealt with headache in three consecutive chapters of his writings. The first chapter was concerned with *cephalalgia*, which Puschmann (1878), in his edition of Alexander's work, translated into the German equivalent of the English *headache*. This chapter was followed by chapters on *cephalaea* (chronic headache) and *hemicrania*. Although Alexander of Tralles is sometimes credited with being the first to accord *hemicrania* the status of a separate headache entity (Labarraque 1837; Allory 1859), some earlier writers in the ancient world seem to have in practice virtually accepted it in that light. Alexander's account, like that of Oribasius, appears rather highly dependent on that of Galen. Superficially, the account appears systematic in its approach, but on closer reading proves to be somewhat disorganized and patchy. Its emphasis was on management, and it contained no more detailed clear formal definition of the three major headache entities.

The reader was told that *cephalalgia* had numerous possible causes and that the one that was operative in the individual circumstances needed to be identified to permit appropriate treatment. The exact natures of the postulated culprit humoral disturbances, and how they produced headache, seem far from completely clear, at least to a present-day reader. Excess heat was said to be responsible for the most severe headaches; headache due to dryness was less severe, and humidity by itself was not sufficient to account for the occurrence of headache unless sharpness was also present. Stagnation and glue-like thickness of the humors were also relevant matters. The chapter on *cephalalgia* contained discussion of varieties of this type of headache: those produced by unusual environmental heat, strong sunlight, hot humors (including those arising from the liver), coldness, gastric dysfunction, bile, fever, and physical injury.

Treatments judged appropriate were set down in some detail in Alexander's text. In relation to *cephalalgia* arising from excess bilious humor, the treatment was to be "effected by means of remedies which purge and draw away the bilious humour" (Liveing's 1873, p. 226 translation).

Cephalaea was very painful and could worsen quickly after relatively minor provocations, such as strong wines, certain smells, smoke, and changes in the intensity of ambient light. The symptom could be due to chronic inflammation of the skull or its membranes, to blockage of humors, or to their excess production or abnormal composition (in regard to their thickness or sharpness). Vapors were considered responsible for *cephalaea* when there was a feeling of heavy weight on the head during the headaches. Alexander went into the management of chronic headache produced by brain inflammation, vapors, sharpness, heat, bile, and abnormal humors. If the underlying problem was excess of a humor, in principle evacuations or bleeding were to be employed. If the temperature of the humors was thought either too high or too low, appropriate countermeasures to cool, or warm, respectively, were recommended.

The cause of *hemicrania* possibly was impure material settling or forming in the affected half of the head. Bile, thick humors, gastric disturbances, or plethora might be the culprits.

Overall, Alexander's was a fairly long account, and probably included modern-day migraine in both its *cephalaea* and *hemicrania* categories. The account incriminated almost every conceivable disturbance in body function, as this was interpreted at the time, as causes of headache. The actual details of the pain production mechanisms that were involved were left vague, to a present-day way of thinking. In principle, from a modern-day standpoint, there was little that was novel and important in the treatments that Alexander recommended.

Paul of Aegina

In the valuable comments that accompanied the section on "headach" in his translation of the *Epitome of Paul of Aegina*, Francis Adams (1844) wrote that Paul (625–690 A.D.) had done little more than abridge the contents of Galen's work on *De Med sec. Loc.* Adams would have had some justification in commenting similarly about the works of Oribasius and Alexander of Tralles if he had been writing about them. The contents of all the Byzantine writings on headache seem to lead back to Galen, and it is likely that even he partly depended on earlier, now lost, sources such as the works of Archigenes.

Concerning headache itself, which Adams may have regarded as tantamount to dealing with *cephalalgia*, in the *Epitome* there were subsections on headache from heat (i.e., a warm temperament), from a cold intemperament, from a bilious humor, from sympathy, from wine, and from a blow. The mechanism of headache lay in disturbances of the humors, sometimes an intemperance, sometimes a redundancy, and sometimes a combination of the two. Heat seemed to cause the worst headaches, while humidity of itself caused no pain unless it was associated with heat, cold, or a fullness of humors. Clear indications were provided as to how the causes of headache were to be recognized. In headaches due to heat, the skin was hotter and drier than normal and the eyes appeared red. The opposite symptoms were present when headache was due to cold, the face then being pale. Bilious headache resembled that due to heat, except that there was in addition gnawing pain in the stomach and pallor of the face. As well, there might be a bitter taste in the mouth. Headaches from sympathy could be due to plethora, particularly venous plethora. There might also be symptoms related to the particular organ in which the sympathy originated. The sufferer's history enabled the diagnosis of headache related to wine intake, and also that resulting from a blow to the head, to be made.

The headaches of *cephalaea* and *hemicrania* were discussed together in Paul's *Epitome*. The pain of these headaches was permanent, might have a throbbing character, and was liable to be increased by noise, cries, bright light, drinking wine, and exposure to strong-smelling things. When the pain seemed to be seated deep within the skull, it extended to the roots of the eyes; when its origin appeared to be outside the skull, it spread around the head. Head pain accompanied by heaviness indicated both plethora and also a fullness present within the membranes of the brain; if headache was accompanied by pungency, there was acrimony of the humors or spirits; if headache was associated with throbbing, there was inflammation of the meninges; if headache was associated with tightness but no heaviness or throbbing, a fullness of a thin and flatulent spirit existed.

The general similarities between Paul's account and those of Galen, Oribasius, and Alexander of Tralles are obvious. However, Paul of Aegina did provide rather more pharmacological detail than Oribasius had. As in the other ancient accounts, treatment of headache appears to have been based on similar therapeutic rationales, such as employing relatively harmless measures locally that were intended to provide comfort, and correcting the postulated underlying humoral disturbance that mediated the headache by removing from the body the relative excess of culprit humor that was believed to be present. Bleeding was recommended, particularly in headache from head injury, but more drastic remedies, such as the use of the cautery, went without mention. At least in relation to the topic of headache, perhaps the most that can be said of the account associated with the name of Paul of Aegina is that it provided a shorter and better organized consideration of its subject than its surviving predecessors had.

Adams's (1844) commentary following each section on aspects of headache in Paul's *Epitome* contains useful observations regarding what both the earlier and also certain medieval authors wrote concerning the symptom. Some of the other surviving earlier Byzantine writings have not been mentioned specifically in the foregoing text. Their contents, insofar as headache is concerned, have been mentioned by Trompoukis and Vadikolias (2007). However, the general conceptual similarity of the accounts produced after the time of Galen suggests that the inclusion of additional material from the often less accessible ancient literature would result merely in a rather tiresome repetition of ideas, with some minor variations in relation to matters of detail. However, there are a few interesting curiosities that might be worth mentioning, for example the recommendation of Scribonius Largus that headache could be treated by wrapping a live black torpedo, with its electric charge intact, around the sufferer's head. Nevertheless, the lack of conceptual advance from a medical standpoint over several centuries would probably make further consideration of headache as described in other surviving ancient writings a relatively unrewarding activity.

Within the ancient Mediterranean world, the general community interpretation of headache may not necessarily have always been along the seemingly primitive medical lines described above. Supernaturally centered interpretations may have been commonplace among the laity, and remedies appropriate to these clearly were in use. Bruyn (1989, p. 35), for instance, cited a third century A.D. protective charm whose translation read as follows:

Against hemikrania

Antaura arose from the sea, she cried out like a stag, she roars like a bull, Artemis Ephesia encounters her and asks 'Antaura, when do you bring the hemikrania?'

THE MEDIEVAL WORLD

The Arabian Physicians

The early medieval Arab physicians Rhazes (860–940), Haly Abbas (949–982), and Avicenna (980–1037) took up the topic of headache at various places in their writings. They were well aware of the medical ideas of the earlier Greek medical authors, particularly those of Galen. Most of the early Arab writings are not readily available in English translation, and the one volume of the *Canon* of Avicenna that is translated does not contain his headache material. Gorji and Ghadiri (2002) have provided an English-language account of headache as it was described in medieval Persian medical literature. Simple and nonrecurrent headache was termed "seda," bilateral prolonged or recurrent headache "bayzeh," and recurrent unilateral throbbing headache "shaqhiqheh," corresponding to the familiar *cephalalgia, cephalaea, hemicrania* triad of the earlier authors. The medieval Persian authors appreciated that headache could be due to diseases such as encephalitis and brain tumor, as well as to certain systemic infections and some general illnesses such as arthritis, gout, and tetanus. They also understood that headache could have psychological causes such as anxiety and depression and that these states could result from passionate (and presumably unrequited) love. Haly Abbas wrote of exertional headache triggered by activities such as weight lifting. This particular author took the view that headache was either seated in the head or was mediated through the agency of sympathy. He thought that headache originating from within the head arose from intemperament, organic disease, flatus, or head injury. Headache mediated by sympathy often arose from biliary matter retained in the stomach. In this case, the headache was relieved by vomiting. Such headache could also originate in the uterus, following miscarriages or retention of the lochia or the menses. The intake of a number of substances—for example, beer, wine, milk, cinnamon, cardamom, garlic, onion, mustard, celery, mulberry, leek, honey, walnut, mushroom, and linseed—could also result in headaches.

The theories of headache production espoused by the Arabian physicians of the early Middle Ages were typical humoral ones similar to those that had already been in vogue for many centuries. Headache sufferers were advised to avoid circumstances known to cause attacks. Those who had overeaten were encouraged to vomit and those who were constipated to use castor oil. Headache sufferers were to avoid wine and to abstain from sour, pungent, salty, or gas-producing foods. Other foods—for example, pomegranate, pear, bread, egg, lettuce, lentil, chicken, beef, unripe grapes, coriander, lime, rhubarb, sweet almond, olives, and squash—were believed to be beneficial from the headache point of view. Bloodletting was regarded as an efficient method for relieving headache, and in the case of obstinate headaches, Rhazes was prepared to recommend opening the temporal artery or applying the heated cautery to the sufferer's head. Numerous substances were applied locally to the scalp, or were swallowed with the aim of providing headache relief. Opium poppy, mandragora, cannabis, and deadly nightshade, all pharmacologically active substances, were used for severe headache. After headache attacks, the sufferer's feet were massaged for several hours, and cold or warm compresses were applied to the head.

The medieval Persian understanding and management of headache were in principle essentially those of almost a millennium before. Some different substances were involved in drug therapy, but that may have been partly a matter of what was readily available locally.

Moses Maimonides

Rosner (1993) published an account of some details regarding headache, which were to be found in the *Medical Aphorisms* of the Hebrew sage Moses Maimonides (1135–1204). Maimonides's ideas were highly dependent on the works of Galen and on humoral concepts of headache pathogenesis. In keeping with these concepts, thick, viscous humors were said to cause headache particularly if these substances were retained in the cavities of the brain, in other words, the ventricles. If thick, cold, white phlegm that had not yet putrefied had accumulated in the brain, headache would develop during deep sleep. Heat or cold could produce severe headache, whereas dryness caused only mild headache. Moisture by itself was not responsible for any headache whatsoever. However, if there was much moisture in the head, a sense of heaviness in that part of the body was experienced. Many of the treatment measures Rosner cited from Maimonides's writings appear to have been concerned with relieving migraine. However, headache in general could be eased by mild pressure on the head, while the humors causing headache required the application of an even degree of warmth to the head. Bathing the head in comfortably warm water was beneficial. Localized headache was managed appropriately by massaging the headache-affected area with oil of roses.

Rosner (1993) also described some other material concerning headache that had appeared in earlier Hebrew writing. In the Talmud (second to sixth centuries A.D.), for instance, the act of blowing away the froth or foam on beverages such as beer or mead was put forward as a cause of headache.

There was little in the material that Rosner cited that suggested that any significant advance had occurred in the understanding of headache that had existed since the time of Galen so long before. Perhaps the theories of headache pathogenesis had become a little more specific in their details, but they still depended on the imagined behavior of the tangible or intangible biological substances variously called humors or vapors.

Jean Fernel

Fernel's account of headache in his *La pathologie ou discours des maladies* (1655), the text originally dating from almost a century earlier, asserted that all head pain arose in the meninges. Sharp, bilious headache resulted from sharp, bilious vapors striking these membranes, heavy headache from cold phlegmatic humors affecting the membranes, and tense headache from flatulence or exuberance of less malign vapors that insinuated themselves between the skin and the pericranium or between the skull and the dura so that the latter membrane was separated from the overlying bone of the skull. Tight, pulsatile headache was caused by subtle bilious blood or a redundancy of spirits that distended arteries and made their pulsation more vigorous so that they had a stronger physical impact on the meninges. As mentioned in chapter 2, Fernel challenged Galen's long-standing idea that head pain arising from the dura tended to be experienced at the roots of the eyes because the dura was continuous with the periosteum at the back of the orbit. He pointed out that the pericranium of the forehead was also continuous with the orbital periosteum. Fernel stated that the ordinary headache that, over many years, commonly affected sufferers at the slightest provocation, was either *cephalaea* or *hemicrania* (the latter a term in the French translation of Fernel's Latin that was rendered as "migraine"). Fernel's account of headache was relatively brief, and, except for the novel explanations of the different characters of the pain of headache, his understanding was basically similar to the ideas of his predecessors.

In the last few pages, an attempt was made to deal with medical thought concerning headache in medieval times. There are clear indications that lay thinking in the same period had not relinquished its affection for supernatural and religious understandings of the symptom, or for employing remedies appropriate to such understandings. Bruyn cited the translation of a 14th-century text:

Concerning hemikrania

In the great name of God Almighty, when hemikrania, the half of *hemikrania*, the *collaborator* of the devil arose from the *depths of the sea*, our Lord Jesus Christ encountered him and asked: where do you go, hemikrania, *half of hemikrania*? And he answered, saying, O Lord, what do you ask me. I go to the servant of God, whose name is [that of the sufferer] to settle in his head, to torture his marrow and *to confuse his eyes*. (1989, p. 37)

As another example, Magnus (1908) quoted from a letter that Martin Luther, while suffering from a violent headache that he did not hesitate to attribute to the Devil, wrote to the elector of Saxony: "My head is slightly subject to him who is the enemy of health and of all that is good; and he sometimes rides through my brain, so that I am not able to read or write." At least until late medieval times, the accounts of headache in medical literature that have survived were largely reiterations and expansions of the accounts of Aretaeus and Galen, particularly the latter. However, as mentioned previously, it is possible that both of these may have originally been derived, at least to some extent, from earlier sources that were subsequently lost.

EARLY MODERN TIMES

Around the very outset of what is usually considered the modern era, Philip Barrough (d. 1600), mentioned as being one of Shakespeare's circle, gave an account of headache in the first set of chapters in book 1 (1583) of his *The Method of Physick*, the first English-language textbook of medicine. Barrough's text contained substantial residues of Galen's account written more than 13 centuries earlier. After referring to the almost inevitable triad of headache types, he subdivided *cephalalgia*, a new (i.e., recent onset) pain in the whole head, into varieties caused by (environmental) heat and cold, (personal) dryness, plentitude of blood, choler, fleame (phlegm?), and windiness, as well as stomach disorders, drunkenness, and fevers. His description of *cephalaea* in the fourth edition is of some interest:

Cephalaea both in Greeke and Latine is the name of headach which is exceeding painfull, continuing long, and hard to cease, which upon light occasions hath very sharpe and great fits, so that the patient can neither abide noise, nor loud speech, nor cleare light, nor drinking of wine nor savours that fill the braine, nor moving but desireth for the greatnesse of the paine to sit or lie quiet in the darke, supposing that his head were broken with a hammer. Also some of them do feele those things that are about their heads, as though they were brused or racked. In many the paine proceedeth unto the rootes of the eyes. This disease sometimes doth continue painfull always, sometimes it hath fits and intermissions, so that for a time they seeme to be perfectly whole. This disease doth vexe women more than men, because of their long haire. (Barrough 1610, p. 15)

It would be hard not to suspect that present-day migraine without aura was the subject of that description. However, Barrough dealt with migraine separately in his book (p. 17): "Hemicrania is a painfull evil remaining in one halfe of the head, either on the right half or on the left from the middle forehead to the hinder part of the head: this griefe in English is called the Migrime." Barrough's material on migraine will be dealt with further in chapters 4 and 5 of the present book.

In 1642 the Dutch physician Johan van Beverwijck still employed the ancient idea that vapors arising from abdominal viscera caused headache, though he also seemed to accept that neural activity originating in the stomach, carried by the vagus nerve, or in the uterus, transmitted via the spinal cord, could be responsible for producing headache (Koehler 1997).

It was in the headache writings of Thomas Willis, and those of some of his contemporaries, at the time of the scientific revolution, that one can find the beginnings of a breaking away from the intellectual confines of Galenism.

Willis

In his *De Anima Brutorum* (1672), Thomas Willis considered headache, particularly in relation to its mechanism, at considerably greater length and on the whole in a more systematic fashion than most previous authors had done. However, the material on headache treatment in some earlier accounts rivaled in its length that of Willis's text. In much of his account, Willis probably had in mind what would now be considered migraine, though he mentioned *hemicrania* only once, and then clearly employed the word in the light of its literal meaning as indicated in chapter 1. Samuel Pordage (Willis 1683) rendered the Latin term into English as "meagrim." Some of the case material Willis described probably represents other modern headache categories. When the modern headache type is identifiable, particularly when it is migraine, the material is considered in the appropriate section of this book rather than here. The general mechanism of headache production that Willis described, with its insight that peripheral nerves were necessarily involved in the production of head pain, can be regarded as constituting his most influential contribution to the understanding of the disorder.

Willis was one of the last of the English Paracelsian iatrochemists, whose philosophies involved rejection of the humoral concepts intrinsic to Galenism. For the humors, the iatrochemists substituted alternative chemical explanations that for the most part also lacked any solid scientific foundation, though in the alternatives can be seen emerging the rudiments of modern chemical knowledge. Willis undoubtedly was familiar with humoral pathology. After all, his task as Sedleian professor of natural philosophy at Oxford was to expound on Galen's doctrines, though in his writings it seems that he may at times have rather fallen short in that obligation. Nonetheless, he did make some use of the ancient idea of circulating humors, though the humors to be found in his writings were more numerous than the traditional ones and sometimes possessed different properties. In a way Willis seemed to invoke the existence of some additional novel humors to subserve particular purposes in his hypotheses of chemical pathogenesis. He did this whenever his line of thought required for some purpose a substance whose actual chemical composition he could not specify. In effect, the words *humor* and *chemical* became virtually synonymous for his purposes. He also invoked the existence of a nervous liquor, the modern-day equivalent of which might be seen in the extracellular and intracellular (or at least intraneuronal) fluid of the nervous system. Willis made considerable use of the old concept of the animal spirits. For him, these spirits moved rapidly along nerve pathways and were the medium through which nervous system activity was mediated. Thus they became in effect largely equivalent to today's nerve impulse. However, Willis also allocated functions outside the neuron to this highly mobile and volatile fluid whose existence he had invoked. He had additional hypothetical chemical ideas about neural activity, which he described in relation to the production of convulsions in his *Pathologiae Cerebri* (1670), but he did not make use of these particular ideas when dealing with headache mechanisms.

Earlier writers on headache mechanisms who had made use of humoral factors to explain the symptom seem to have thought that qualitatively or quantitatively abnormal humors produced head pain by direct effects. Willis disagreed with this rather simplistic idea. In its place, he proposed that his culprit humors acted on cranial tissues that contained nerve fibers to cause these tissues to contract or convulse. These contractile events distorted and irritated the nerve fibers in the tissues. Such a process resulted in nerve activation, which produced the pain experienced in the distributions of the nerves involved. Thus, to Willis, mechanical distortion of nerve fibers as a result of humoral (i.e., chemical) or direct mechanical effects was the immediate mechanism of headache production.

The parts of the head that Willis believed could give rise to headache, basically those in which nerve fibers could be found, have been mentioned in chapter 2. From almost the outset of his writing on headache, he made his readers aware of his difficulty in providing a fully satisfactory explanation for headache:

> The Headache, though it be a most frequent Distemper, hath so various, uncertain, and often contrary original, that it seems most difficult to deliver an exact *Theorie* of its appearance, containing the solutions of so manifold, and often opposite things. (Willis 1672/1683, p. 105)

He tried to find his way to a satisfactory basis for designating subtypes of headache. It had usually been accepted by his time that headaches were either extracranial or intracranial in their site of origin. Willis stated that extracranial headaches were milder than the intracranial variety unless they were experienced frequently. Intracranial headaches arose from the meninges, which were more sensitive and more highly vascularized than the extracranial tissues. However, he commented that there were other possible criteria by which headache phenomena could be categorized, namely, their clinical characteristics or their mechanism of production. Clinically,

> there are many other differences of this Disease, to wit, That the pain is either light or vehement, sharp or dull, short or of continuance, continual or intermitting; its approaches sometimes periodical and exact, sometimes wandering and uncertain. (Willis 1672/1683, p. 106)

Mechanistically,

> also by reason of the Conjunct Cause, which (as shall be declared by and by) sometimes is the Blood, sometimes certain excrements of it, as either the Serum, or nourishing juice, or vapours, or wind; sometimes it is the nervous liquor, sometimes a congression or striving of it with the bloody liquor: The Headach may be called, either bloody, and that either simple, or else serous, vaporous, or otherways excrementitious; or else Convulsive, from the humour watering the nerve Fibres, and irritating them into painful Corrugations.

Proceeding methodically, Willis subdivided headaches into types based on a mix of clinical patterns and cause. Thus to him headache was either (1) accidental, with an identified solitary immediately preceding cause but with no underlying predisposition, or (2) occasional and habitual, in which there was a continuing underlying cause, though individual headache attacks could occur without any obvious immediate provoking cause.

Occasional and habitual headache could be present continuously, when there might often be intracranial pathology present even though it could not be recognized until autopsy. Alternatively, this type of headache could occur intermittently, sometimes periodically, sometimes irregularly. There are clear similarities between Willis's accidental headache and the old concept of *cephalalgia*, though Willis's classificational criterion was the existence of a known cause for the headache. There are also similarities between his occasional and habitual headache and the then conventional category of *cephalaea*. Willis's classification seemed to leave no place for the by then well accepted medical entity of *hemicrania*.

Willis wrote of his accidental headache (p. 107) that it "happens almost to all men after drinking of Wine, Surfetting, lying in the Sun, or vehement exercise, also in the fitts of Feavours." His occasional and habitual headache had two main causes. It might be due to "an evil or weak Constitution of the affected part," which sometimes was "innate and inherited ('because the Disease is so often delivered from the Parents to the Children')" (pp. 106, 107). More often, it was due to cold

> taken by reason of the Northern winds, Snow, or Rain, the Pores of the skin in some
> regions of the Head, yea, and the nerve fibres themselves are closed up, or otherwise
> perverted or weakened, that they are not able to bear the outward air, or the agitation of
> the Blood or Humours, but presently the Headach arises (Willis 1672/1783, p. 107)

or to local structural pathology, damage to neural tissues, being produced by vascular factors, "vehement Passion, Surfeit, Drunkenness, also a blow, wound or contusion of the Head," inflammation, impostumes, scirrhous tumors, and other pathologies demonstrable only at autopsy.

"Morbific matter" (one of those nebulous entities whose existence Willis was prone to invoke but whose actual or presumed nature he avoided specifying) tended to heap up at the vulnerable sites in the head to cause pain. This morbific matter could be present in the blood, serum, nourishing juice, or nervous liquor (i.e., in latter-day intravascular and interstitial fluids). Willis went on to provide examples:

(i)   Sometimes the circulating blood itself caused the pain if it distended blood vessels at the site of pain production in the meninges, and this distension mechanically distorted and consequently activated the local nerve fibers.

(ii) Sometimes serum leaked into the meninges after the influx of more arterial blood than the venous outflow from these membranes could accommodate. The extravasated serum from the blood then mechanically distorted the meningeal tissue and thus activated its nerve supply.

(iii) Various serum constituents might activate meningeal nerve fibers directly. These serum constituents "infectious Recrements, as sulphureous, saline, sharp, acid, bilious or melancholic, or of some other kind" (Willis 1672/1683, p. 108)—a mix of iatrochemistry and residual humoral pathology—were formed in increased quantity elsewhere in the body and released into the circulation in circumstance such as "great and sudden mutation of the Air, the season of the year, excess heat, cold or moisture, plentiful feeding, drinking of Wine, Bathing, immoderate Venus, violent passions" (Willis 1672/1683, p. 109). Such excessive formation of serum constituents could also occur for no apparent reason. The stomach, spleen, mesentery, liver, and other parts of the body were the usual sites of their formation. Headaches that appeared to be related to abnormal activity of these organs were in Willis's time regarded as "sympathetic." Willis rejected the then commonly held idea that vapors could rise from the spleen to cause headache. He attributed any association between the two either to the existence of nerve connections between spleen and head or to an evil ferment (this time a "Melancholic humour") that was degenerated so that it assumed a vitriolic nature and was released into the blood by the spleen. He applied an analogous line of thought to headache that was attributed to consent with the liver, mesentery, or womb. For him, sympathy could be neurally mediated, or could depend on circulating chemical substances of various natures:

(iv) Circulating dietary nutrients of abnormal composition might also act at vulnerable parts of the head to produce periodic headache. The time of occurrence of such headache would be related to the time of intake of the culprit food.

(v) Defective nervous liquor might accumulate in the nerves of the head and irritate them, particularly if they were already constitutionally vulnerable. Headache produced by this mechanism was more likely to occur in the morning after a long sleep, because this gave nerve fibers more time to take in excessive amounts of the defective nervous liquor.

In the above array of hypothetical headache-producing mechanisms, Willis invoked only a single humor in relation to each item. However, Willis also speculated that if two abnormal humors were involved simultaneously, and if they interacted chemically, more severe meningeal distortion might occur, and as a result even more severe headache would be present. In such combinations of humors, the nervous juice was likely to be the main head-ache-producing agent.

In these hypothetical possibilities that Willis raised, one may see little more than speculation gone rather wild, with perhaps unintended lapses into humoral concepts. Nevertheless, if one is prepared to work one's way through the ideas sympathetically and carefully, and is conscious of the primitive state of chemical knowledge of the time (Willis was a contemporary at Oxford of Robert Boyle, the father of modern chemistry), some quite significant insights can be perceived to reside in them.

In his account, Willis mentioned a particular type of headache that began with a feeling of prickling in the hypogastrium or in a limb, and which then ascended to the head. Such a headache had traditionally been ascribed to the effects of rising vapors. However, Willis postulated that it was the consequence of a convulsive process that moved centripetally along nerves. If this neural activity reached the head, it might cause the meninges to convulse, distorting the local meningeal nerves, and in this way produce headache. Whether this particular headache situation represented migraine with a sensory aura, or headache following an epileptic seizure of focal cortical origin, must remain a matter for speculation.

Willis explained the association between headache and vomiting as being mediated through nervous connections that linked the brain and the stomach. Presumably these were the same nerves that provided one of his alternative mechanisms for explaining the sympathy between the stomach and the head that was responsible for headache (see above).

Willis's interpretation of headache pathogenesis, originally lengthy and somewhat repetitious, was considerably condensed and reordered in the above account to clarify it for the reader. One could massively simplify Willis's concept of the mechanism of headache by stating that he believed headache was produced by mechanical distortion of meningeal nerves, and that this distortion resulted from changes in cranial blood vessel caliber or from the effects of various circulating chemical substances. Admittedly, doing this would result in the loss of considerable conceptual material, some representing insights almost prophetic in their import. Willis not only provided a more detailed set of observations about circumstances relating to headache than any that had gone before, but in proposing a role for sensory nerves, he devised one that involved a significantly different interpretation of the mechanisms whereby headache was produced. It abandoned almost entirely the concept of vapors and their effects, retained the ancient idea of humors but under that guise gave some of them a more physiologically plausible though primitive chemical basis, and developed a more detailed conception of the pathogenesis of headache than any previous account had done. Of course, Willis's ideas would have been more persuasive if they had been founded on actually demonstrable rather than on imagined entities, but that same criticism could be leveled at previous hypotheses of headache production. Perhaps rather sadly, Willis's speculative interpretation of headache pathogenesis found little sympathy among his contemporaries and immediate successors. It was too different from the then current long-established ideas, and Willis's iatrochemical concepts were not congenial to much of the conventional thinking of his time.

Willis permitted himself some observations on the prognosis of particular types of headache. In an otherwise healthy person, headaches attributable to definite external causes (e.g., wine drinking, immoderate exercise) were safe. If episodes of headache occurred repeatedly over long periods of time, the disorder would not easily be cured. If headache went on continuously, there was risk of serious underlying intracranial pathology being present. Headache associated with vomiting, vertigo, convulsive manifestations, or drowsiness was also likely to be due to serious pathology.

Willis went into headache treatment at some length. He related the measures he recommended to the attempted correction of headache mechanisms as he interpreted them, but nevertheless finished up recommending the conventional treatments of his day. However, he did make someone critical comments about the lack of efficacy of some of the more drastic measures that had been described.

He noted that his accidental headache with evident causes tended to settle down spontaneously but could be relieved by bleeding, rest, and induced sweating. For habitual headache, whether continual or intermitting, his principles of treatment were to (i) suppress the formation of the headache-evoking chemicals at their source and also prevent any convulsive activity at their source that might subsequently be transmitted to the head via neural pathways, and (ii) cure the sites in the head where a predisposition to headache existed. For the first of these aims, "medicinal fortifications" were to be instituted. For the second, if it appeared that excessive blood in the meninges was responsible for the headache, bleeding was to be carried out, epithemes applied to the head, and the body cooled and kept "soluble" by the use of clysters. Various items of diet were recommended. If the headache still persisted, venesection or the use of leeches was to be considered. Willis's rationale for phlebotomy was not the conventional one, namely, that it would remove excess pathogenic humor. Instead, he stated that the emptying of blood vessels resulting from the bleeding would enable serum that had leaked into the meninges to return into the vascular compartment, and thereby make the meninges less tight.

Willis proceeded to provide wise advice in relation to prescribing head-ache treatment for the individual sufferer:

Medicines fit for this purpose may be everywhere found in Books: which notwithstand-ing are not to be made use of by *Empericks* rashly with, and without distinction; but ought to be designed according to the judgment and skill of a prudent Physician, always having a respect to the Constitution, the temperament, and proper disposition of the Patient, and to other accidents and circumstances, and to be compounded or altered according as the matter requires. (1672/1683, p. 115)

He provided some examples of such commendable treatment principles, and then commented somewhat critically in relation to the class of medi-cines called *Cephalicks* because they were believed to render the nervous liquor "more friendly and benigne to the Membranes of the Head." He fur-ther indicated that "these kind of Remedies, although they are not always effectual, yet they oftentimes take away some Headaches not much inveter-ate, and in some, help sometimes how pertinacious soever they be." Such an observation, preferably expressed in slightly more modern English, could be made with justification in relation to headache therapy a third of a millennium later.

Willis's account contained much additional pharmaceutical and thera-peutic advice, some of it a little quaint and its rationale elusive:

We ought not to omit, or postpone the use of Millepedes or Woodlice, for that the juice of them, wrung forth, with the distilled Water, also a Powder of them prepared, often-times brings notable help, for the Curing of notable and pertinacious Headaches. (1672/1683, p. 118)

In subsequently dealing with the problem of intractable headache, but under the designation of surgical remedies, Willis discussed the use of plas-ters, including blistering plasters, "linaments of oils," ointments, fomenta-tions, and head bathing, all which he thought of little use. He mentioned the burning or cutting of issues in the limbs or inserting setons into the back of the neck to draw off issues, and the use of the cautery. Of the latter he commented:

If we should measure this practice by the fruit or success, it will appear to be rarely ben-eficial, but more often unlucky. For I never knew any healed, but many troubled with Headaches, to be much the worse for it. (Willis 1672/1683, p. 119)

While Willis knew that trephining the skull had been recommended for intractable headache, he was not aware that it had ever been attempted.

In his experience, another surgical measure claimed to be useful in this situation, the opening of an artery, often failed. He saw no logical reason to prefer it to venesection as a means of removing blood from the body.

The significance of Willis's interpretation of headache does not lie in any immediate consequences it had for the understanding of disease or the practice of medicine. Rather, it was the first reasonably comprehensive attempt at what by modern standards could be seen as a scientific interpretation of the disorder, an attempt that substantially but not completely discarded ancient ideas and venerable terminology. Willis's thought was too far ahead of its time. Consequently, his ideas were not particularly influential in the advance of contemporary medicine, but in retrospect their originality, conceptual greatness, and intellectual daring warrant latter-day admiration.

Wepfer

Willis's Swiss contemporary Johan Jakob Wepfer provided accounts of headache and other head pains, as they were manifested in individual patients, in nearly 100 pages of his *Observationes medico-practicae de affectibus capitis*, published posthumously in 1727 through the efforts of his grandsons Bernard and George. He included commentary on each case report. The types of headache he dealt with were, in terms of today's headache classification, a mix of primary and symptomatic varieties. Some of the former are reasonably easily equated with present-day types of headache, and if so are considered further in the relevant parts of the present book. Because Wepfer's interest seemed to be in his individual headache examples, his overall interpretation of headache and of its mechanisms of production and treatment is not readily apparent. It would seem that he was attempting to present a range of individual examples of headache, rather than a balanced survey of the topic, and therefore his headache writings probably are probably better analyzed on a case-by-case basis.

Hoffman

In one section of Lewis's (1783) English-language translation of Frederick Hoffman's work (which appeared in Latin in 1739), the topic of "*cephalaea* or headache" was discussed. The *cephalaea, cephalalgia, hemicrania* triad continued to be mentioned in Hoffman's text, together with that highly localized pain at the crown of the head called *clavus hystericus*, initially so named by Willis's contemporary Thomas Sydenham (as mentioned in chapter 1). The text of Lewis's translation tends to read like a series of semidisjointed observations that fail to coalesce into a coherent overall picture. Accumulation of blood in the cavities of the frontal bone was reported to produce an obstinate fixed continuous pain in the forehead. Subsequently, local pus formation might occur. Pain arising in the meninges was said to be associated with redness of the eyes, vertigo, stupor, forgetfulness, and decreased hearing. Headache from immoderate influx of blood produced a red, humid, hot face, turgid vessels, dry nostrils, and strong pulsation of the temporal and "jugular" arteries. Collected serous humors caused a heavy head pain. Headache could be a symptom of illness, such as measles, smallpox, intermittent fever, menstrual obstruction, or indigestion; it could be due to eating flatulent food, and it also could have a venereal basis.

There were some observations about headache prognosis. Continuing headache that prevented sleep, if associated with fever, might go on to a state of frenzy. Headache of sudden onset that occurred in hypochondriacal and melancholic persons, who experienced impaired hearing and internal pulsation of the blood vessels, could result in madness, while frequent headache in youth tended to be associated with gout late in life.

As to treatment, accumulated blood or humors were to be diverted from the head. Strictures of the meninges that obstructed the circulation should be relaxed. (How this was to be achieved is not readily apparent.) Offending matter should be expelled from the body, and measures should be undertaken to strengthen the head and the nervous system. If there was an immoderate influx of blood, venesection should be carried out near the part affected, and the gastrointestinal tract should be emptied by the use of clysters and infusions of rhubarb and senna. Sedative mixtures were prescribed to restrain "orgasm" of the blood. Drugs were used to produce blistering.

Hoffmann's account obviously dealt with both primary headache and symptomatic headache. In translation, it was rather reminiscent of late medieval and even earlier accounts of the disorder and seemed to contain little that was new. It failed to provide any balanced and comprehensive view of its topic.

Boissier de Sauvages

Inspired by Linnaeus's classification of the plant kingdom, François Boissier de Sauvages attempted a similar exercise in relation to the known diseases, classifying them in terms of a hierarchy of classes, orders, and species in his *Nosologie Méthodique* (1772). Order 2 of his "Class of Pains" included the category of head pains. As mentioned in chapter 1, this category embraced not only eye, ear, and dental pains but also the headache entities *cephalaea*, *cephalalgia*, and *hemicrania*.

At first, Sauvages dealt with head pain in general. He attributed it to vascular engorgement or to stagnation of blood or lymph in the affected part. The engorgement could be a primary event or be secondary to inflammatory processes. Head pain, as well as having such local causes, might occur as a manifestation of sympathy in relation to a morbid process that was present somewhere in the body apart from the head, for example in the stomach or womb. Sauvages made almost no mention of humors or vapors, or of temperaments, in his consideration of the causes of head pain.

He seemed to consider that the word *cephalalgia* referred to headache both in general and in the old more particular sense of the Latin term. He described its character as being a heaviness of the head or a sensation of discomfort resembling that of the distension of the inside of the head. He believed that such headache arose from engorgement of the meninges. *Cephalalgia* could be distinguished from *cephalaea* because the latter was a more severe pain that affected the membranes outside the skull, whereas *hemicrania* was experienced in the forehead or in parts of the head that received a sympathetic innervation. Sauvages proceeded to subdivide *cephalalgia* into 13 types, beginning with *cephalalgia* related to (vascular) plethora. He indicated that his second and third types, catamenial and hemorrhoidal *cephalalgia*, were really subtypes of his plethoric *cephalalgia*. His interpretation of the relation between the remainder of his 13 types of *cephalalgia* and the plethoric kind is not particularly clear. The other 10 types were those related to the stomach, to fever, to pulsation (in the temples), to pregnancy, to inflammation, to catarrh, to hysteria, and to metallic intake or exposure, or were intermittent or anemotropic. His catamenial *cephalalgia* was headache occurring at the time of suppressed or delayed menses rather than headache occurring at the time of normal menstruation. The hemorrhoidal *cephalalgia* seemed to be simply *cephalalgia* in persons who also had hemorrhoids. His subdivisions of *cephalalgia* proved to hold no lasting interest for medicine. Several of the categories appear to have been based on reports in the literature of single cases, but this is understandable when Sauvages was attempting to fit all known examples of disease into his grand organizational scheme.

When he turned to *cephalaea*, Sauvages invoked the point of differentiation that was known to Caelius Aurelianus more than 1000 years before, namely that *cephalaea* was a chronic headache whereas *cephalalgia* was an acute and temporary one. The pain in *cephalaea* was severe and continuous. Nonetheless, Sauvages wondered whether *cephalaea* was fundamentally different from *cephalalgia* except in the matter of its degree of severity. He again designated a number of varieties of *cephalaea*—such as those associated with syphilis—with acrimony of the humors, with arthritis, with fever, and with melancholy, and also nominated the existences of a *cephalaea polonica* and a *cephalaea* serosa, the latter allegedly arising from accumulation of serum in various parts of the head. Again, some of these categories were based on single case reports or on associations that might easily have been coincidental.

Turning to *hemicrania*, under which he included the very localized head pain referred to in French as "clou," Sauvages (or his translator) began with the curious statement that its principal symptom was severe periodic pain of both sides of the head, often situated in the temples, the forehead, or around the eyes. Thereafter he dealt with one-sided head pain, designating 10 varieties: an ocular one, a dental one, a sinus one, one associated with coryza, a hemorrhoidal one, *clavus hystericus*, a purulent type, a *hemicrania* from infection, a *hemicrania* associated with kidney disease, and one associated with the phase of the moon. Clearly within his concept of *hemicrania* he took in unilateral head pain causally associated with a number of forms of local infective or other types of disease process, as well as *hemicranial* pain that was probably coincidentally associated with abnormalities present elsewhere in the body.

Sauvages did provide some information concerning the suggested treatment of several of his major subvarieties of headache and also for what he believed were their causes. What he wrote was often merely a reiteration of what others had previously described in relation to single reported cases that were perhaps unusual or even unique. He provided no systematic account of headache therapeutics. In his ideas concerning pathogenesis, Sauvages broke away almost completely from the old humoral doctrines, substituting the notions of blood flow abnormality or of sympathy, the latter an effect that occurred at a distance from its presumed site of origin. On the whole, Sauvages's *magnum opus* did not seem to lead to useful ends in relation to the understanding of headache. Nor did it remain influential for very long. William Cullen, the more or less contemporaneous sober-minded Scot, of Glasgow and later Edinburgh, may have been wise in failing to include headache as an item in the nosology that he devised shortly after Sauvages.

Heberden

In his posthumously published *Commentaries*, the London physician William Heberden gave an account of *capitis dolor* and *capitis dolor intermittens*:

> The most violent headache will frequently harass a person for the greatest part of his life, without shortening his days, or impairing his faculties, or unfitting him, when his pains are over, for any of the employments of active or contemplative life. (1802, p. 75)

Although he did not plainly state that it was the case, nearly all of Heberden's account reads as if he were dealing solely with periodic headache, probably mainly of migrainous type. He did not mention the terms *cephalaea* or *cephalalgia* and did not discuss mechanisms of headache production.

While medicine was in the process of throwing off the last constraints imposed by Galenistic concepts of headache pathogenesis, there is little doubt that the more educated sections of the community were tending to give less credence to supernaturally based understandings of disease. However, such notions certainly had not died out. Indeed, Bruyn (1989) stated that this type of interpretation persisted in Yugoslavian folk medicine in the 19th century, and Quave and Pieroni (2005) described its existence in rural communities in southern Italy even in the latter part of the 20th century.

By the end of the 18th century, continental, and particularly French, authors were beginning to devote increasing attention to the topic of migraine. There was a corresponding decrease in the relative portion of publications that dealt with headache as a whole, even though English-language authors in the first half of the 19th century still tended not to accord migraine any substantial place in their considerations of headache (e.g., Vaughan 1825; Weatherhead 1835). Probably more than anything else, it was the publication of Samuel Tissot's *Traité des Nerfs* in the late 1770s, and in its subsequent editions, that saw migraine become the predominant entity among medicine's categories of headache. Consequently, after close of the 18th century, it becomes practicable to consider the modern varieties of headache individually as distinct entities, and to take up their histories.

However, recognition of the importance of migraine among headache types also raises the question of where the accounts of this disorder may have been present in the older literature that has already been surveyed. The ancients simply did not know present-day migraine as a discrete headache entity (Lebarraque 1837; Chaumier 1878). The matter arises at various places in the next chapter of this book.

CHAPTER 4
Migraine

Clinical Phenomena

The French word *migraine*, or its English equivalent *megrim*, or variants of the latter, seems to have come into popular use in Western European and British communities around the middle of the second millennium A.D., or even earlier, well before the word found a respectable place in medical terminology. For instance, according to Wilkinson (1992), John Calvin used it in 1552 when writing of his own headache attacks. Barrough (1610) in the fourth edition of his *The Method of Physick*, and probably in earlier editions, used "migrime" as the synonym for *hemicrania*. A definition of *migraine*, not *megrim* or another variant such as *mygrame* or *mygrane*, appeared in the 1616 version of Bullokar's *An English Expositor*: "a disease coming by hrs, either in the right or left side of the head, caused by distempered humours or vapours, brought thither from the veines or arteries at uncertaine times." It is almost as if members of the laity discerned something distinctive about this particular pattern of head pain and became aware of how frequent it was. They came to regard it as an important type of head pain well before medicine was able to free itself from the mental shackles imposed by adherence to the long-hallowed headache type triad of *cephalalgia*, *cephalaea*, and *hemicrania*. Even as late as 1854 Edward Sieveking, a substantial figure in the London neurology of the mid-Victorian era, could write at length on chronic and periodic headache, and describe patently obvious instances of migraine, without mention of that name. Four years later, Copland (1858) did not employ the word *migraine* in the account of *headach* in his *Dictionary*. Nor did Shuldham (1876) use the word *migraine* in his classification of headache. Interestingly, migraine does not exist as an entity in traditional Chinese medicine (Garcia-Albea Ristol 1997).

Admittedly, one cannot now be sure as to exactly what type or types of headache fell within the early modern era lay notion of *migraine*, though in medicine for a long time the word was often taken simply as a vernacular synonym for its own preferred term *hemicrania*. However, the category of *hemicrania* could include not only recognizable migraine but what would now be considered nonmigrainous unilateral head pains of various types (Labarraque 1837; Allory 1859). As well, and as already mentioned, what would now be regarded as migraine was included within the entities of *cephalalgia* and *cephalaea* (an instance of the latter, from the writings of Galen, was cited in chapter 1). In the older accounts of *cephalalgia, cephalaea,* and *hemicrania*, there usually is uncertainty in knowing whether the writer was dealing with instances of what would now be diagnosed as migraine unless some characteristic feature of the latter disorder happened to be mentioned. The feature that, above all others, permits the recognition of migraine in the old accounts is the description of a reasonably typical migraine visual aura. The diagnostic importance of an aura is reflected in the contemporary International Headache Society Classification of Headache (2004), in which at least five attacks of characteristic headache without aura are required before the diagnosis of migraine can be sustained, but the diagnosis is acceptable after only two headache attacks with aura. Unfortunately, the older descriptions rarely contain sufficient detail of the character of head pain, and of its accompaniments, including any aura, to allow confident recognition of migraine.

Until comparatively recent times, medicine did not seem to pay appropriate attention to the natural histories of disorders that occurred in episodes over long periods of time. Each individual episode often seemed to be regarded as a separate illness. As a result, the headache accounts in the older medical literature usually do not provide information about the time courses of disorders that feature recurrent headaches, but merely describe individual headaches. This denies the reader the time-pattern data that might have permitted a reasonably confident diagnosis of migraine without aura. However, information is sometimes available about the time courses of recurrent headache in biographical accounts intended for a general readership. Instances of probable migraine without aura can sometimes be recognized in such writing. One example in the general classical literature, dating from 167 A.D., can be found in book 1 of the *Meditations* of the second-century Roman emperor Marcus Aurelius, who, after a long recital of the numerous virtues possessed by his father, wrote that "after his paroxysms of headache he came immediately fresh and vigorous to his usual occupations" (1906, p. 16). Although these headaches could have been some much less frequent type of recurrent head pain, simply on statistical probability migraine would be the likely diagnosis.

Another such example, a perhaps more persuasive one, is to be found in the recurrent pattern of headache described in some of the letters of John Churchill, first Duke of Marlborough (1650–1721). The texts of the relevant letters were reproduced in a biography written by his great linear ancestor Sir Winston Churchill (1933) during the latter's years in the political wilderness between the two world wars of the 20th century.

Testimony to the duke's headaches is available in 33 of his surviving letters written to the 10 years younger Sarah Jenyns, the woman he courted from 1675 onward, married, and then spent his life with. Many of the letters were written during the times of their separation while he was involved in political or military activities. During their three-year courtship, a few of his letters mentioned his headache (Churchill 1933, vol. 1, pp. 110–128). Thus on one occasion, possibly to enhance his standing in her eyes, he wrote "My head did ache yesterday to that degree that I was so out of order that nothing should have persuaded me to have gone abroad but the meeting of you who is much dearer than all the world beside to me" (p. 110). On another occasion, his tone was more tentative, perhaps seeking sympathy, possibly attempting to make peace after some discord between them: "I have been so extremely ill with the headache all this morning that I have not had the courage to write to know how you do" (pp. 124–124). To this Sarah responded as follows, perhaps mischievously, perhaps exasperatedly, perhaps having in mind the intention of inflicting some mild punishment:

At four o'clock I would see you, but that would hinder you from seeing the play, which I fear would be a great affliction to you and increase the pain in your head, which would be out of anybody's power to ease until the next new play. Therefore, pray consider, and without any compliments to me, send me word if you can come to me without any prejudice to your health. (p. 124)

Marlborough's headaches continued during the early years of their marriage. When he was in Edinburgh with his patron James, Duke of York, while Sarah remained in London with their child, on January 29, 1680, he wrote, "About an hour after I had written to you by the last post, I was taken ill of my old fits, and last night I had another of them so that for this two days I have had very violent headachings as ever I had in my life" (Churchill 1933, vol. 1, p. 147).

Over the next two decades there were no further letters, but during the years of Marlborough's great command of the Anglo-Dutch armies in their struggles with the armies of the marshals of France, he mentioned headaches on a number of occasions in his letters to the duchess. At 11:00 A.M.

on May 24, 1706, during the pursuit of the fleeing French army following his victory at Ramilles on the previous day, he paused to pen this note:

> I did not tell my dearest soul in my last letter the design I had of engaging the enemy if possible to a battle, fearing the concern she has for me might make her uneasy: but I can now give her the satisfaction of letting her know that God Almighty had been pleased to give us a victory. I must leave the particulars to this bearer, Colonel Richards, for, having been on horseback all Sunday, and after the battle marching all night, my head aches to that degree that it is very uneasy for me to write. (Barnett 1974, p. 169)

Five days later, he reported on the situation again: "I have been in so continued a hurry ever since the battle of Ramilles, by which my blood is so heated, that when I go to bed I sleep so unquietly that I cannot get rid of my headache" (Barnett 1974, p. 170). During the morning after his victory at Oudenarde in 1708, he informed his friend the Lord Treasurer Godolphin, "My head aches so terribly that I must say no more."

In the years of his retirement, he suffered a fate to which the migraine sufferer may be more susceptible than those not so afflicted, when in 1766 he fell victim to a stroke. His duchess described its effects:

> Though he had many returns of his illness, he went many journeys, and was in all appearances well, excepting that he could not pronounce all words, which is common in that distemper, but his understanding was a good as ever. But he did not speak much to strangers, because when he was stopt, by not being able to pronounce some words, it made him uneasy. (Barnett 1974, p. 270)

Six years later, another stroke carried off this man, who is often regarded as one of the greatest army commanders in all recorded history. The evidence from Marlborough's private correspondence constitutes a typical enough account of the way many a life has been lived out in what, in retrospect, can be seen as having been an overall tolerably satisfactory equilibrium with the limitations imposed by recurrent migraine.

In the two examples cited above, the descriptions of the headache features themselves might scarcely justify a diagnosis of migraine. It is the time pattern, with headache recurrences over long periods without neurological complications, which suggests that migraine probably was the disorder that was responsible. There are, of course, numerous other recorded examples of prominent persons who, over the ages, have almost certainly suffered from migraine. Lennox (1946), for instance, mentioned Woodrow Wilson, Richard Wagner, George Eliot, Nietzsche, Haller, Linnaeus and the poet John Greenleaf Whittier. Friedman (1972) named as probable migraine sufferers Alexander Pope, Heinrich Heine, Edgar Allen Poe,

Guy du Maupassant, Leo Tolstoy, Frederick Chopin, Peter Ilich Tchaikovsky, and Virginia Woolf. Jones (1999) wrote about Julius Caesar, Saint Paul, Thomas Jefferson, Ulysses Grant, Harry Truman, Charles Darwin, Karl Marx, Freud, and (as already mentioned) Calvin, while Diamond and Franklin (2005) added further mainly literary names such as those of Rudyard Kipling and Lewis Carroll in an account of written descriptions of headache phenomena to be found in the general literature. Macdonald Critchley (1986), in writing of some famous migraineurs, introduced further names: Blaise Pascal and Max Muller; and elsewhere in his book *The Citadel of the Senses,* he briefly described his own experience of scintillating scotomas. Pearce (2003) dealt with the migraine of Sigmund Freud. It almost seems as if those interested in migraine and in reading biography have little difficulty in coming across migraine sufferers in the material that they read. As well, there are numerous accounts of migraine in the general, and particularly in fiction literature, some so realistic that it seems likely that the authors had personal experience of the phenomena that they described. E. M. R. Critchley (1996) published a small collection of these writings, and in so doing incidentally provided evidence that Rudyard Kipling was a self-confessed hemicranial migraine sufferer.

MIGRAINE IN THE MEDICAL LITERATURE

The Ancient World

As mentioned briefly in chapter 3, there is a description of what almost certainly was an attack of migraine with visual aura in one of the later writings of the Hippocratic corpus. The material appeared in largely similar wording at two separate places in the Hippocratic writings on *Epidemics* (5. 83 and 7. 88). The latter account reads, in the words of Smith's translation, as follows:

> Phoenix's problem: he seemed to see flashes like lightning in his eye, mostly the right. And when he had suffered that a short time, a terrible pain developed toward his right temple and then around his whole head and on to the part of the neck where the head is attached behind the vertebrae. And there was tension and hardening around the tendons. If he tried to move his head or opened his teeth, he could not, as being violently stretched. Vomits, whenever they occurred, averted the pains I have described, or made them gentler. (1994, p. 207)

Apart from this, there seems to be no convincing account of migrainous auras in the available literature from ancient times. Perhaps people in those days were reluctant to put such experiences on record if they occurred, fearing that their sanity might be questioned. Another possibility is that migrainous visual auras may have been interpreted as visions emanating from supernatural influences. It has been suggested that the blinding light experience associated with St. Paul's conversion on the road to Damascus may have a physical explanation in the form of a visual aura of migraine (Göbel et al. 1995).

The Medieval World

Singer (1917, reprinted 2005) suggested that the visions of the famous female medieval mystical philosopher Hildegard of Bingen (1098–1179; figure 4-1), abbess of a Benedictine convent in the Rhineland, were manifestations of migraine auras. He cited the translation of her description of one such vision:

> I saw a great star most splendid and beautiful, and with it an exceeding multitude of falling sparks which the star followed southward. And they examined Him upon His throne almost as something hostile, and turning from Him they sought rather the north. And suddenly they were all annihilated, being turned into black coals. (Singer 1917, p. 78)

The falling sparks, part of the illustration that accompanied this portion of the text, and thought to have been drawn by her own hand, seem to resemble what migraine sufferers sometimes describe in their auras. However, the remainder of the drawing includes a reasonably well executed sketch of a human-like figure, and this is a far more realistic and complex component to the hallucination than migraineurs usually seem to describe as having occurred in their auras. One might wonder whether the abbess drew from personal experience of the visual auras of migraine and added representations of human figures that were of religious significance for her.

The Scientific Revolution

At the end of the 16th century, when Philip Barrough in England discussed *megrime* briefly, taking the word as a synonym for *hemicrania*, he did not add anything of significance to details of clinical phenomenology. However, his description of *cephalaea* (Barrough 1610) made it likely that he also included instances of what would now be considered migraine within the latter category (see chapter 3).

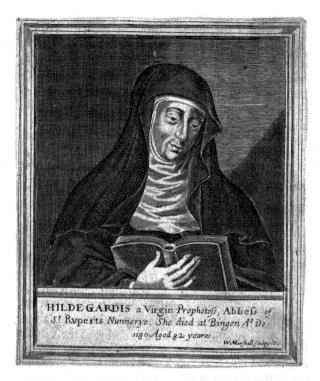

Figure 4-1 The Abbess Hildegard of Bingen (1098–1179), whose mystical visions suggest that she may have experienced migraine visual auras. Courtesy of Wellcome Library, London.

The next reasonably unequivocal account of migraine with aura appears to be that provided by Charles Le Pois (Carolus Piso; 1563–1633), who had described at some length his own headache experience in the section on *hemicrania* in his *Selectiorum observationum et consiliorum de praetervisis hactenus morbis affectibusque praeter naturam* (Le Pois 1618). He also described an instance of what he termed *hemicraniae insultus* (hemicranial onslaught), which occurred in a black-haired 12-year-old girl of noble birth whose aura was a one-sided sensory one. No visual disturbance was mentioned. A sense of formication (prickling or crawling sensations) began in the little finger of her left hand and spread to her ring and middle fingers, then over the hand to involve the forearm, upper arm, and neck on the left side. It was associated with severe pulsatile headache in the left forehead, and eye, ear, and teeth regions. The episode culminated in the vomiting of bile. Consciousness was unimpaired throughout. Subsequent attacks occurred, but were less severe. This would seem to be the first account of the sometimes loosely termed, for clinical purposes, *hemiplegic migraine*.

Thomas Willis's account of headache phenomena, described in chapter 3, very probably included instances of migraine, but will not be considered further at this point because of uncertainty as to when he was dealing exclusively with that type of headache. At much the same time as Willis wrote, though its publication was delayed until the following century, Johann Jakob Wepfer described a 23-year-old woman who saw moving objects that resembled flies, first in her right eye and then in both eyes, as the pain of an attack of a *hemicrania* grew worse (Observation 54 in his *Observationes*, 1727). Wepfer provided descriptions of 14 instances of *hemicrania* in this work. Not all were definite instances of migraine, though some, such as that outlined immediately above, and his account of *Hemicrania alternatim nunc dextrum, nunc sinistrum latus occupans*, very probably were. He also included an account of *Apoplexia metus* (Observation 108), which Isler (1987-a) thought may have been the first account of what was later termed *basilar artery migraine*. However, the sufferer described in that Observation had experienced an episode of right hemiplegia a year before, and one may wonder whether the brain stem symptoms that Wepfer described may have been manifestations of organic basilar artery disease rather than of migraine.

The Modern Era

From the end of the 17th century onward, almost until the time of Tissot, late in the 18th century, migraine headache with aura again largely escaped description in the literature, though there continued to be occasional, not unambiguously recognizable, accounts of the entity without aura. In Diderot's *Encyclopedia*, dating from 1765, there was a section dealing with migraine. The contents of this section seem to have gone largely unnoticed in the medical literature until reproduced by Isler et al. (2005), together with an English-language translation. The author of the section on migraine, who was identified only by the letter *m* at the end of the section, was thought by Isler et al. to be a Montpellier medical graduate Jean Jacques Ménuret de Chambaud. In the account, the word *migraine*, and not *hemicrania* or *cephalalgia*, was used throughout. The pain was described as acute, vivid, and lancinating and was only sometimes confined to one side of the head. Intolerance to light and noise was noted, but there was no mention of nausea, vomiting, or any aura phenomena. It was recognized that the disorder was sometimes inherited, and various provoking causes were nominated. The natural history of the condition was dealt with rather superficially, both in relation to the individual attacks and to the longer term course of the disorder. It was appreciated that the attacks were not life-threatening and that the disorder tended to die out in old age. The account in the *Encyclopedia* was shorter and a good deal more superficial than that of Tissot, which appeared soon afterward.

Samuel Tissot's writings in the latter part of the 18th century, more than anything else, deserve credit for beginning to make the Western European medical profession aware of migraine as a major clinical entity. As mentioned above, the word *migraine* had been used earlier by both the medical profession and the laity, particularly the latter, and its clinical features had been described and its nature and management discussed. Indeed, as previously pointed out, much of the earlier literature on headache probably dealt with what would now be considered migraine, if sufficient clinical detail had been recorded to permit the diagnosis. Nonetheless, it appears to have been Tissot's account, both by virtue of its quality and its timing, and his self-appointed role as educator of the contemporary European medical profession, that served to make at least its French-speaking component widely aware of the disorder. This probably stimulated the outpouring of French doctoral theses dealing with the topic of migraine that occurred during the course of the following century. Tissot's account was longer, more detailed, more comprehensive, and more systematically organized than any that had gone before. It also contained a new and more plausible interpretation of migraine pathogenesis than its predecessors, though it was one that soon proved inadequate. Furthermore, the account was written in the vernacular, rather than in the Latin that was fading from use in scientific writing, and was explicitly intended for the education of the laity as well as for professionals.

Samuel Auguste André David Tissot was born in 1728 in a Swiss village near Lausanne, educated in the home of his uncle, a Calvinist pastor, and then at the Geneva Academy, from which he graduated with an MA in 1745 (Emch-Dériaz 1992). Four years later, he earned an MD from the University of Montpellier, where he had been influenced by Boissier de Sauvages. Tissot then worked as a country doctor in his native Switzerland before commencing practice in Lausanne itself. There he held appointment as a physician to the town's poor, with a right of private practice. He initiated a campaign to vaccinate the local community against smallpox, described in his *L'inoculation justifée* (1754). As the years passed, his fame spread, and he became successively professor of medicine at Lausanne (1766), professor of practical medicine at Pavia (1780), and ultimately the first vice-president of the College of Medicine at Lausanne (in 1787). He died, probably from long-standing tuberculosis, in 1797. By the latter stages of his career, he had come to be regarded as probably the most famous physician in all continental Europe.

Tissot published 25 books and monographs. His *Avis au peuple sur sa sante* was intended to educate laypeople about illness and proved enormously influential for subsequent generations. Tissot's *L'onanisme* dealt with his views on male masturbation. Both works were translated into several European languages and appeared in a number of editions. He also translated into English Albrecht von Haller's 1755 study *De partibus corporis humani sensilibus et irritabilibus* and wrote a long scientific introduction to it. With the exception of this latter work, all of Tissot's writings appeared to be intended to improve the health of the wider community by making the laity and their medical attendants better informed about important illnesses and their management. Tissot's largest single work was his *Traité des nerfs*, dealing with psychological as well as neurological illness. It was published in stages, between 1778 and 1780, and translated into several European languages, though not into English.

At the beginning of his account of migraine, Tissot defined the place of the disorder in the then accepted spectrum of headache types, of which there were four: *cephalalgia, cephalaea, migraine* (the former *hemicrania*), and *le clou ou l'oeuf.* Tissot regarded the quite localized *le clou ou l'oeuf* (the nail or the egg) type headaches either as migraine variants or as symptoms of the "vapors." To Tissot, migraine was a unilateral headache not associated with detectable organic disease. He thus appreciated that every unilateral headache was not necessarily true migraine. As well, toward the end of his account, he mentioned that he had seen instances of headache that resembled migraine in all respects except that the pain was not restricted to one side of the head. He thought that Wepfer had probably described two cases of this same phenomenon under the designation of a "*cephalalgia* resembling migraine" (in Wepfer's *Observationes medico-practicae de affectibus capitis internis et externis*, 1727). Tissot's preparedness to mention this matter marks another of the stirrings of a realization that the essence of migraine might be something other than merely the location of the head pain.

Tissot's account of migraine brought together in one place more of the commonly encountered clinical phenomena of the disorder than any earlier account had. The pain of the disorder was by definition restricted to part or all of one side of the head. It involved mainly the frontal region: the area around the eye and the temple. However, the pain could extend downward to the teeth, and backward as far as the shoulder and the arm on the same side. The pain tended to be mild when it began, and to increase to its maximum over an hour or an hour and a half. Typically, it persisted at its maximum intensity for several hours before fading away. The pain always became severe at some stage, and the whole attack often lasted some 25 to 30 hours, or longer. The character of the pain could be "splitting," but there was no mention that it sometimes had a pulsatile character. During attacks, sufferers found it preferable to rest. They tried to avoid speaking, seeing, or hearing. These latter observations suggested that Tissot may have been aware of the experience of photophobia and phonophobia during the attacks. The eye on the affected side sometimes looked red during migraine attacks, and the eyes might weep. The arteries in the forehead and temple on the affected side could be tender to pressure during the attacks and the face swollen and hypersensitive to touch. Blood could sometimes be extravasated into the painful area. Nausea and vomiting were often present during attacks, and the vomiting sometimes seemed to relieve the headache, though this desirable outcome did not occur consistently. Errors of vision, visual hallucinations such as bright lines and scintillations, and noise in the ears might occur in relation to the attacks, though Tissot did not make clear that such disturbances usually preceded the headache itself. He mentioned an instance of hemianopia that occurred during a migraine attack, and another of what he described as the sort of visual alteration that can be experienced after looking too long at the sun. He remarked that deranged stomach function (presumably nausea and anorexia), occurred with some frequency before migraine attacks, and referred to Willis's account (in De anima brutorum) of a woman whose headache attacks were preceded by a greatly increased appetite. In his account, Tissot proceeded to describe two patients who had developed a hemisensory disturbance prior to the onset of their headaches: a 32-year-old officer in the Austrian service who experienced visual, unilateral upper limb and facial sensory symptoms and speech disturbance; and a 12-year-old girl who simultaneously experienced the sudden onset of severe migraine involving her left eye, ear, and temple, and a sense of formication beginning in the little finger, subsequently extending to the forearm, upper arm, and neck. In the latter, there was an accompanying occasional spasmodic neck retraction and jaw spasm. Consciousness remained unimpaired. The attack culminated in the vomiting of bile. (It appears likely that this is the case that Le Pois reported in 1618.)

Tissot believed that all migraine attacks in a given patient tended to be similar in character and to affect the same side of the head. However the attack frequency, severity, duration, and pattern of periodicity varied considerably between sufferers. The disorder was often inherited. Typically the attacks commenced between the ages of 8 and 20 years, but could begin earlier or later in life. Nevertheless, an onset after age 25 was unusual. The attacks tended to recur with a degree of periodicity. The individual sufferer's earlier attacks often were relatively mild, but their severity subsequently increased. There was a tendency for attacks in women to occur around the time of menstruation. At menopause, the attacks could become more severe, but in both sexes after the age of 55 to 60 years they usually became milder and less frequent, and in old age might cease altogether.

Following intercurrent illness, migraine could become more severe, or milder, or could even cease.

Tissot mentioned various apparent complications of migraine attacks and also the possibility that migraine might be replaced in the affected individual by other disorders. Nearly all the examples he cited of both these phenomena were single instances drawn from the literature. The complications that he mentioned included scotomas, blindness, and other visual impairments; squint; ecchymoses at the headache site; convulsive movements of the face; shoulder and arm pain; paralysis; impaired memory; aphasia; wasting of one temporalis muscle; a sense of chest constriction and restricted breathing; and memory impairment. Migraine attacks might be replaced by indigestion or by asthma. Tissot seemed not entirely unaware of the possibility that some of the associations he had reported might have been matters of chance or of the presence of additional undiagnosed pathology, but he raised such reservations in only a few of the instances he described.

Thus Tissot's account of the clinical features of migraine was more detailed and thorough than any previous one. It took in not only most of the phenomena commonly described by sufferers, but included the hitherto largely neglected visual and other cortical phenomena that are often encountered as elements in the migraine aura. However, Tissot did not seem to perceive that these visual and sensory abnormalities usually preceded the headache itself, but simply recorded them as components of the overall clinical phenomena. Therefore, the idea that there are two main varieties of migraine—namely, the disorder with, and without, aura—could not have been derived readily from his account. The migraine aura was still to find its place as perhaps the most distinctive element in the spectrum of migraine phenomenology. Early 19th-century writers on *hemicrania*, or migraine, did not touch on it (e.g., Petroz 1817) until Piorry took up the matter in 1831.

At this stage some purpose may be served by tracing the story of the migraine aura from its beginning to the late 19th century, even though this involves returning to some ground already covered.

The Aura of Migraine

Probably the first, albeit brief, account of the visual aura of migraine is that which occurred in the writing on *Epidemics* in part of the Hippocratic corpus that is thought to have emanated from later members of the Hippocratic school. The relevant wording appears earlier in this chapter (see p. 77). In Francis Adams's translation of Aretaeus, the section on *cephalaea*, in which *heterocrania* (to most other writers *hemicrania*), was dealt with was followed immediately by a portion of text dealing with scotoma (or vertigo). In the latter, there was mention that *cephalaea* can be followed by *scotoma*. The proximity of these two sections may be responsible for the idea that Aretaeus described migrainous scotomas. However, the description of the experience of scotoma in Aretaeus reads very much more like that of present-day vertigo with tinnitus than any present-day scotomatous defect in vision. Therefore the Hippocratic school's description of a migrainous visual disturbance seems the only one that is even moderately confidently identifiable until the early years of the 18th century.

In 1723, before the (1727) publication of Wepfer's Observation 54 (though the account must have been written in the previous century), Abraham Vater and J. Christian Heinicke of Wittemberg described what would pass as instances of reasonably definite migraine visual auras, though without mention of related headache. Their accounts appeared in the publication *Dissertatio qua visus vitia duo rarissima, alternum duplicati, alterum dimidiati physiologice et pathologice considerata exponuntur* ("Two extremely rare faults of vision are explained, one of them double vision, the other halved vision, considered as to physiology and pathology"). Rucker published a translation of the relevant part of the Latin text:

> A plethoric young man, endowed with a noble, frank, and agreeable spirit, and well-born, accustomed to continual companionship, decided several years ago to stay some while in a place remote from the pleasing intercourse of friends and adverse to the inclination of his nature. Our friend, in no wise used to being alone, bore this discontentedly and wearied his spirit greatly with fretfulness and sad meditations. Falling, moreover, into the abuse of sour and harsh new wine, he found himself afflicted by a hypochondriac disposition, obstruction of the bowels, and precordial anxiety to such a degree that hardly through a quarter of an hour had he power to read attentively or meditate on anything, even though standing at the time. A state of things came about that he, who from other days had devoted himself to painting miniatures, while occupied with painting a picture so tiny as hardly to exceed the size of a penny [obole], strained his sight too much; the vision suddenly became disordered, and he perceived darkness spreading before his eyes. By this all objects which his eyes observed were divided in half as if cut through the middle, so that whether he looked at anything with both eyes together or with one or the other closed, he saw but half, the other half entirely escaping his sight. His spirit was not a little perturbed by this strange and uncommon condition, especially when he found it continuing for some time. The symptom persisted hardly beyond an hour or two, however, and afterwards vanished of itself, without use of any remedy. (1958, p. 98)

The second instance was that of

> a noble lady from whose own mouth we heard, at that same time we were engaged in
> preparing this dissertation, that she herself was very often affected in such wise that she
> saw all objects only as halves of themselves, especially in such time as she was with child;
> the symptoms nevertheless did not persist long, but soon passed.

In the light of subsequent knowledge that migrainous visual auras can occur without involving any positive illusory element, and also without accompanying headache, the circumstances in which the first instance described above occurred, and the repetitions of the disturbance in the second one, make it likely that these accounts are the earliest descriptions of migrainous visual auras that have so far been traced in modern times.

Fothergill

More or less simultaneously with Tissot's publication of the *Traité des nerfs*, John Fothergill (1712–1780; figure 4-2), in London, described his own migraine headache with aura:

> It begins with a singular kind of glimmering in the sight; objects swiftly change their
> apparent position, surrounded with luminous angles, like that of a fortification.
> Giddiness comes on, head-ach and sickness. (1784, pp. 120–121)

Ware

There was a further British report of what may have been a migrainous aura associated with a mild headache in 1814. James Ware presented to the London Medico-Chirurgical Society an account of three instances of persisting *muscae volitantes*. After discussing his views on their pathogenesis, almost as an after thought he added, but did not discuss, his Case 4. The description of this sufferer's disorder, as it was recorded, read as follows:

> About ten years ago, when about forty-eight years of age, I experienced the first attack of
> the malady which I mean to describe; and it has repeatedly returned at irregular periods,
> from that to the present time. The first notice that I have of the attack is a peculiar inde-
> scribable sensation at the bottom of the eye, which does not amount to pain, and is so
> slight that its reality is not to be determined, unless I direct my attention very particu-
> larly to it. After a few seconds the objects, in a small point, nearly in the centre of the field
> of vision, become indistinct; and, shortly afterwards, invisible; . . . In a few seconds

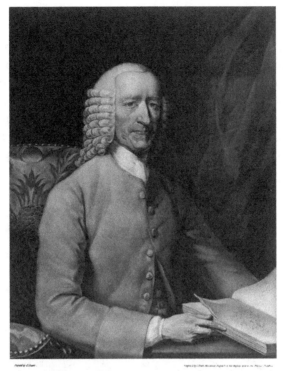

JOHN FOTHERGILL MDFRS.SA..

Figure 4-2 John Fothergill (1712–1780). Courtesy of Wellcome Library, London.

more, that is, in about half a minute from the commencement of the attack, the point that was invisible becomes lucid, appearing to be a circular spot, about the eighth of an inch in diameter; in which a yellow flame seems to undulate from the centre to the circumference with almost coruscating quickness and splendor. This spot increases by the extension of the undulating flame until it acquires an apparent diameter of about three quarters of an inch, which takes place generally in about six or eight minutes. The fiery veil, which conceals objects, becomes then thinner in the centre, and objects are there seen through it. The vision increases until at length a ring of light only remains, which continues to enlarge until it is lost by seeming to extend beyond the field of vision. . . .

At first no pain was felt; but during the last twelve months, a slight uneasiness under the forehead, on, the opposite side to that of the affected eye, has generally accompanied and succeeded the attack. (Ware 1814, pp. 274–275)

At the time when Ware published this, the functional anatomy of the visual system was not fully appreciated. This probably explains why he thought the disturbance in sight involved only one eye.

In the mid-1820s, further reports of temporary visual disturbances, some accompanied by headache, began to appear in the English-language literature. William Hyde Wollaston (in 1824), then vice-president of the Royal Society of London, described his episodes of short-lived homonymous hemianopia affecting either side of his visual fields on different occasions. He made no mention any associated experience of headache. He deduced that the episodes represented disturbed function of the visual pathway central to the decussation of the optic nerves.

Parry

In the following year, Caleb Hillier Parry (1755–1822; figure 4-3; Larner 2005), of Bristol, described an occurrence of repeated episodes of the visual phenomena of the migraine aura in a 30-year-old woman (Parry 1825-a).

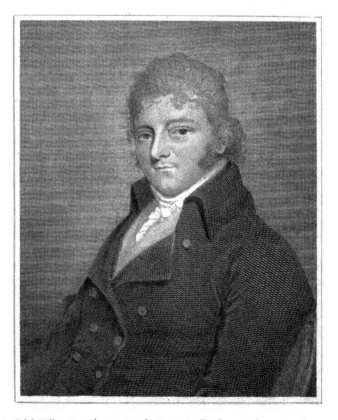

Figure 4-3 Caleb Hillier Parry (1755–1822). Courtesy of Wellcome Library, London.

The visual disturbance was followed by decreased sensibility in her right hand that ascended to the right side of her face and tongue, with inability to speak and some mental confusion. Severe headache then developed. Parry's account also contained the description of another possible instance of the phenomena.

Abernethy

A year after Parry, Mr John Abernethy (1764–1831), surgeon at St Bartholomew's Hospital in London, recorded his own experience of a vision disturbance. No positive visual phenomena were noted, and there also was no mention of any associated headache. His account in the *Lancet*, comprising part of an anatomical lecture he had given, was recounted in a somewhat more robust style than became the norm in latter-day medical literature. Abernethy described his experiences after having fallen from his horse and being driven home by coach:

> I then perceived, for the first time in my life, an imperfection in my sight. I could not see more than two-thirds of an object. First of all, however, I should tell you, my vision was indistinct, but I found it arose from the eclipse of the *third* of every object on the right hand. I ascertained this particularly as I went home, because if I saw such a long name as my own, for instance, *A-ber-ne-thy*, in a *bookseller's* shop window, or any such place, I could see *A-ber-knee*, but I could not see the *thigh* at all. *(Loud laughter.)* Well, I looked with one eye, then I looked with the other, but still I perceived that the third of every object was eclipsed, on what I may call my right side. Now this sort of case is alluded to by Dr. Wollaston, and he contends that it might be a defect in the optic nerves. (Abernethy 1826, p. 1170)

Abernethy then proceeded to describe the conversation he had with a medical friend concerning the matter, before going on:

> But since that time I have been entertained with it often, and often without having had any blow. . . . And let those who can account for it from a decussation of the nerve, do it; my own opinion is, that it arises from the *irregular actions of the retina*.

Abercrombie

In 1828 John Abercrombie, of Edinburgh, wrote of the familial incidence of migraine with aura. He described a 25-year-old woman who, for several years, had suffered episodes of blurring and then loss of vision that appeared to involve her right eye (the anatomy of the central visual pathway and its functional correlates were then still imperfectly understood). This disturbance was followed by a numbness that began in the right fifth finger and spread to the hand, the arm, and the right side of the face and the trunk. There was no associated weakness, but confusion and speech difficulty were present. As these symptoms began to resolve, severe headache and vomiting developed. Each episode lasted, in all, around 24 hours. Her younger brother, aged 22, suffered similar episodes.

Babington

Benjamin Babington (1794–1866), a physician at Guy's Hospital in London, in a paper dealing with epilepsy and in relation to the epileptic aura, recorded the following:

> A near relative of mine furnishes an example. He is much subject to headache, dependent on a disorder of the stomach. . . . These attacks are often ushered in by a sensation of tingling in one arm, which mounts up from his fingers' ends, and gradually advances towards the face on the same side, affecting one half of the tongue, palate and lips. (1841, p. 10)

It is impossible to know whether a visual component to the aura phenomena may have also been present, as a sufferer may have been reluctant to mention so peculiar an experience, and physicians at the time probably were not conscious of its significance and therefore may not have asked about it.

Despite these sporadic English-language observations of migrainous, mainly visual, auras, it was Tissot's French-speaking successors who first took a major and sustained interest in the phenomenon of the migraine aura.

Piorry

In Paris, in 1831 and again in 1835, Pierre Adolphe Piorry (1794–1879; figure 4-4), published what became an influential account of a particular variety of migraine, which he termed "iridal" or "ophthalmic" migraine, tantamount to migraine with a visual aura, and described the visual phenomena in some detail. Piorry was both physician and poet (Labarthe 1868), and became a professor of medicine at the Hôpital de la Pitié. He attempted to seek a fame similar to that of Laennec, the inventor of the stethoscope,

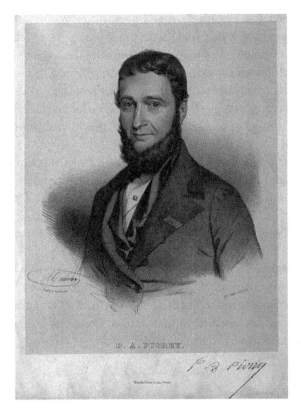

Figure 4-4 Pierre Adolphe Piorry (1794–1879). Courtesy of Wellcome Library, London.

by devising the pleximeter in 1826 (Sakula 1979). This was an instrument intended to refine the accuracy of the location of pathology in the internal organs of the body by percussion of the surface of the chest and other parts of the body.

Migraine with and without Aura

Following Piorry's (1831) publication, the French literature increasingly referred to visual disturbances immediately preceding the headache of migraine (Labarraque 1837; Calmeil 1839; Allory 1859). Several French doctoral theses and other accounts in the latter part of the century were devoted to the topic of the aura (e.g., Tamin 1860; Dianoux 1875; Galezowski 1878, 1882; Baralt 1880; Charcot 1882; Féré 1883; Babinski 1890). Calmeil's (1839) section on migraine in the second edition of Adelon's *Dictionnaire de Médicene ou Répertoire Générale* reinforced the impact of Tissot's account of the visual aura of migraine and augmented it with mention of the relatively subtle personality, mood, and alimentary tract function changes that sometimes preceded migraine attacks. Calmeil also noted the dilatation of the temporal arteries that could be seen during the headache episodes. Despite all this attention being given to the migraine aura in the French literature, it is curious that there was no clear mention of any visual aura preceding migraine headache in, for instance, the Paris MD thesis on migraine submitted in 1870 by the Englishwoman Elizabeth Garrett Anderson (Wilkinson and Isler 1999).

In contrast to the situation in France, the entity of migraine with a visual aura, as distinct from isolated instances of the phenomenon, was slow to find its way into the German- or English-language medical literature of the first six decades of the 19th century. Romberg (1853), in the second German edition of his *Manual*, wrote of premonitory symptoms of migraine attacks, such as yawning, irritability of temper, anorexia, and bulimia but did not mention visual or sensory prodromes. Apart from the isolated reports already mentioned, little was still being written specifically on the topic of migraine in the English-language medical literature until 1870. The tempo and the content of publications concerning migraine in that language then began to accelerate rather quickly.

George and Hubert Airy

On June 5, 1865, Sir George Biddell Airy (1801–1892), the British Astronomer Royal, wrote to the editors of *Philosophical Magazine* a letter that was subsequently printed under the title "The Astronomer Royal on Hemiopsy." The letter had been written in response to a recent paper titled "On Hemianopsy" that had appeared in the same journal. The latter paper (Brewster 1865) had been written by Sir David Brewster, the principal of Edinburgh University. In his letter, George Airy stated that he had suffered more than 20 episodes that began with an indistinct mist at the central point of his vision. Then short lines that changed direction and situation appeared in his visual fields, followed by a progressively expanding arch made up of trembling zigzags of brightness with slight scarlet edges. These tended to occupy one upper quadrant of his visual field. The central part of his vision became clear as the zigzags expanded, the episodes ending within 20 to 30 minutes of their onset. Airy provided a drawing of the pattern his visual disturbance (figure 4-5) but stated that he could not tell whether the phenomenon involved one or both eyes. The apparent side of his visual disturbance varied from episode to episode. Airy wrote that he knew of two friends with similar visual problems, but in each the visual disturbance was followed by headache, whereas in Airy it was not. However, in an episode

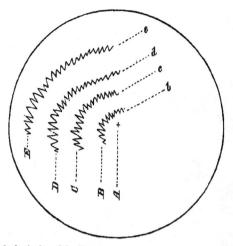

A, the beginning of the disease.
B*b*, C*c*, D*d*, E*e*, successive appearances, as the arch gradually enlarges.

Figure 4-5 The illustration of a scintillating scotoma published by the British Astronomer Royal, Sir George Airy, in *Philosophical Magazine* in 1865.

on one occasion, he "had not the usual command of speech" and feared he "might be talking incoherently."

Following the Astronomer Royal's account, in the 1870 *Philosophical Transactions of the Royal Society* there appeared a paper titled "On a Distinct Form of Transient Hemianopia." Its author was Airy's son, Hubert Airy (1838–1903), a Cambridge medical graduate who later worked in the public health field (Eadie 2009). Hubert Airy's paper began with this sentence:

> It is certainly matter of surprise that a morbid affection of the eyesight, so striking as to engage the attention of Wollaston, Arago, Brewster, Herschel and the present Astronomer Royal, should have received but little notice from the profession to whose province it exclusively belongs. (p. 247)

Over the previous 15 years, Hubert Airy had experienced a total of perhaps 100 episodes of scintillating scotoma of a pattern and duration similar to those experienced by his father, but in the son's case followed by the gradual onset of diffuse headache and slight nausea. The visual change was described in detail in the paper, and illustrated by a colored drawing which has subsequently been reproduced in a number of places in the medical literature (figure 4-6).

In his paper, Hubert Airy reviewed the available literature, though he seemed not to be aware of the accounts of Tissot and Piorry, or of the earlier

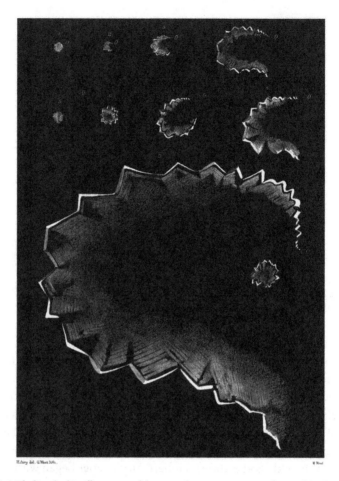

Figure 4-6 Black-and-white illustration of the expanding migrainous visual aura of Sir George Airy's son Hubert Airy, published in the *Philosophical Transactions of the Royal Society* in 1870.

isolated case reports. He also recorded the descriptions that several eminent contemporary British men of science had provided regarding their own visual auras. He concluded that two patterns of visual disturbance had been described under the designation *hemiopia* or *hemiopsia*. One pattern, experienced by Wollaston (1824), Arago (1858) and Brewster (1865), and also described earlier by Pravaz (1825), comprised brief episodic fully reversible partial or complete hemianopic impairment of vision without any added illusory visual phenomena. The other pattern, that of the mathematician and astronomer Sir John Herschel, the physicist Sir Charles Wheatstone, the Astronomer Royal himself, and the Lausanne physicist professor Louis Dufour, involved the illusory pattern of visual disturbance described above. Hubert Airy, dissatisfied with the terms *hemiopia* and *hemiopsia* that had been used to describe the phenomenon and, recalling Fothergill's statement that the appearance resembled that of a fortification, coined for it the term *teichopsia* (town-wall vision), a word that continues to be used today to describe it.

Latham

The publication of Hubert Airy's paper was followed within the next three years by the appearance of papers, and then monographs, on migraine authored by two other Cambridge men, P. W. Latham (1872, 1873) and Edward Liveing (1872, 1873). In the span of less than half a decade, those in English-language medicine had received the information that would enable them to become familiar not only with the phenomenon of the migraine aura, but also with the spectrum of clinical manifestations of the entity of migraine itself, often termed in the contemporary literature "sick headache." One of the two monographs on migraine that appeared, that of the long-lived Peter Wallwork Latham (1832–1923), then deputy for the Downing Professor of Medicine at Cambridge and subsequently Downing Professor, in its own right seems to have held little sustained interest for the medical profession. However, Latham's ideas about migraine pathogenesis were novel and important and will be discussed at some length in chapter 5. Latham's *On Nervous or Sick-Headache, Its Varieties and Treatment* appeared in 1873. It was based on two lectures that he had given, and ran to some 71 pages. Within that compass, it contained a reasonable but not exhaustive description of migraine, including a good deal of material drawn from Airy's paper. Latham seemed to accept that the headache of migraine did not necessarily have to be exclusively one-sided, though it might be predominantly so.

In contrast, the monograph on "megrim" written by Edward Liveing achieved enduring fame as a medical classic.

Liveing

Edward Liveing (1832–1919; figure 4-7) was a Cambridge medical graduate who expanded his MD thesis into a substantial monograph that exceeded 500 pages. Published in 1873, it was titled *On Megrim, Sick-Headache and Some Allied Disorders* (figure 4-8). Liveing held a physician's appointment at King's College Hospital in London, and for many years served as registrar of the Royal College of Physicians of that city. Some further details of his career have been made available by Pearce (1999). Like Latham, Liveing

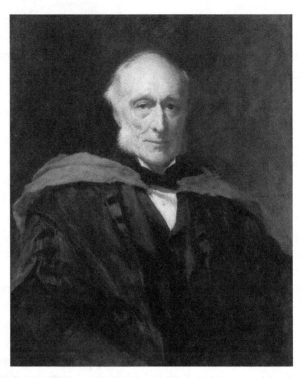

Figure 4-7 Edward Liveing (1832–1919). Courtesy of the Royal College of Physicians of London.

did not insist that the headache of migraine must be unilateral, indeed writing of the word *migraine* that

> its etymological signification of *Half-headedness*, having so very restricted an application, that its use has rather cramped than extended our knowledge of this class of disorders. We shall see that a unilateral character is a common but by no means a constant feature of the maladies which we are about to consider, and that they are otherwise intimately allied. (Liveing1873, p. 2)

Liveing did not pursue the history of the disorder in any consecutive fashion, but he was well aware of the relevant earlier literature and provided an organized systematic and detailed account of the condition, written in the rather more leisurely style of a bygone day. He included some statistics that applied to his own patients and to certain case series from the literature and overall provided an excellent source of reference not only for his contemporaries but for future generations. He developed a concept of migraine pathogenesis that differed from the one that Latham published almost simultaneously (see chapter 5). Apart from throwing off the intellectual shackles imposed by the requirement that migraine headache must be one-sided,

ON MEGRIM, SICK-HEADACHE,

AND

SOME ALLIED DISORDERS:

A CONTRIBUTION

TO THE PATHOLOGY OF NERVE-STORMS.

BY

EDWARD LIVEING, M.D. Cantab.

HONORARY FELLOW OF KING'S COLLEGE, LONDON;
FORMERLY ASSISTANT PHYSICIAN TO KING'S COLLEGE HOSPITAL;
EXAMINER IN MEDICINE, UNIVERSITY OF CAMBRIDGE, 1870-71.

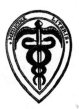

LONDON:
J. AND A. CHURCHILL, NEW BURLINGTON STREET.
1873.

Figure 4-8 The title page of Liveing's *On Megrim, Sick Headache, and Some Allied Disorders* (1873).

as others had begun to do at least since Tissot, Liveing's descriptions of migraine phenomenology contained little that had not previously been available in the literature, if searched for. However, Liveing brought together conveniently and in an eminently readable form much previously published material. After his monograph appeared, Liveing seemed to show little interest in taking knowledge of the subject of migraine further.

It has already been mentioned that there was a veritable outpouring of French-language doctoral theses on aspects of migraine in the second half of the 19th century. Data from some of these have been made use of in the present book, but they contain large amounts of material that are repetitive, so much so that Edmond Chaumier (1878) chose to end the first sentence of his own historical thesis on the subject with the words "Tout est dit." From the late 19th century onward, the majority of material that was published concerning migraine phenomenology appeared in the English language, irrespective of its country of origin.

Wilks

Airy, Latham, and Liveing were not the only English physicians who wrote on migraine and headache in the last three decades of the 19th century. Sir Samuel Wilks (figure 4-9), pathologist and physician at Guy's Hospital in London, was an even more considerable figure, a man sometimes credited

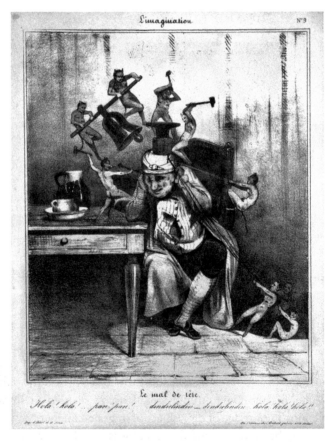

Figure 4-9 Cartoon of a headache sufferer whose head is being repeatedly hammered by demons, reflecting the throbbing and hammering character of the pain in some migraine attacks. Courtesy of Wellcome Library, London.

with being the greatest scientific clinician of his day in Europe. Wilks was the first to provide evidence that syphilis affected the internal organs of the body, and to recognize that the diseases ulcerative colitis and primary systemic amyloidosis existed. Moreover, several years before John Hughlings Jackson, he had suggested that all epilepsy arose in the cerebral cortex (Wilks 1866), though he did not develop that insight further. Wilks described with heartfelt intensity his sufferings from migraine in a paper published in the *British Medical Journal*:

> I need scarcely describe a sick-headache—how one rises in the morning more dead than alive, perfectly unable to swallow the smallest particle of food, and often perhaps actually sick; how the head throbs, and the pain increased by the slightest movement; how speaking or doing is a burden beyond bearing; how one prays to be left alone in the utmost quiet, so that he may, if possible, sleep. . . . The only remedies which are of any avail are those which act on the nervous system, such as hot tea and coffee or, after the stomach is quieter, and the more urgent symptoms have passed off, a little wine or ammonia. If the headache take more the form of hemicrania, then remedies are occasionally useful. (1872, p. 8)

There was even more detail in Wilks's volume of *Lectures on Diseases of the Nervous System* (1878). He may have added little that was factual and important concerning migraine to what his British colleagues had already written, but his writing was more vigorous in style and, because of his already great reputation, more likely to have reached a wider readership. And Wilks did emphasize the throbbing character that is often inherent to the migraine headache, a matter that was not given much emphasis in many earlier accounts:

> Its great peculiarity is the throbbing that occurs with each beat of the heart, aggravated by every movement of the body, and more especially of the head itself. . . . The sufferer walks slowly, since everything which makes his arteries beat a degree more violently adds to his misery; in his head he perpetually hears or feels "throb," "throb," "throb," and his only relief is to support his head against a pillow or rest it on the hand, and avoid all possible excitement. (1878, p. 426)

Gowers

William Gowers (1845–1915), Liveing's next-door neighbor on Queen Anne Street, London, was one of the very great figures in the history of neurology, arguably the greatest neurological clinician of all (Critchley 1949). He possessed remarkable powers of observation and documentation and very considerable ability to analyze and interpret clinical data. His writings were prolific, though at times somewhat repetitive, and his prose style unusually simple and direct in an age more prolix than the present one. His enduring fame rests chiefly on his two-volume *A Manual of Diseases of the Nervous System*. This work ran to nearly 2000 pages of text and illustration, and in at least some circles was regarded as the bible of neurology. It was substantially based on extensive personal experience and is fairly widely accepted as the greatest large textbook on the subject ever written, and ever likely to be written, by a single author. In the first edition of the *Manual* (1888), Gowers devoted 19 pages to the topic of "paroxysmal headache or migraine." After the lapse of more than a century, Gowers's account of the clinical manifestations of migraine contains almost everything that one would expect to find in a present-day comprehensive description of the disorder. Gowers began his account with an elegant *de facto* definition of the condition:

> Migraine is an affection characterised by paroxysmal nervous disturbance of which headache is the most constant element. The pain is seldom absent and may exist alone, but it is commonly accompanied by nausea and vomiting, and is often preceded by some sensory disturbance, especially by some disorder of the sense of sight. The symptoms are frequently one sided. (Gowers 1888, p. 776)

Thus he perceived migraine not simply as a matter of headache but as a nervous system disturbance whose most frequent manifestation was headache. Perhaps because of this interpretation of the nature of the condition he devoted a good deal of attention to the sensory manifestations of the disorder. He pointed out that these manifestations could occur in the absence of headache, though this was rare. As well, the same migraine sufferer could at different times have headache with, and without, the occurrence of sensory symptoms. The pattern of the manifestations could change during the course of the sufferer's life. Gowers indicated that migraine sufferers might at other times experience lesser degrees of headache. Factors that provoked migraine attacks included fatigue, excitement, digestive disturbances, particularly those occasioned by certain items of diet, visual impressions, bright light, or changes in the intensity of ambient light. There could be premonitory symptoms before the actual migraine attack commenced, including a heavy head, somnolence, and slight headache. The pain of the migraine was not necessarily unilateral, but if it was bilateral it tended to be more severe on one side than on the other. If they were present, the sensory symptoms of the attack itself usually involved vision, and comprised spectral changes, or loss of part of the visual field, or were combinations of these. Occasionally there were hemisensory symptoms with or without a mild degree of hemiparesis, and aphasia. He thought the latter usually was sensory rather than motor in nature, and occurred if the dominant side of the body was affected by the sensory changes. There could also be slight mental changes and a vague sense of disequilibrium and, very rarely, sudden deafness and tinnitus. Elsewhere, in his Bowman Lectures on subjective visual sensations (Gowers 1895), in his book on *The Borderland of Epilepsy* (1907), and in a lecture on the prodromes of migraine (1909), Gowers provided even more detailed accounts of the visual and somatic sensory disturbances that might occur in the disorder. In particular, he emphasized the features of the somatic sensory symptoms of migraine that permitted their differentiation from the consequences of epileptic discharges that arose in the sensory cortex of the brain.

Gowers observed that in a given individual, the attacks tended to be reasonably similar in their features, though over time the attack character could change. At one stage of life, an individual could have more than one pattern of migraine attack. In attacks, the pain usually began relatively mildly and at first was localized but later became more widespread and could possibly change in predominance from one side of the head to the other during a single attack. Nausea and vomiting in the attack usually occurred after the pain had reached its zenith. At that stage the pain might resolve fairly quickly after vomiting had occurred. However, if nausea and vomiting developed early in the attack, the act of vomiting did not seem to be able to bring about the termination of the attack. Indeed, vomiting then might temporarily increase the headache. Bright light also could increase the severity of the headache. Gowers said little about the character of the headache except that, at its onset, the pain might be "boring." During the headache the sufferer's face usually was pale and the extremities cold, but later in the attack the pallor might be replaced by flushing. Rarely the sufferer's face was flushed from the outset of the attack. Sometimes at the end of an attack a diuresis could occur. If the patient could sleep, the attack might have resolved by the time he or she woke again.

The frequency of migraine attacks in a given individual varied, but there was often a degree of inexact periodicity in their timing. In women, there was a tendency for attacks to occur around the times of menstruation. There was often a trend for the attacks to tend to diminish in frequency and severity as the sufferer grew older.

In all, Gowers provided a wonderfully clear description of migraine manifestations. In a way, his account largely completed the process of making the English-speaking medical profession of the late 19th century aware of the clinical pattern and behavior of the disorder, a little over a century after Tissot had begun the process. However, there were certain aspects that did not find their way into Gowers's account. Thus there was no clear description of the intolerance to light that is relatively frequent in migraine attacks, though Gowers did mention that light made the headache worse. The reasonably often noted intolerance to noise during the attacks received no mention. Although Gowers wrote of the site and severity of the pain of migraine, he said very little about the pain's character. In particular, he did not mention that the headache was often throbbing in nature. However, this point often seemed to escape notice in the 19th-century migraine literature and was barely mentioned in Living's monograph. In Gowers's writings, there was no indication that frequently recurring migraine could merge into a situation of continuing headache that persisted over long periods of time. Nor was there mention of some of the complications of the disorder that sufferers occasionally experienced. These latter matters will be dealt with later in this chapter. Gowers may have been unaware of them because of the nature of his medical practice; being a consultant may not have allowed him to follow individual migraine sufferers over long periods of time.

During this late 19th-century British surge of interest in migraine, on the Continent there had continued to be, at least in French-speaking regions, the publication of a number of theses (some mentioned above) and other substantial writings on migraine. Under the authorship of Louis Hyacinthe Thomas, a 137-page monograph on the subject appeared in 1887. In this work, Thomas divided the topic into *migraine vulgaire* (i.e., common migraine, or migraine without aura) and *migraine ophthalmique* (more or less equivalent to migraine with aura, the so-called classical migraine). This pattern of distinction has been preserved down to the present time.

By the end of the 19th century, the clinical spectrum of migraine had by and large been described in, and disseminated throughout, the medical community, by virtue of the influential writings of Gowers and others. However, since that time, and during the 20th century, aspects of migraine not touched on in Gowers's account have come to notice. In addition to Thomas's two major clinical types, other less common but clinically recognizable patterns of migraine phenomenology have since been recognized. The designations of these additional entities have sometimes proved to have a continuing clinical utility, though the entities themselves have come to be regarded as not fundamentally different from the two major subtypes of migraine. They have therefore been embraced within the ambit of the two major types in contemporary classifications of the disorder. Various complications of migraine, and various associations of other conditions with the disorder, have also been described in the literature. These matters will now be considered, from a historical viewpoint.

Clinical Subtypes of Migraine

Migraine Ophthalmoplégique

Some aspects of the history of migraine with a visual aura (*migraine ophthalmique; iris migraine*) have already been described, but the French-language literature around the end of the 19th century sometimes referred to a different entity with a rather similar name, the *migraine ophthalmoplégique* of Charcot. In 1890, and again in 1897, the great French clinician Jean-Martin Charcot, occupant of the world's first chair of neurology (at the Hôpital de la Salpêtrière in Paris) described instances of external eye muscle palsy that developed during attacks of headache in migraine sufferers. The resulting double vision might persist beyond the duration of the attack, though it ultimately disappeared. For his 1897 paper, Charcot collected a total of some 32 cases from the French-language literature and implied that he might have been able to find further instances if he had carried out a more careful search. In Britain, even earlier than Charcot, Saundby (1882) and Paterson (1890) had reported probable instances of eye muscle palsy occurring during migraine attacks.

It should perhaps be noted at this point that the Parisian clinician Charles Féré (1897), one of Charcot's pupils, had described an instance of what he called *migraine ophthalmospasmodique*. In his patient, at the peak of a left frontotemporal headache, there had occurred involuntary contraction of the muscles of the eyeball and the eyelids. The condition does not seem to have attracted any subsequent continuing interest, and is mentioned here partly because, at a quick glance, its name may easily be mistaken for that of *migraine ophthalmoplégique*.

Retinal Migraine

Since a report by Galezowski (1882), occasional accounts of the entity of so-called retinal migraine have appeared in the literature. The condition comprises a temporary or sometimes permanent disturbance of the vision of one eye that develops during a migraine attack. The literature on the topic was reviewed by Grosberg et al. (2006). These authors added a further six instances to those they found in the literature and commented that continuing visual limitations were much more frequent in this subset of migraine sufferers than in those with the very much more frequent variety of migraine in which the aura involved the vision of both eyes, in other words, classical migraine.

In 1961 the Birmingham (United Kingdom) neurologist Edwin Bickerstaff reported a series of 34 patients, mostly female and nearly all under the age of 23, who had experienced episodes of a rather characteristic disorder (Bickerstaff 1961-a). The episodes began with a visual disturbance that comprised either positive visual manifestations or a total loss of vision in both visual fields. This was followed by vertigo, ataxia of gait, dysarthria, and occasionally tinnitus. There was tingling and numbness in all the extremities of both sides and sometimes also around the lips and on both sides of the tongue. These symptoms lasted from 2 to 45 minutes. They then subsided rapidly and fully. In each case, subsequent severe throbbing headache developed, usually at the back of the head and often associated with vomiting. There was a family history of migraine in close relatives in 28 of the 34 patients. The pattern of symptoms was interpreted as being consistent with a disturbance of neural function throughout the territory of supply of the basilar artery. Nearly 12 months later, Bickerstaff (1961-b) reported four further instances of such basilar artery migraine, all in young females. In one of these women there was gradual loss of consciousness on several occasions during the episodes, irrespective of whether the sufferer was standing or recumbent. No convulsing occurred, and there were no sequelae. All relevant investigations available at the time provided no explanation for the episodes of impaired consciousness. It was considered that they were not likely to be syncopal in nature. Bickerstaff pointed out that Gowers (1907) had described an 18-year-old female who began to have right-sided migraine attacks. After 10 years, her pattern of attack changed. She began to suffer bilateral distortions and losses of vision, followed by severe vertigo and dysesthesiae in the arms, legs, and jaw that went on for 10 minutes. She then became unconscious for some 15 minutes. After recovering consciousness, she had severe headache at the back of her head which went on for about two hours. Bickerstaff thought that Gowers's case might well have been an earlier instance of the disorder to which he had drawn attention in his publication half a century later. Since Bickerstaff's account, there have been further reports of the syndrome, for example that of Swanson and Vick (1978).

Familial Hemiplegic Migraine

The earliest description of this pattern of migraine may well be that of the sister and brother reported by Abercrombie in 1828 (see pp. 89–90). In 1910, J. Michell Clarke, professor of medicine in the University of Bristol, described a family in which recurrent episodes of fully reversible hemiplegia or, in one case, tetraplegia accompanied attacks of migraine. There was often associated loss of speech. The disorder was traced through three generations and appeared to have an autosomal dominant pattern of inheritance (Clarke 1910). Later, Charles Whitty (1953), at Oxford, described six cases of what he called familial hemiplegic migraine (one in an appendix to his paper). Two of Whitty's cases were siblings whose father had similar attacks. Of the remaining four cases, only one had a family history of similar hemiplegic attacks. Whitty noted that, since Clarke's report, Dynes (1939) and Symonds (1970, originally 1951) had described examples of the condition. Bradshaw and Parsons (1964) published a pedigree in which several members had hemiplegic migraine and others had different clinical patterns of the disorder. The hemiplegic manifestations were sensory, rather than motor. A little while later, Heyck (1972) published a collection of 45 instances of hemiplegic migraine. There was a family history of migraine with, or without, aura in some 60 percent of his patients. In 13 of the 45, all attacks were of the hemiplegic type. The genetic basis of the familial disorder, the presence of mutations within the CACNA1A gene, is now known (Tournier-Lasserve 1999).

Persisting Neurological Deficits after Migraine

Charles Féré (1881) stated that Charcot had predicted that the temporary neural dysfunctions of migraine with aura might possibly persist and become permanent in some instances, and went on to cite examples of this happening. Hermann Oppenheim (1894) described a woman with long-term migraine who, four months after childbirth, had a typical headache attack accompanied by aphasia and then developed a hemiparesis, which went on to coma and death. At autopsy, her left middle cerebral artery was thrombosed. Subsequently, occasional instances of survival with persisting neurological deficits that followed migraine attacks were described by Infield (1901) and Thomas (1907). The relevant literature was reviewed by Dunning (1942), while Connor (1962) published the details of 18 instances of clinically localized and persisting retinal, cortical (mainly visual cortex), and brain stem defects that had followed migraine attacks. A more recent careful evaluation by Bogousslavsky et al. (1988) indicated that migrainous stroke tended to involve the cerebral arterial territory from which neurological manifestations arose during migraine attacks, namely the posterior cerebral artery, in most instances. Evidence has become available that migraine itself is also associated with an increased risk of the occurrence of ischemic stroke (Spector et al. 2010).

There have also been very rare accounts of death from ischemic damage to the brain that occurred during migraine attacks and in which at autopsy there was no evidence of abnormalities in the intracranial arteries (Peters, 1934; Selby and Fryer 1984), and also none in the great arteries of the neck (Guest and Wolff 1964). The mechanisms responsible for the infarctions remain unknown.

Migraine Equivalents

The issue of the existence of migraine "equivalents," and the limits that should be set to the range of phenomena that might validly be included within such a concept, are both contentious. On the one hand, in a given individual the recurrence of typical migrainous visual auras over long periods of time without accompanying headache and without the appearance of evidence of underlying brain or eye disease, would probably be accepted as a migraine visual equivalent by most people interested in the matter. The link between such isolated episodic visual disturbances and migraine is made more probable by the existence of individuals who at different times experience the same pattern of visual aura with or without headache. On the other hand, should the concept of migraine equivalent extend to someone who has recurrent episodes of a symptom that might in theory arise from the brain and for which no cause can be demonstrated after appropriate investigation, and where there is no association between the episodes and headache? The answer would probably be "No." But there are intermediate situations, for example when the individual with otherwise unexplained episodic neurological symptoms had a past history of migraine or a family history of the disorder, or when otherwise inexplicable episodic neurological disturbances without headache that occur in infants and children prove to be associated with the appearance of migraine later in the life of the affected individual, such as cyclical vomiting of children (Langmead 1905; Li et al. 1999) or recurrent bouts of otherwise unexplained abdominal pain (Buchanan 1921; Symon and Russell 1986). And if the idea of a migraine equivalent is valid in these situations, to what extent can it also be applied with justification to similar symptoms in those who lack past or family histories of migraine?

One of the perhaps more convincing examples of a migraine equivalent is the rather aptly named "Alice in Wonderland syndrome" described by Todd (1955). Lewis Carroll, the pseudonym adopted by the Oxford academic Charles Dodgson, the author of *Alice in Wonderland*, was a migraineur. He conferred on his literary creation Alice episodes of an illusory disturbance in her perception of her own body image. Todd reported six patients who experienced episodic illusory body image distortions. Most either had migraine at other times or came from families in which other members suffered migraine attacks.

In the more recent literature, an interest has been taken in the relationship between migraine and vestibular disturbances (Stahl and Daroff 2001). There are accounts of vestibular migraine (migraine-associated vertigo) in which otherwise unexplained bouts of nonpositional rotational vertigo are ascribed to migraine, with or in the absence of migraine-associated features (Lempert and Neuhauser 2009). There is also the perhaps related disorder named by Slater (1979): benign recurrent vertigo. This comprises recurrent bouts of vertigo without symptoms of cochlear disturbance that last from one minute to 24 hours and are followed by positional vertigo. Some sufferers have personal or family histories of migraine. However, it should be noted that at an earlier time, experienced clinicians such as Symonds, in 1950 (Symonds 1970), were well aware of the idea of vestibular migraine.

Chronic or Continuous Migraine

Gowers and other writers of his time made little or no mention of it, but migraine attacks in the individual sometimes increase in frequency and severity until a state of continuing headache prevails. This situation has been variously termed transformed migraine (Mathew et al. 1987), mixed headache, chronic migraine, or chronic daily headache. The history of the concept, under the designation of chronic migraine, was traced by Manack et al. (2009). It has gradually come to be appreciated that continuing and frequent (usually at least daily) intake of headache-relieving medications plays a significant role in the etiology of the phenomenon.

However, migraine developing into more or less continuous headache had been described long before these recent accounts. Thomas Willis (1672) in his *De Anima Brutorum*, described an often cited example in a patient identified by Critchley (1964) as Anne, Countess of Conway and Killultagh (1631–1679). Anne Conway (Hotton 2004) was a philosopher of some note and author of the posthumously published *Principia philosophiae antiquissimae et recentissimae* (1690). Her headaches had begun at the age of 12. Willis recorded her experiences as follows (in the words of Pordage's "Englishing" of the Latin):

Some years since, I was sent for to visit a most noble Lady, for above 20 years sick with an almost continual Headach, at first intermitting: She was of a most beautiful form, and a great wit, so that she was skilled in the Liberal Arts and in all sorts of literature, beyond the condition of her sex; and as if it were thought too much by Nature, for her to enjoy so great endowments, without some detriment, she was extremely punished with this Disease. Growing well of a Feavour before she was twelve years old, she became obnoxious to pains in the Head, which were wont to arise, sometimes of their own accord, and more often upon every light occasion. This sickness being limited to no one place of the Head, troubled her sometimes on one side, sometimes on the other, and often thorow the whole compas of the Head. During the fit (which rarely ended under a day and a nights space, and often held for two, three, or four days) she was impatient of light, speaking, noise, or of any motion, sitting upright in her Bed, the Chamber made dark, she would talk to no body, nor take any sleep, or sustenance. At length about the declination of the fit, she was wont to lye down with a heavy and disturbed sleep, from which awakening she found her self better, and so by degrees grew well, and continued indifferently well till the time of the intermission. Formerly, the fits came not but occasionally, and seldom under 20 days or a month, but afterwards they came more often: and lately, she was seldom free. Moreover, upon sundry occasions, or evident causes (such as the change of the Air, or the year, the great Aspects of the Sun and Moon, violent passions, and errors in diet) she was more cruelly tormented with them. (1672/1683 pp. 121–122)

Such an account could scarcely represent any disorder other than migraine that had developed into virtually continuous headache whose course was punctuated by further migraine exacerbations. Anne Conway described the intensity of her suffering in a letter to the Cambridge philosopher Henry More:

I have formerly given you some intimation of the great increase of my distemper. . . . Which doeth not yet abate upon me but contrarily I have been so much worse than I was when I writt last since good fryday I have not been able to goe abroad, and am very little off my bed. I find myself very faint and weak, but yet as little strength as I seeme to have. I still endure these violent paines (which I always thought would be accounted intolerable by a stronger body than I ever had), and that more frequently than ever. I cannot dissemble so much as not to professe myself very weary of this condition. (Skwire 1999, p. 9)

There are further references to episodic migraine evolving into a persisting headache situation in the earlier 20th-century literature, for example Oppenheim (1904) and Collier (1922). Later the relationship between such headache and the continued and frequent intake of headache remedies began to be described, though it had been observed much earlier. Georget and Calmeil (1834), in their article "Cephalalgia, cephalée" in *Adelon's Dictionary*, had written that medications called "céphaliques" had acquired a certain reputation as anticephalics. They had stimulant and antispasmodic actions, but their long-term continued use might "augmenter la maladie."

Ergotamine-overuse headache was reported by Peters and Horton (1951), though there had been earlier intimations in the literature that such an event might have occurred (Boes and Capobianco 2005). Also, in the 1950s, it had been noted in Switzerland that continued use of simple, readily obtainable analgesics, especially phenacetin, could be associated with the development of chronic headaches (Isler 1986). It has become apparent that the phenomenon is not confined to intake of any particular class of headache-relieving drug (Diener and Limmroth 2004). Nor does it seem related to the drugs' known mechanisms of action. Further, lest it be assumed that at least the headaches of Anne, Countess of Conway, were a pure evolutionary stage in her migraine uncontaminated by the consequences of drug therapy, it should be noted that Willis had gone on to record the following:

> For the obtaining a Cure, or rather for a tryal, very many Remedies were administered, thorow the whole progress of the Disease, by the most skilful Physicians, both of our own nation, and the prescriptions of others beyond Seas, without any success or ease: also great Remedies of every kind and form she tried, but still in vain. Some years before, she had endured from an ointment of Quicksilver, a long and troublesome Salivation, so that she ran the hazard of her life. . . . There was no kind of medicines both *Cephalicks, Antiscorbutics, Hystericals,* all famous *Specificks,* which she took not. (1672/1683, p. 122)

Willis forbore indicating how he managed the situation in the countess, and with what measure of success. His silence concerning the matter, and experience of the same situation more than 300 years later, suggests that he may not have obtained the success he sought.

Status Migrainosus

In 1892 Charles Féré described an "état de mal migrainuex." It comprised frequently recurring migraine attacks without recovery from torpor and stupor between consecutive episodes. He saw a phenomenological parallel between it and status epilepticus. In his own cases, there were reversible defects in neurological function that were present during the *status migrainosus.*

CHAPTER 5
Migraine

Pathophysiology

Until the stage when a sufficient understanding of the mechanisms of the body's normal functioning had been achieved, thinking about the processes of disease tended to be concerned with causation rather than with the ways disease manifestations were produced. Causes tended to be sought simplistically in some unusual event that had impacted on the sufferer's life or body shortly before or at the onset of symptoms of the underlying disorder. If no such causal event could be identified, its existence was usually assumed, and some name was often found for it. That name might reflect some unproven and perhaps unprovable internal or external influence, or it might merely reveal, or conceal, ignorance as to its nature. To some extent, present-day lay thinking about disease still tends to linger in such a state. However, over the centuries, medical interpretations of disease have gradually become more sophisticated and more complex. It has been increasingly recognized that several layers of causation, as well as alterations of various aspects of bodily function, may be involved in the overall process that results in the manifestations of illness.

Migraine is an episodic disorder in which there may be predisposing factors as well as factors that precipitate the occurrence of individual attacks. At the present time, these causal factors are often termed, respectively, the remote or predisposing causes, and the immediate or precipitating causes, though other terms may also have been applied to them in the past. An adequate interpretation of the pathophysiology of migraine should explain not only any underlying tendency to the disorder and how causal factors initiate the events of the individual migraine attack, but should also define the subsequent alterations in body function that are responsible for the full gamut of the disorder's manifestations. Thus, in relation to the migraine attack, a fully satisfactory explanation of the phenomena should take in not only the mechanisms of headache production, but also those of the various aura phenomena, any premonitory symptoms and body disturbances that herald the attacks, the various associated manifestations such as nausea, vomiting, intolerance of light and sound, and any recognized complications that do not appear to have independent causes.

In the account that follows, it may be useful to keep these considerations in mind when thinking about the adequacy of the various explanations of migraine that have been produced over the course of many centuries. The literature of the history of the disorder is replete with hypotheses and concepts that may have appeared to explain with some adequacy particular aspects of the causation or mechanism of symptom production in migraine, but that failed to account for other well-established aspects of the whole migraine process. Blau (1992) pointed out that the desired comprehensive interpretation of migraine pathogenesis remained elusive. Despite subsequent advances in knowledge, it continues to do so at the time of writing.

THEORIES OF MIGRAINE PATHOGENESIS

Over the course of the centuries, a number of theories of the causation of migraine have appeared in the literature. These theories can be seen to fall into two major broad types: those that see the disorder as arising from influences extrinsic to the sufferer's body, and those based on the notion that migraine arises within the sufferer's body. The extrinsic causal factors have included supernatural influences, and various external physical, chemical, and psychological circumstances; the intrinsic causes embrace various genetic, neural, vascular, chemical, and psychological factors. Theories based on extrinsic causes often fall short of explaining how the proposed cause produces the clinical phenomena of migraine, whereas those based on internal causes often fail to explain how external attack triggering factors may activate the disease process, and also may not account for the totality of the internal disturbances involved in the disorder.

Turning to the matter of the altered body mechanisms responsible for the symptoms of the migraine attack, there have again been two main classes of theory: those that regard the pathogenic mechanism as primarily vascular, and those that consider the process as primarily neural. Subdivisions, as well as hybrid versions, can be discerned within each of these two categories of theory. There have also been other, less often proposed and shorter lived theories: dietary-, endocrine-, and eyesight-based ones, for example.

In the light of those introductory comments, the story of the interpretation of migraine across the centuries may be taken up.

Ancient and Medieval Times

It has already been pointed out that ancient and medieval authors nearly always dealt with headache in general, or with types of headache that do not correspond at all closely with the modern categories of the disorder. Many of the pre-1600 A.D. accounts would have inevitably included instances of migraine, perhaps at more than one place in the one account. Unfortunately, it is often impossible to be sure if or when in those accounts the mechanisms of what would now be regarded as migraine were being dealt with specifically. As explained in previous chapters, it seems to have often been the practice of latter-day authors to regard earlier material dealing with *hemicrania* as providing accounts of the entity of present-day migraine. However, it was also pointed out that the *hemicrania* category of the past probably often included nonmigrainous one-sided headache, and did not include the nonunilateral migraine that found its place, together with other types of headache, in the categories of *cephalalagia* and *cephalaea*. Therefore, apart from a few instances, one must assume that what ancient and medieval authors wrote about the causes and mechanisms of headache (see chapter 3) would probably have also been their views about the causes and pathogenesis of migraine, had they recognized the present-day entity. Where it is possible to recognize probable migraine in the early headache accounts, for example in the Hippocratic corpus (chapter 4), there sometimes was no material concerning the cause and pathophysiology to be found in the text near the account. Aretaeus in the second century A.D. did follow his description of *heterocrania*, the features of which make it likely that he had present-day migraine in mind, with the brief observation that "the cause of these symptoms is coldness with dryness" (Adams 1856). It seems that one has to come down to the time of the 17th-century scientific revolution and Le Pois, Willis, and Wepfer before one can be reasonably sure that an author has been discussing the pathogenesis of probable migraine in his account of headache. Even then, the matter may have arisen almost incidentally and in only part of the author's overall account of headache. Only from Tissot (1780) onward is there substantial material in the literature that can confidently be related to the cause and mechanism of reasonably definite modern-day migraine.

Despite the above reservations, because the Englishman Philip Barrough, when discussing *hemicrania*, chose to write of "migrime" in the vernacular, his views on its pathogenesis, based on humoral concepts, are quoted below.

They comprise part of the background traditional medical thought from which Willis had later to liberate his own thinking:

> This paine cometh often by fits, and in some the griefe is felt within the skull, in some within deepe in the braine, and in some other nigh to the temples in the muscles there. This paine is caused by ascending and flowing of many vapours or humors either hote or cold, either by the veines, or by the arteries, or by both. Sometimes they oneley proceed from the parts contained in the skull, that is, from the brain and his films, which thrust out their excrements and superfluities from them; and sometimes from the parts of the body beneath the head which send up corrupt vapours and humors from themselves to the braine. (Barrough 1610, p. 17)

In those words one can perhaps see, by virtue of a degree of stretching of the imagination, forerunners of both the neural and the vascular types of hypotheses of migraine pathogenesis that others would develop in the future.

The Scientific Revolution

The great William Harvey (1578–1657), in his *Anatomical Lectures*, delivered in 1615–1616, briefly, and almost incidentally, touched on the pathogenesis of "*hemicranea.*" In describing the innervation of the stomach, he stated baldly, in Witteridge's (1964) translation of his Latin, that "because of these nerves there is great sympathy between the stomach and the brain and vice versa, wherefore if the brain be injured vomitings and migraine ensue." Unfortunately, Harvey provided no additional information regarding brain injury as a cause of migraine, and did not venture further into the question of the headache's mechanism.

Le Pois

At much the same time as Harvey wrote, Charles Le Pois (1618), who may have been interested in migraine because he himself was a probable sufferer (chapter 4), dealt with the topic in the section on *hemicranias* within his broader category of internal head affections from serous impurities. In the words of Isler's (1987-a) translation, Le Pois ascribed *hemicrania* to "an aqueous humour that flows over the head, but is agitated and fermented by some sudden aerial storm and perturbation." Le Pois had indicated that an acrimonious vapor that originated in the stomach ascended to the head, where it distended the cerebral membranes. This distension caused them to contract and thus produce headache. He postulated that the contracted brain membranes then produced an insipid serosity that entered the cerebral blood vessels and by this means calmed and comforted the membranes, thus bringing the headache to an end. In writing on *hemicrania*, Le Pois did not make clear why the headache that was produced was one-sided. He reasoned that the vomiting was produced by the headache, rather than that a gastric upset caused both the vomiting and the headache:

> Since the headache invariably precedes the abdominal pains and spasms, as I have experienced in my own case and that of others, and as will appear from the following narrative, it may be hence inferred that the head suffers idiopathicaly, but the stomach and bowels by sympathy with the head. (in Liveing's 1873, p. 239, translation of the Latin)

Le Pois's was an explanation that simultaneously incorporated remnants of humoral pathology, Paracelsian iatrochemistry, and possible supernatural intervention by intangible external powers to account for the initial abnormality in the humors from the stomach. If the idea seemed satisfactory in its own time, at least part of it would probably be almost meaningless to most people today. At least Le Pois did identify the meninges as the site of origin of the pain of migraine.

Willis

Though Thomas Willis wrote on "headach" in general in his *De Anima Brutorum* (1672), he did provide an explanation for the mechanism of what he termed *"hemicrania,"* a word that Pordage translated as "meagrim":

> Secondly, The other kind of Headach, to wit, within the skull, is more frequent, and much more cruel, because the Membranes, cloathing the Brain, are very sensible, and the Blood is poured upon them by a manifold passage, and by many and greater Arteries. Further, because the Blood or its Serum, sometimes passing thorow all the Arteries at once, both the *Carotides* and the *Vertebrals*, and sometimes apart, thorow these or those, on the one side or the opposite, bring hurt to the Meninges, hence the pain is caused that is interior; which is either universal, infesting the whole Head or its greatest part, or particular, which is limited to some private region; and sometimes produces a Meagrim on the side, sometimes in the forepart, and sometimes in the hinder part of the Head. (Willis 1672/1683, p. 106)

Thus, at least the now usually read English-language translation of Willis would suggest that he related the type of headache that he was considering to increased arterial blood flow within the skull. Further, he proposed that the flow increase, and the pain, might be restricted to the territory of a particular artery, or number of arteries. Hence he explained localized head pain in *hemicrania*. It is noteworthy that to Willis, and consistent with the word's derivation, *hemicrania* was not necessarily unilateral, as mentioned in chapter 1. The mechanism of headache production that Willis proposed was one that others would invoke in the future.

Elsewhere in *De Anima Brutorum*, Willis provided two case histories that are undoubtedly those of migraine sufferers. The first, that of Anne, Countess of Conway, was described at some length in chapter 4. After his account of her headaches, which had begun following a fever when she was 12 years old, Willis went on to provide a record of the treatments to which she had been subjected, and then proceeded to explain the basis of what had become her chronic daily headache. He also traced the development of the mechanism of her recurrent headaches from their beginning:

> If we should inquire into the *Aetiology* or the Causes of this inveterate Disease, we can suspect nothing less than that the *Meninges* of the Brain, being from the beginning more lightly touched, had afterward contracted an habitual and indelible vice. It appears by the History, that the distemper first arose from a Morbific matter which was translated into the head, after an ill cured Feavour. Then perchance, by reason of some hurt brought to the Membranes, the tone of the Fibres was so much endamaged, that afterwards, the Humors flowing in them, both the nervous and others, being heaped up to a fullness, or growing hot by more aggravation, raised up the fits of the Headach. But at length, the diseased cause growing worse, by reason of the frequent fits, it seems that the unity of those Fibres, were so much broken, that from thence little Tumors, or Scirrhous knots or swellings, being raised up in all the exterior *Meninge*, or in a great part of it, produced pains almost continual, and those apt to be made worse by or embitter'd upon every light occasion. (Willis 1672/1683, p. 122)

Here Willis provided what seems to be a different explanation of the mechanism of the countess's episodic migraine headache, proposing that there was an initiating humoral or chemical cause ("Morbific matter") that predisposed her to further headaches by altering the physical state of her meninges. Her migraine attacks occurred when there was an additional buildup or alteration of the (imagined) fluids present in her meninges. The repeated episodes of damage to the meninges led to permanent alteration of the dura mater, and therefore to chronic headache. There was no explicit mention of any brain artery blood flow alterations being responsible for the headache at any stage.

Willis recounted a second case history:

> A beautiful and young Woman, indued with a slender habit of body, and a hot Blood, being obnoxious to an hereditary Headach, was wont to be afflicted with frequent and

wandering fits of it, to wit, some upon every light occasion, and some of their own accord; that is, arising without evident cause. On the day before the coming of a spontaneous fit of this Disease, growing very hungry in the Evening, she eat a most plentiful Supper, with an hungry, I may say greedy appetite; presaging by this sign, that the pain of the Head would most certainly follow the next Morning; and the event never failed this Augury. For as soon as she awaked, being afflicted by a most sharp torment, thorow the whole forepart of her Head, she was troubled also with Vomiting, sometimes of an Acid, and as it were a Vitriolick, Humor, and sometimes of a Cholerick and highly bitterish; hence according to this sign, this Headach is thought to arise from the vice of the Stomach.

That I may render a reason of this, first it appears, that a Vomiting will succeed a hurt of the Head, to wit, after a blow, or wound, or a fall; yet a pain of the Head rarely or never follows, upon Vomiting, the pain of the Heart, of the Stomach, any otherways labouring, unless the Blood comes between. Wherefore in the aforesaid case of this sick Person, as it appears plainly that the *Meninges* of the Brain were before disposed to Headaches, its fits were stirred up by every agitation of the Blood; hence it is obvious to be conceived, when the heterogeneous particles are heaped up in a fullness, in the bloody Mass, by reason of the vice of the Chyle, presently a flux of it arising, for the expulsion of the trouble, those being but evilly match'd, being separated by the Blood, and partly poured forth out of the Arteries into the Ventricle, do raise up its Ferment, and so produce hunger; and partly rushing into the predisposed meninges of the Head do there dispose the tinder, or rather incentive of the Headache about to follow. (1672/1683, p. 125)

Such reasoning may not be easy to follow for someone unfamiliar with Willis's iatrochemical thinking. He seems to have tried to indicate that his beautiful young woman had inherited a vulnerability to probable migraine without aura, and that the site of this vulnerability lay in her meninges. In her, an abnormality in the absorbed contents of a meal resulted in a chemical disturbance (heterogeneous particles) in the blood. The circulating abnormal chemicals then not only caused vomiting but entered the stomach and there underwent a chemical reaction that led to hunger (in this regard, Willis's time relations between events seem to have gone a little astray). Part of the abnormal circulating chemicals also activated the headache-producing mechanism in the predisposed meninges. It is all highly fanciful, unprovable in Willis's own time, but ingenious. Taken in conjunction with his other interpretations of a probable migraine mechanism, it provides a reasonably comprehensive interpretation of the pathogenesis of the disorder in terms of entities whose existences he could do no more than postulate. Basically, Willis had devised a chemical interpretation of the initiation of a migraine attack and of the basis of a predisposition to the disorder. Elsewhere in his account, as mentioned above, he had invoked vascular factors to explain why the pain of migraine might be localized to part of the head. Those prepared to accept that part of Willis's other writing on "headach," which also happened to deal with migraine (and this is probably true), can also argue that he had also produced the idea that scalp nerves were involved in the production of headache—"a painful pulling of the (nerve) Fibres (in the meninges)." Partly on that basis, it has sometimes been asserted that Willis also devised a neural theory of migraine pathogenesis, but that claim depends on what he meant by "fibres" in relation to the meninges. Whether or not he devised such a theory, he also raised the possibilities that altered vascular behavior and chemical changes played roles in migraine pathogenesis.

The whole content of Willis's account of headache suggests that he was thinking mainly of migraine throughout, but there are clear indications at places in his text that other headache entities were included in his thinking. The material cited above provides some reasonably representative information about his thinking on the mechanisms of probable migraine and also takes in many of his ideas on headache production. However, there is a great deal of additional detail in his full account, and much nebulous iatrochemistry. Some of it, which seems not to be related to migraine, has been dealt with in chapter 3 in relation to his views on headache in general.

Wepfer

The volume of Johann Jakob Wepfer's *Observationes medico-practicae de affectibus capitis internis et externis* appeared in 1727, more than three decades after his death. His ideas about the pathogenesis of migraine were reasonably similar to some of those of Willis. With the deferred publication of his concepts, it is sometimes difficult to know whether certain of his ideas were dependent on Willis, or vice versa. Wepfer outlived Willis, and his account of various ideas relevant to headache often seems rather better organized than Willis's, but this does not necessarily mean that the ideas originated with Willis and were subsequently refined by Wepfer.

As mentioned previously, sometimes there is difficulty in being sure as to when Wepfer in his *Observationes* was dealing with what would pass as present-day migraine. He used the venerable *cephalalgia, cephalaea, hemicrania* classification of headache types, and his *hemicrania* category contained examples of unilateral headache associated with other diseases. The *Observationes* themselves comprised a series of case histories dealing with a gamut of the clinical manifestations of particular diseases, and each observation had Wepfer's commentary affixed to it. His Observation 54 described the course of what was almost certainly hemicranially distributed migraine with a recognizable probable visual aura that occurred in a young woman who was ill with what was likely to have been a urinary tract infection.

Unfortunately, in this case of clear-cut migraine, Wepfer did not go into the mechanism of the headache production in detail, though he mentioned that, in consent with the stomach, a chylous humor was responsible for producing head pain that originated in the meninges. Wepfer held the view that the headache of hemicrania was of vascular origin, and that the vascular disturbance was due to postulated defective serum, or overfilled vessels. Isler (1985) stated that Wepfer considered that brain disturbance accounted for the migraine visual aura and vomiting in the attacks.

For more than a century after Willis and Wepfer, there was no real advance in the understanding of the pathophysiology of what was recognizably migraine. Most medical authors continued to write in terms of *hemicrania*, and the ambiguity remains as to how that term would equate with present-day migraine.

Fordyce

John Fordyce, in his *Dissertatio de hemicrania*, published in 1758, had considered that that disorder was "generally an idiopathic affection." He rejected the idea that the attacks were provoked by disorders of the abdominal viscera. Presumably he would have regarded the present-day entity of migraine in the same light.

Whytt

Robert Whytt, professor of the theory of Medicine at Edinburgh, stated that headache arose from the nerves of the forepart of the head, which were activated by changes in the diameter of the local blood vessels (Whytt 1768). He thought that a viscid or acrid "humour" might affect both the blood vessels and the nerves to bring this situation about. Thus, remnants of the old humoral pathology lingered in his thought, linked to a plausible postulated mechanism that could account for both the production of pain, and for the site where it was experienced, which might be unilateral. Again, he did not apply these ideas specifically to migraine, as he did not seem to recognize that entity per se, but he enunciated the idea that an altered cranial vascular caliber might affect local nerves to produce headache.

Sauvages

In his attempt to classify all human disease, as indicated in earlier chapters, Boissier de Sauvages (1772) defined several types of *hemicrania* (migraine).

Some of them were clearly symptoms of local pathological disorders, and indeed Sauvages seemed to have gone to some pains to nominate varieties of pathology that might conceivably explain all his different types of unilateral head pain. As a consequence, present-day migraine cannot be identified with confidence in any member of Sauvages's *hemicrania* category, though examples of it probably would have found their way into his *cephalalgia* group of head pains, which he in general attributed to vascular engorgement of the meninges.

At much the same time as Sauvages, the unnamed writer on "migraine" in Diderot's *Encyclopedia* of 1765 (Isler at al. 2005) proposed the view that migraine originated outside the skull, probably in the pericranium. In the account, it was mentioned that spastic contraction of the pericranium and its blood vessels was the cause of the headache.

Tissot

Samuel Tissot, in his *Traité des nerfs* (1780), dealt at some length with migraine, and migraine alone, as a specific topic. In his section on the cause of the disorder, Tissot said that he could not accept the opinion held by Charles Le Pois, Wepfer, and others that migraine was due to the accumulation of an acid serosity. He had more sympathy for the view of LePois's father Nicolas who, while he accepted that migraine sometimes depended on a sharp serosity, thought that more often it arose as result of consensus with the stomach and the lower abdominal viscera. Nicolas Le Pois may have also been the first to suggest that in females who experienced migraine when lactating, the disorder arose from a consensus with the breasts or was sometimes due to retained or abnormal milk. Tissot himself believed that the stomach was the usual primary source of migraine, and that the head symptoms arose as the result of a process of sympathy with that abdominal organ.

Tissot advanced several sets of observations from the literature to support his view. First, he stated that all migraine sufferers noted that their stomachs were upset at the approach of their attacks; if they ate something that upset them, the subsequent migraines were likely to be more severe and to occur more frequently. Tissot sought support from the ancients to promote this line of evidence. Thus he pointed out that Caelius Aurelianus (Drabkin 1950) had sometimes tried to induce vomiting to relieve migraine. This to Tissot suggested that Caelius (or rather Soranus of Ephesus, whose ideas Caelius repeated) believed that the stomach played an important role in producing the disorder. Alexander of Tralles in the fifth century A.D.

had chosen remedies that depended on a consensus with the stomach in managing migraine. Second, Tissot observed that measures that rehabilitated the stomach tended to relieve migraine. He cited the example of Haller (some of whose writings he had previously translated and edited). Haller had a bad stomach and suffered frequent migraine, but after giving up wine found that his stomach recovered and his migraine settled. Third, Tissot noted that factors that made other head maladies worse often did not influence migraine, yet anything that deranged the stomach produced migraine attacks. Fourth, and finally, Tissot cited the observation that during migraine attacks, at the moment the stomach contents were removed by vomiting or by the effect of purging, migraine headache subsided. Tissot then referred to several older authors who had provided examples of the latter phenomenon in their writings, for example Bianchi, van Swieten, and Rivierius.

Tissot reasoned that the effects of the stomach disturbance that initiated migraine were transmitted by nerves (presumably the vagus) to branches of the trigeminal nerves, in particular the supraorbital ones. Therefore the pain site usually corresponded to the territory of distribution of the latter nerves, though the pain could be present more extensively in trigeminal innervated territory. Other features of the migraine attack were related to neural activity that originated in the stomach and spread to other parts of the central nervous system. Thus spread of the activity to the site of the brain mechanism that was responsible for vomiting resulted in the latter symptom. The vomiting then removed the stomach contents from the body and thus relieved the headache. Variation in the degree of involvement of nervous system components in the different stages of the pathogenic mechanism explained why all the migraine attacks in a given individual did not necessarily result in identical manifestations.

The frequency of migraine attacks would be altered by factors that worsened or mitigated derangements of the stomach, and also by factors that made nerve function more delicate or more robust. Thus diet, drinks, movement, inactivity, excessive sleep, passions, anger, evacuations, and changes of season had marked influences on migraine. In females, attacks tended to occur at times of menstruation, and the pattern of attacks tended to change at menopause. Hemorrhoids also had effects on migraine. Most of these factors acted via Tissot's postulated mechanism of sympathy (neurally mediated).

Late in his account of the causation of migraine, Tissot mentioned that plethora sometimes caused attacks. He cited the instance of a young man who had had numerous headache attacks over at 12-year period until he began to have frequent nosebleeds. Thereupon the migraine disappeared until the age of 19. His nosebleeds then ceased. His migraine returned about six months later. Tissot cited another example from the literature where deliberate therapeutic bleeding led to gradual improvement in migraine.

Tissot abandoned all notions of humoral factors playing a part in the pathogenesis of migraine and found no role for a vascular element. Essentially, he envisaged migraine as a neurally mediated scalp (mainly supraorbital territory) neuralgia that was initiated by disturbances of stomach function. His ideas about the cause of migraine were, at the time of his writing, reasonably comprehensive. They might have proved persuasive had the observations of the instigating stomach disturbance on which they depended represented anything like the universal experience of sufferers. Unfortunately, the latter was far from the case.

Writing on *hemicranias* at much the same time as Tissot, Schobelt (1776) considered that *hemicranias* were a special form of rheumatism, brought about by an ascent of humors. The introduction of the notion of rheumatism involved a degree of novelty. The humors retained a substantial place in Schobelt's thinking, and his ideas overall were not specifically related to migraine.

Fothergill

In 1778, John Fothergill, the London Quaker physician (Rose 1999-a), tried to attract the attention of English readers to the frequency of "sick headach" (Fothergill 1784). In doing this, he attributed the disorder to "inattention to diet," without attempting to explain the mechanisms through which this produced headache. Thus, like Le Pois and Fordyce, he considered that migraine was idiopathic in nature and originated from the region of the stomach. However, he also observed that often no symptoms of alimentary tract disturbance were experienced before the headache of migraine began.

Parry

Caleb Hillier Parry of Bristol, in 1789 (Parry 1792), observed that unilateral carotid compression on the headache-affected side temporarily relieved *hemicrania* and bilious headache. It was an important and sometimes still overlooked observation, or rather the rediscovery of a much more ancient observation dating back to the first century A.D. (chapter 3). The pain response to the arterial compression has significant bearing on the interpretation of the pathogenesis of migraine and in particular on the role of vascular factors in headache production in the disorder.

Heberden

At the very end of the 18th century, the English physician William Heberden (1802) continued to maintain the view that migraine usually arose from the stomach, and that the head became involved secondarily through the medium of "sympathy." In addition, Heberden seemed to allow the possibility that, in migraine, the head could be affected primarily. His view scarcely represented an advance over Fothergill's ideas in relation to migraine.

Martin

Prosper Martin (1829), in France, regarded migraine as a result of nervous irritation, abundance of blood, or, frequently, a bad state of the stomach or intestines. He had written at a time when medical thought was on the verge of attributing the disorder to a primary disturbance of nervous system function, and his views straddled the older and the emerging concepts.

Piorry

Pierre-Adolph Piorry's main contribution to the literature on migraine lay in his emphasis on the recognition and characterization of the visual aura of the disorder (Piorry 1831). In the paper in which he first described this visual phenomenon, he also put forward a novel hypothesis regarding the mechanism of both the aura and the ensuing headache. He stated that migraine or *hemicrania* was at that time accepted as a neuralgia involving one side of the head. Piorry then proceeded to add his own refinement to this concept. He proposed that an exciting cause, whose nature he did not specify but which probably was ambient light, acted on the retina and the iris diaphragm of the eye to cause a local alteration in nervous activity as well as pupil constriction. This combination of effects produced a kind of vibration or oscillation of the iris. When the iris was contracted, the image of a small luminous circle with irregular margins was produced. This image became larger as the iris then dilated progressively. However, if the pathological process (still of unspecified nature) subsequently extended into neighboring branches of the trigeminal nerve, particularly the supraorbital, pain would be experienced in the territories of these nerve branches. Through anastomotic neural communications, the sympathetic nervous system and vagus might become involved, resulting in nausea and vomiting. It was also possible that the disturbance might spread into the nerve supply of the tongue, face, and limbs to explain pain and other disturbances experienced in these parts of the body during migraine attacks. Thus Piorry regarded migraine with a visual aura as an ocular or ciliary neuralgia. The latter term was later to be applied to a rather different type of headache (chapter 7).

Forty years afterward, near the end of his long life, Piorry returned to the topic of migraine, though in a publication in which he was writing primarily on vertigo (Piorry 1875). He tried to bring out analogies between the experience of vertigo and the features of the common pattern of visual aura of migraine. Both disturbances involved oscillation: the former of the eyeball itself, the latter of some of the contents of the eyeball. This seems a rather far-fetched idea. Despite all that had happened in relation to the understanding of the mechanism of migraine in the interval, Piorry reiterated his earlier interpretation of the mechanism of migraine production, though he added a little further detail to it by explaining that after the disturbance extended to the frontal and temple branches of the trigeminal nerves, it spread through anastomoses with the spheno-palatine ganglion to the vagus and so produced nausea and vomiting. Migraine remained for him an "irisalgia."

The neuralgia idea of the nature of migraine headache that Piorry had utilized had been present earlier in the literature, for example to some extent in the writings of Willis (1672), Wepfer (1727), and Whytt (1768). It continued to appear in Romberg's *Manual* (1853), in Symonds in his Gulstonian lectures (1858), in Woakes (1868), and in Elizabeth Garrett Anderson's doctoral thesis of 1870 (Wilkinson and Isler 1999). All of these authors appeared to regard migraine as a neuralgia that involved trigeminal nerve branches. Over the same period of time, there were additional, and perhaps sometimes more important, contributors to the same idea.

Pelletan

One year after Piorry's hypothesis appeared, Jules Pelletan de Kinkelin (1832) designated several varieties of migraine on the basis of the body organ from which he believed the headaches arose. His main varieties were the (i) *migraine stomacale*, as Tissot had indicated, (ii) *migraine irienne*, or *ophthalmique* of Piorry, (iii) migraine uterine (i.e., menstruation-related migraine), and (iv) *migraine plethorique*, a category that reflected the idea that migraine arose from excess "determination" of blood to the brain, in other words, cerebral congestion. Pelletan accepted the idea that there was a consensus (a "sympathy") between the stomach and the brain, and that the consensus was mediated via nerve connections (whose details he did not specify). He proceeded to extend this idea of consensus so that it applied between the brain and the other body organs from which he postulated migraine originated, and also between the brain and the supraorbital nerve, or the whole ophthalmic division of the trigeminal nerve. Thus he neatly explained how disturbed functioning of a distant part of the body could produce localized head pain. Unfortunately, the hypothesis depended on the assumed existence of anatomical pathways. Ultimately it would have perished because of inability to demonstrate these pathways. However, his interpretation was overtaken by other events.

Calmeil

Soon after the time when Piorry first drew attention to the visual aura of migraine, his fellow countryman Louis-Florentin Calmeil (figure 5-1) added to the literature the insightful comment that most of the factors that appear to bring about migraine attacks must act via neural pathways in the brain if they are to produce their clinical expressions in the nerve pathway connecting the brain to the face and the muscles of the head (Calmeil 1839). The headache of migraine itself he regarded as a rheumatic type of neuralgia that involved branches of the trigeminal nerve. Calmeil suggested that the neural disturbance of migraine could spread to the nerve supply of the stomach, rather than vice versa, and considered that the visual aura symptoms of migraine were of cerebral origin. In some sufferers he noted that, during attacks, there was visible evidence of increased local blood flow in the painful area (conjunctival injection, facial warmth, hair standing on end, increased arterial pulsation, and sometimes local spontaneous hemorrhages). He thought that such manifestations must have a neural basis, but it was one whose nature and site of origin he could not specify. An answer to the nature and site of a neural disturbance capable of producing the vascular disturbance that Calmeil had mentioned was not to be forthcoming until another quarter of a century had gone by.

In these and other French-language writings of the fourth decade of the 19th century, there can be seen a progressive tendency to explain the pathogenesis of migraine in terms of altered nervous system function, with Calmeil rapidly disposing of Piorry's hypothesis that there was an ocular basis for the visual aura of the disorder. Instead, Calmeil located its site of origin within the brain itself. These writings marked a high point in the development of one type of neural hypothesis of migraine pathogenesis

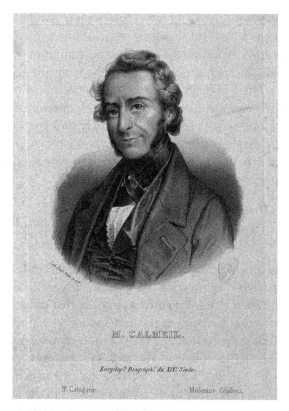

Figure 5-1 Louis-Florentin Calmeil (1798–1895). Courtesy of Wellcome Library, London.

before the focus of interest in the mechanism of migraine began to shift in the direction of vascular factors.

Marshall Hall

In the wake of his discovery of the mechanism of the mechanism of the reflex arc, Marshall Hall (1833) located the site of origin of migraine head-ache to the sensory nerves (of the head). Later (Hall 1849) he used his reflex arc mechanism to suggest that peripheral irritation of the afferent limb of the arc could reflexly cause neck muscle spasm, and that this spasm obstructed the jugular venous blood return from the cranium. He proposed that the resulting cranial venous congestion (Hall's *phlebismus*) brought about migraine headache. This idea was perhaps more an example of Hall's capacity to develop theories based on his discovery of a highly important neural mechanism than a satisfying explanation of the basis of migraine.

It ignored both the aura and the already available evidence pointing to cranial arterial changes during the headache attacks.

Auzias-Turenne

The possibility that cranial venous congestion might be a mechanism of migraine production also occurred to Auzias-Turenne (1849-a, 1849-b), in Paris, at much the same time that Hall made use of it. However Turenne developed the idea into a much more persuasive and comprehensive hypothesis of migraine pathogenesis than Hall had. Curiously, his idea has largely been ignored ever since, possibly because Turenne did not help his future reputation by later proposing that syphilis could be prevented by immunizing uninfected individuals with material taken from chancres.

In brief, Turenne suggested that distension of the various venous sinuses near the base of the skull could cause compression of the trifacial (i.e., trigeminal) nerve in the cavernous sinus, and in particular compression of its first division. The nerve compression often occurred mainly on one side, and thus produced predominantly anterior unilateral headache. In synchrony with the heart beat, there would be pulsation of the carotid artery within the cavernous sinus and this would produce pulsatile compression of the venous blood in the sinus. As a result, the headache would increase and decrease in time with the arterial pulse. Venous blood, either in the foramen lacerum or in the distended jugular vein within the carotid sheath in the neck, could compress the vagus nerve to cause nausea and vomiting. Congestion of the ophthalmic vein would cause redness of the eye, and perhaps blurred vision. A head position that favored blood draining from the intracranial venous sinuses, as when sitting upright, would tend to relieve the headache. The venous sinuses within the skull become more dilated with aging, and therefore more able to accommodate venous blood, so that migraine would tend to die out as the sufferer aged. Turenne put forward the idea that migraine became less active during the reproductive years of the sufferer's life because more of the body's venous blood was diverted to the pelvic organs and away from the head during reproduction. He explained how dietary indiscretion might provoke migraine attacks. The culprit food caused formation of bad chyle. This led to the production of "vitiated" blood that was responsible for languid blood flow in the venous sinuses of the skull, distending them, and this distension became the basis of the headache production. Compared with earlier explanations, and despite a few peculiar and fanciful elements, Turenne's hypothesis for its time offered an ingenious and unusually comprehensive explanation for the clinical features of the migraine attack. However, it did not seem to account adequately for the positive phenomena of the visual aura. Unfortunately for Turenne, no convincing confirmatory evidence for the proposed pathological basis of the hypothesis ever became available.

Anstie

In his Lettsomian lectures of 1866, the London physician Francis Anstie, when dealing with trigeminal nerve pains that occurred during the period of body development, stated the following: "The most frequent of the painful affections of the fifth nerve which are traceable to this source is *migraine*, or sick headache." Thus he regarded migraine not only as a neuralgia but, unlike most of his predecessors, as a neuralgia that originated in the trigeminal nerve itself instead of somewhere else in the body. Although he still expressed the same view of the nature of migraine in his accounts of *Neuralgia* that appeared in Russell Reynolds's *System of Medicine* (Anstie 1880), and in his own monograph with the title of *Neuralgia* (1882), in the interval (Anstie 1873) he had put on record that "migraine is a neuralgia and depends on inherited defects in nutrition of the medulla oblongata." He indicated that he had held this view for several years, and that he was pleased that Liveing (1872, 1873; see later in this chapter) had come to the same idea independently.

Du Bois-Reymond

The great Berlin physiologist Emil Du Bois-Reymond (1818–1896; figure 5-2) published an interpretation of the altered body physiology that he believed could explain the features of his own migraine. He was at some pains to stress that his view applied only to his own particular situation, but his writings were very influential at that time. The paper in which he described his interpretation was translated into French (Du Bois-Reymond 1861) and English (Liveing 1873). Inevitably, his caveat about the limited applicability of his interpretation tended to be lost sight of and his interpretation came to be applied to migraine in general.

Du Bois-Reymond wrote his paper at a time when there was considerable interest in the function and dysfunction of the sympathetic nervous system, and when Claude Bernard had recently described the consequences of dividing the cervical sympathetic trunk on one side. Since the age of 20, Du Bois-Reymond had experienced attacks of headache in the right temple of moderate, but not incapacitating, severity. The pain was increased by coughing or bending down. It also increased with each beat of the superficial

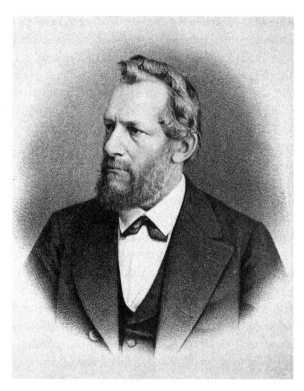

Figure 5-2 Emil Du Bois-Reymond (1818–1895), the Berlin physiologist who interpreted the features of his migraine in terms of altered sympathetic nervous system activity. Courtesy of Wellcome Library, London.

temporal artery, and the vessel itself during the attack felt like a hard cord in comparison with its fellow on the opposite side. His face became pale and drawn, and his right eye appeared a little injected when the attacks were present. At the peak of the pain, he might experience nausea. Near the end of an attack, his right ear became red and his skin warmer. Once Du Bois-Reymond had reasoned his way to the probable mechanism of his symptoms, he looked in a mirror during an attack to see if his right pupil was dilated. It was, and an independent witness confirmed his observation.

Du Bois-Reymond stated that he would make no attempt to explain the periodicity of his attacks or the associated gastric disturbance. His interest lay in the pain and its relation to circulatory disturbance. He argued that the pain was due to a tetanus (i.e., a painful spasm) of the muscle coat of the arteries present in the part of his head where the pain was experienced, and that the tetanic contraction resulted from overaction of the right cervical sympathetic trunk. He assumed that the ophthalmic, internal carotid, and vertebral arteries on his right side were also contracted during his attacks, and that this contraction involved alternate shortening and lengthening of the muscle coats of the intracranial arteries, leading to cerebral blood pressure fluctuations that caused nausea. Decreased blood pressure in the visual apparatus might explain the visual aura phenomena that others sometimes experienced during migraine attacks. Ultimately, fatigue of the cramping arterial wall muscle caused the arteries to relax. The facial skin then became warmer because of the resulting increased blood flow. Du Bois-Reymond admitted that this interpretation did not account for his right eye appearing injected during the headaches, and speculated that perhaps the muscle coats in the arteries that supplied blood to the surface of the eye fatigued much more quickly that the muscle coats of the other involved arteries.

Because the cervical sympathetic trunk arose from the upper thoracic portion of the spinal cord (the cilio-spinal region), he suggested that his migraine resulted from an affection of the upper dorsal region of his spinal cord, and that this led to unilateral cervical sympathetic overaction. He concluded his paper by writing that in many, perhaps in most, sufferers, migraine might be neuralgic in nature. He then hinted that within the known spectrum of migraine phenomena there were to be found other examples of what could be regarded as *hemicrania sympathotonica*.

Du Bois-Reymond's views really took in mainly the question of pain production during migraine attacks, and deliberately did not consider the provocation of attacks or their tendency to recur. His interpretation did not long go unchallenged. Brown-Séquard (1861) rapidly rejected the idea that arterial wall muscle spasm could be painful, pointing out that stimulation of the cervical sympathetic trunk in experimental animals, particularly in cats and dogs, did not appear to cause pain. He raised some other objections and then, in concluding, commented that in most of the cases of migraine that he had observed, there had been signs of cervical sympathetic paralysis, rather than sympathetic overaction, during the headaches.

Möllendorf

Brown-Séquard's latter point was made more emphatically in 1867 by the Berlin author Möllendorf, whose avowed aim was to show

> that Hemicrania is a partly typical partly a-typical one-sided loss of power in the vaso-motor nerves governing the carotid artery, whereby a relaxation of the artery and a flow of arterial blood towards the brain are established. (in Liveing's 1873 translation, p. 307)

Möllendorf did not restrict himself to an analysis of the phenomena of migraine as it occurred in a single individual. Instead, he tried to account for many of the described features of the disorder, though perhaps he did not pay sufficient attention to the aura. He claimed that he had seen oph-thalmoscopic evidence of increased retinal blood flow in the eye on the affected side during a migraine attack, but his strongest item of evidence was the fact that carotid compression on the side of the headache relieved the pain, and did so only while the compression was maintained. This, of course, was simply the phenomenon reported by Caleb Hillier Parry a century before (Parry 1792), and noticed long before that.

Möllendorf proposed that the increased cerebral blood flow caused irri-tation of the brain and distension of the intracranial contents. The postu-lated brain irritation interfered with normal intellectual activity during the attacks and altered the functioning of the olfactory, optic, and auditory nerves. It also produced an overresponsiveness in trigeminal nerve branches and, by irritating the vagus, caused nausea and other disturbances of func-tion of the upper alimentary tract. The distended brain within the inexpan-sible skull affected the nerves at the base of the skull, including the optic ones, thus explaining vision alterations in the attacks.

Jaccoud

Möllendorf's was a more inclusive hypothesis than that of Du Bois-Réymond, but one that depended on an almost contrary set of observations. Some of Möllendorf's postulated mechanisms seemed to have difficulty in accounting for one-sided cranial phenomena in migraine. The differences between the two sets of contrary observations, Du Bois-Reymond's and Möllendorf's, certainly need reconciliation. Another German contempo-rary made an attempt to achieve this, but before he had done so, the Swiss Sigismond Jaccoud (1830–1913; figure 5-3) suggested in 1869 that the difference between the two interpretations might be no more than a matter of the two sets of observations on which they depended being made at dif-ferent stages in the course of migraine attacks. Jaccoud (1869) proposed that a phase of cervical sympathetic function overactivity might be fol-lowed by a phase of sympathetic exhaustion. This was probably the first mention of a concept that achieved some popularity over a number of years, but one for which later writers rather than Jaccoud seem to have received the credit.

Eulenburg

Another contemporary investigator of the sympathetic nervous system, Albert Eulenburg (1840–1917), who at the time held the chair of medicine

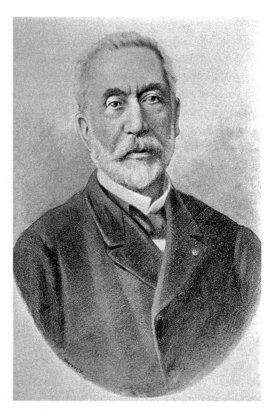

Figure 5-3 Sigismond Jaccoud (1830–1913). Courtesy of Wellcome Library, London.

at the University of Greifswald, wrote on *hemicrania* (migraine) for von Ziemssen's *Cyclopaedia* (Eulenburg 1877). He recognized that neither Du Bois-Reymond's idea nor Möllendorf's *hemicrania neuro-paralytica* could explain the situation of migraine sufferers who exhibited no marked vaso-motor disturbance during their headaches. Eulenburg therefore suggested that any rapid onset change in arterial diameter, whether it involved con-striction or dilatation, might irritate nearby trigeminal nerve endings, and so produce the pain of migraine. This allowed him to accommodate nearly all the features of the two earlier sympathetic nervous system–based but contrary hypotheses within one concept:

> Probably, in migraine, the local anomalies of circulation, without regard to their special mode of origin, are to be regarded as the essential and universal causal condition, while, on the other hand, tetanus or relaxation of the muscles of the vessels exercises rather an indirect influence, confined to single cases, and acting through the local anaemia or hyperaemia of which it is an important cause. (1877, pp. 20–21)

It was another neat solution, but it and Jaccoud's interpretation became perhaps rather overtaken by the results of studies carried out in England in the early 1870s. This work seems to have been set in motion by Hubert Airy's (1870) publication on migraine aura phenomena that played an appreciable role in shifting interest in the site of origin of migraine from the cranial vasculature back to the brain itself.

Wilks

In the year before Hubert Airy's well-known paper appeared in 1870, that great and versatile scientific clinician of Victorian England, Samuel Wilks, proposed an interpretation of the mechanism of migraine headache very similar to that of Möllendorf (Wilks 1869). In his textbook, based on the content of his earlier lecture course at Guy's Hospital, London, Wilks later put the matter thus:

> The fact is, that in this distended throbbing carotid and its branches lies the source of the trouble. The vaso-motor nerve on one side seems for the time paralysed, the vessels of the head dilate, more blood is sent to it, hence the increased heat, throbbing, and pain which the patient must suffer till the tone of the nerve is restored. (1878, p. 427)

It seems unlikely that Wilks was aware of Jaccoud's suggestion or of Möllendorf's paper when he originally produced this idea. At some time between 1872 and 1873, after Latham (1872) had first published his ideas on the mechanism of migraine (see later in this chapter), Wilks made Latham aware that he had already expressed a reasonably similar view in print (Latham 1873). Wilks did not seem to set any great store on his own priority in medical discovery (though he did in relation to the discoveries of his great predecessors at Guy's Hospital, Bright, Addison and Hodgkin), but he would scarcely have bothered to raise the matter with Latham if he had already known that others had priority over them both.

Airy

Although Hubert Airy did not put forward an explanation of the migraine mechanism in his account of the migraine aura, he did raise three pertinent questions (1870, p. 263). First, was the visual disturbance in migraine due to a "temporary suspension of function, propagated by continuity, among the nerve cells of the visual sensorium (wherever that may be)"? Second, did the headache that followed the visual disturbance "tell of further propagation of the nervous disturbance into parts of the brain where disturbance is ache"? And third, did the disturbance of speech and hearing that occasionally occurred in migraine attacks imply further extension of the initial disturbance into "the regions of brain-substance appropriate to these functions"?

Airy made no plain statement to this effect, but it is clearly implicit in these questions that he thought that migraine must have its origin somewhere in the brain itself and that there was localization of function within at least that part of the central nervous system. It should be remembered that Airy posed these questions in the very year that Jackson (1870) first mooted in public the idea that there was localization of motor function in the cerebral cortex. It was also the same year in which Fritsch and Hitzig (1870) in Berlin provided experimental evidence that this indeed was the case. However, it would be some time before the cortical locations of the representations of aspects of brain function, apart from speech and motor control, were known.

Latham

Peter Wallwork Latham, a Cambridge academic, in 1872 and again in 1873, and well aware of the contents of Airy's paper, published his own hypothesis of the mechanism of the migraine attack. He suggested that factors such as fatigue, anxiety, or other depressing causes made the brain less able to inhibit the sympathetic nervous system. The resulting cervical sympathetic overactivity produced cerebral artery constriction. This led to a decreased cerebral blood flow, which in some sufferers caused the aura, whether or not this aura was visual in nature. However, the sympathetic nervous system became increasingly fatigued and exhausted from its overactivity. As a result of this exhaustion, a state of sympathetic underactivity supervened, with cranial artery dilatation and consequent headache. Latham's explanation was, overall, a mix of Du Bois-Reymond's and Wilks's ideas, and was similar to Jaccoud's and Eulenburg's concepts, and may have been devised earlier than that of Eulenburg. It appears to have been thought out independently, without awareness of the ideas of these other writers. It, or Eulenburg's theory, seems to mark the origin of the so-called vascular (arterial) line of hypothesis of migraine pathogenesis, though the concept had been foreshadowed to an extent in the thinking of Willis and Wepfer 200 years before. However, Latham did not see the matter as primarily that of a vascular disturbance. He indicated that he regarded migraine essentially as a nervous system disorder. He probably held this view both because he believed that the initiating factor in the attacks usually acted via the central nervous system and because the sympathetic nervous system was the agency whose altered activity was responsible for the postulated vascular alterations. These, from his point of view, were secondary.

Liveing

Almost simultaneously with the appearance of Latham's publications, Edward Liveing in a paper that appeared in the *British Medical Journal* (1872), and in his classical monograph *On Megrim, Sick Headache, and Some Allied Disorders* (1873), proposed a rather different theory of the migraine attack mechanism.

Liveing began his account of the causative mechanism of migraine by providing an extensive and critical discussion of earlier theories of the pathogenesis of migraine attacks. His account was interlaced with a consideration of the mechanisms of various episodic brain disorders, particularly epilepsy, but also took in disorders such as asthma, hiccup, angina pectoris, myoclonic jerks, and sneezing. Out of this background, Liveing put forward the idea that migraine was the result of a "nerve storm." At much the same time, John Hughlings Jackson had been prepared to consider a similar wide array of episodic disorders as consequences of possible paroxysmal brain disturbances arising from his "discharging lesions" that were responsible for epileptogenesis (Jackson 1873). Latham's nerve storm resembled to an extent the concept of an explosive copula that Willis had created two centuries earlier to explain the basis of a set of disorders similar to those about which Liveing had later written. Liveing's nerve storm did not seem as conceptually violent an event as the explosive discharge of Willis's copula (Willis 1670) or the eruption of Jackson's "discharging lesion." Liveing's idea seems to have been that of an inherited tendency to irregular accumulation and subsequent discharge of nerve force, a "neurosal seizure" that could occur anywhere along a portion of the central nervous system that extended from the optic thalamus rostrally to the vagal nucleus in the lower brain stem caudally. The thalamic disturbance accounted for the visual aura—in 1872 the course of the visual pathway beyond the lateral geniculate bodies of the thalamus was not established. Vagal nuclear disturbance explained the nausea and vomiting of migraine, while paroxysmal disturbance somewhere in between apparently accounted for the headache.

Liveing's was a reasonably adequate hypothesis that took in many of the features of the migraine attack. However, it required acceptance of the idea that the occasional dysphasic speech alteration that occurs in migraine auras had a thalamic origin at a time when the role of Broca's (1861) area in the cortex in relation to speech production had already been known for several years. Further, Living's hypothesis failed to accommodate the cranial circulatory changes that had already been described too often in migraine attacks to allow them to be disregarded. Nonetheless, and despite the earlier intimations in the writings of Willis and Wepfer, Liveing's publications are often taken to mark the origin of the neural line of hypothesis of migraine pathogenesis. If this is accepted, and Jaccoud's and Eulenburg's attempted reconciliations of the hypotheses of Du Bois-Reymond and Möllendorf are ignored, the two main subsequent lines of approach to the understanding of the mechanism of migraine, the neural and the vascular, developed almost simultaneously in Victorian England as result of the writings of two Cambridge men, neither of whom during his subsequent career seemed to exhibit any further major sustained interest in neurological matters.

In the 1870s, apart from that of Liveing, there was some speculation by others that migraine arose in the brain. As mentioned above, John Hughlings Jackson was beginning to explore the ramifications and intellectual limits of his vision of epileptogenesis as a cerebral cortical process and for a time included migraine within the ambit of his concept. His ideas are discussed further a little later in this chapter. One J. L. Teed, of Kansas City in the United States, in 1876 proposed an interpretation of migraine based on what now seems a somewhat idiosyncratic understanding of neurophysiology, even after allowing for the fact that the mechanism of the nerve impulse was not then understood. He suggested that the pain of migraine arose from a primary central nervous system disturbance and did not originate at the sites where it was felt. Teed explained:

> In migraine the true seat of pain is central; it is by no means probable that the terminal nervous fibrillae in the apparent and external seat of pain are involved, only as they are recipients of prolonged force waves from the central neurine, which waves meeting with a point of resistance at the end of the nerve, there produce the effect felt as pain, and diffused tenderness; just as the pulse wave when resisted produces the effect felt as throbbing; and this seems the more probable, as in slight attacks, many of the central or psychical symptoms are present the pain being absent; and in somewhat more severe attacks, the pain is often not felt while at rest. (1876, p. 243)

Late 19th- and 20th-Century Developments

During the remaining years of the 19th century and much of the first half of the 20th, there appear to have been few new ideas about the mechanisms of migraine that both substantially advanced the medical understanding of the disorder and survived the scrutiny of time.

William Gowers (1888) in volume 2 of his *Manual of Diseases of the Nervous System* accepted the idea that a cerebral cortical disturbance was responsible for both the aura and the pain of migraine. However, he was cautious regarding the nature of the cerebral process that initiated these events. His interpretation may have been influenced by a hypothesis of migraine and epileptic seizure pathogenesis that was produced by his colleague at University College, London, Sidney Ringer, the professor of therapeutics. On the basis of his concept of the mechanism of experimentally produced tetanus, Ringer (1877) conceived the notion that migraine was not due to any sudden excesses of nervous system energy (i.e., Liveing's "nerve storm"). Instead, he suggested that it originated in a relatively sudden loss of local nervous system "resistance." Such resistance was in most ways largely tantamount to the later concept of inhibition. Ringer proposed that the loss of resistance, presumably resistance to the passage of pain impulses, began in the "nucleus of the supra-orbital nerve." By the latter term, he probably meant part of the trigeminal nuclear complex in the brain stem. In this way, he explained the possible unilateral site of the headache of migraine. The loss of resistance might then spread more or less selectively to the vomiting center, to cause the nausea and vomiting. It could also extend to involve other parts of the brain and there release their functions, thus accounting for various aura and other migrainous phenomena. In effect, Ringer's idea was similar to that of Liveing, except that Liveing invoked primary neural overaction to produce the events of migraine, whereas Ringer proposed a decrease in normal function of a brain region that allowed another region to escape from restraint. In either case, the clinically observable result of the proposed mechanism would have been the same.

With the beginnings of the measurement of the concentrations of endogenous substances in body fluids near the end of the 19th century, there appeared suggestions that qualitatively or quantitatively altered biological materials, or exogenous toxins, might cause headaches. Haig (1893), in particular, but also others, postulated that there was a causal relationship between uric acid, gout, and migraine, Haig going so far as to term migraine "uric acid headache." Campbell (1892) raised the possibility that the long-accepted relationship between stomach disturbance and migraine might be mediated not via neural connections or humors, but by toxins (of unspecified chemical nature) that were absorbed from the stomach.

Moebius (1894) suggested that an initial brain disturbance in the migraine attack caused altered cervical sympathetic tone, with the resultant change in cranial blood flow producing the headache. In this way, he linked the neural and the vascular types of hypothesis concerning migraine pathogenesis.

However, Latham (1872, 1873) had earlier proposed a reasonably similar idea.

By the end of the 19th century, the suggestion that migraine was primarily a cerebral disturbance was again becoming the dominant explanation of its mechanism. The idea that the disorder was a cranial neuralgia had largely disappeared from the contemporary literature, and the vascular or hybrid autonomic dysfunction-vascular disturbance hypotheses were on the whole passing from favor. However, the London physician Lauder Brunton, at the turn of the century, still saw fit to state the following:

> In ordinary cases migraine depends on some spasm of the vessels outside the head, but not infrequently there may be spasm of the vessels inside the head, and then the functions of the brain may be affected. (1899, p. 1242)

This was an interpretation that was appealing in its simplicity, but not really adequate in regard to the then current belief about the relationship between the caliber of the extracranial vessels and the headache. Wilfred Harris (1907), a British authority on aspects of head pain, remained content to accept Latham's vascular-based concept of the pathogenesis of the disorder. Oppenheim's (1911) large textbook seemed almost to evade committing itself to any definite hypothesis of migraine pathogenesis. Twelve years later, Jelliffe and White (1923) set down a strange notion that appears to have been predominantly autonomic and vasomotor in its nature. However, it contained an echo of the ancient and long-discredited notion that the cerebral ventricles played a role in brain functioning, for these writers indicated that migraine was due to a variety of stimuli that acted on the autonomic nervous system to produce "vasomotor spasms and paralyses with hyperemia and pressure on the brain substance and cerebral ventricles."

By the third decade of the 20th century, vascular hypotheses of the migraine mechanism began to find favor again. Edwin Bramwell (1926) avoided issues about the presence of visible effects of extracranial artery dilatation or constriction during attacks with his refinement of the earlier autonomic nervous system based vasospasm-vasodilatation hypotheses of Eulenburg and Latham. Bramwell suggested that the headache of migraine arose while the meningeal arterial spasm phase was passing off, whereas cerebral artery spasm and consequent cortical ischemia accounted for the aura. Seven years later, Critchley and Ferguson (1933) took a similar view. Kinnier Wilson (1940), in his posthumously published textbook, tried to explain as many features of the migraine attack as possible on the basis of asynchronous and asymmetrical vascular changes affecting the cerebral cortex and also possibly occurring in the meninges. These ideas could explain many features of the migraine attack, but before such a hypothesis could be accepted, there needed to be verification that the proposed arterial alterations were present during the attacks.

Several further hypotheses also appeared in the early 20th-century period, proposing alternative mechanisms for the production of the manifestations of migraine. One suggested that episodic pituitary swelling caused the headache in some migraine attacks (Timme 1926; Thompson 1932). If the swollen pituitary expanded upward and came in contact with the optic chiasm, visual disturbance could be explained. If the gland temporarily bulged laterally into the cavernous sinus, it might involve various cranial nerves, including the first and second divisions of the trigeminal, and so account for both the headache and the very much more uncommon cranial nerve disturbances that may appear during attacks. Pathological confirmation of this ingenious proposal, which provided an explanation for many migraine manifestations, could not be obtained. Consequently the idea perished, as had Auzias Turenne's somewhat similarly anatomically sited venous hypothesis many years before.

James Collier (1928), when writing on epilepsy, attributed the headache of migraine to postulated brain swelling. He invoked the possibility that part of a swollen cerebral hemisphere might protrude downward through the tentorial orifice in migraine attacks (a mechanism of his "false localizing signs" of cerebral tumor). The herniated portion of brain might cause compression of various cranial nerves in the region of the orifice and thus explain the temporary cranial nerve palsies that rarely complicate migraine attacks.

Several contemporary authors seemed almost bemused by Spitzer's (1901) suggestion that migraine occurred when a portion of the choroid plexus of one lateral ventricle protruded into an already congenitally narrow foramen of Munro and temporarily blocked the CSF outflow through it. This block would result in acute but reversible unilateral distension of the appropriate lateral ventricle, and thus cause unilateral headache. The idea perished for want of confirmatory pathological evidence, as well as from its other deficiencies.

There were also hypotheses of migraine causation proposed that attempted to explain mainly, or solely, the instigation of the attacks and that tended to ignore the subsequent events that produced the symptoms of the attacks. For a time, allergy was invoked as a major precipitating cause of migraine, on the basis of anecdotal and circumstantial evidence only, without there being any real scientific proof. Subsequent reasonably adequately designed experiments failed to demonstrate the assumed association (Loveless 1950). Similarly, the underlying cause of the disorder was ascribed to defective vision or vision refractive errors, claims strongly asserted by Hurst (1924) and others. The latter idea was fairly soon afterward rejected by Bramwell (1926). Sigmund Freud himself proposed a psychodynamic interpretation of the origin of the disorder (Karwautz et al. 1996), but this suggestion could not be validated by scientific methods that were independent of Freud's own underlying psychodynamic concepts.

Wolff

To this stage in the development of knowledge, around the mid-20th century, hypotheses regarding the mechanism of the migraine attack had been based on interpretations of clinical observations of migraine sufferers during their attacks. From the 1940s onward, experimental data from animals and humans, some in the latter obtained during actual migraine attacks, and findings from the various forms of human ancillary investigation that had become increasingly available, began to illuminate the situation.

Harold Wolff (1898–1962), of New York, in association with colleagues, carried out a considerable amount of research into migraine mechanisms in the period from the 1940s onward until his death (Goodell 1967). Two editions *Headache and Other Head Pain* appeared under his authorship, the second posthumously. The second edition contains a long account of the various investigations related to the mechanism of migraine in which he had been involved. It also contains other experimental data relevant to headaches. The experimental material is much too extensive for detailed discussion in the present text. However, it may be useful to cite selected portions of the summary of Wolff's interpretation of the migraine mechanism and to then offer some comment on the experimental data from which his views were derived. To Wolff, the events of the migraine attack were as follows:

> An initial local vasoconstriction of cerebral arteries produces visual and other non-painful, sensory, preheadache phenomena. As the vasoconstrictor preheadache phenomena recede, vasodilator headache manifestations begin. . . . In most patients the headache arises in one or another of the distended branches of the external carotid arteries, although any or all of the major cranial arteries may be involved at one time or another in headache of the migraine type. . . . Vasodilatation sustained during several hours leads to a thickening or edema of the affected artery wall and often to edema of the adjacent tissues. Because of transient thickening of their walls, the soft, readily collapsible arteries become rigid and pipe-like. Further, the pulsating pain becomes a steady ache, and the artery itself becomes tender on palpation.
>
> Secondary to such prolonged pain and distension of cranial arteries, skeletal muscles of the head and neck contract. Prolonged muscle contraction in itself becomes painful, and adds a component to the migraine headache which may outlast the vascular pain. (p. 682)

This account reads rather like a description of the vascular component of the hypotheses of Möllendorf, Eulenburg, and Latham, except that it omits the sympathetic nervous system mechanism that they invoked. However, Wolff added an element that had not appeared previously in the literature, the notion of posterior neck muscle contraction that developed during the headache and seemed to coincide with a change in the pain's character from its earlier throbbing nature. Later, Boquet et al. (1982), by means of electromyography, demonstrated the existence of the postulated excessive contraction of the trapezius muscle on the side of hemicranial migraine in 50 percent of a group of headache-free migraineurs.

Wolff worked in a hospital environment where he could make continuous observations on patients during their headache attacks, and obviously on some occasions was able to follow patients from before the onset of their headaches through the course of the attacks. The particular aspect of the preheadache phase that he studied experimentally was the visual aura. In a number of subjects he showed that this could consistently be shortened or even abolished by the administration of the vasodilator drug amyl nitrite, or by having the subjects breathe carbon dioxide (which was another way of achieving vasodilatation). On this basis he concluded that intracranial vasoconstriction was present during the preheadache phase and was responsible for any neurological manifestations that occurred during it. During the early headache phase, he noted that pressure on the ipsilateral common carotid artery in the neck consistently relieved unilateral headache, that pressure on the occipital artery relieved posterior headache, and that pressure on the superficial temporal artery relieved frontal headache on the affected side. He was able to measure increased amplitudes of pulsation of these arteries during the early stages of the headache and observed that as the headache progressed, these arteries tended to become rigid and pipe-like. The vessels then were more difficult to compress and were tender when they were compressed. At this stage of the attack, the earlier throbbing pain was changing into a steady ache. In the early stages of the headache, pain relief could be secured by injecting the drug ergotamine. In parallel with the ergotamine-induced relief of headache, the amplitude of the scalp arterial pulsation lessened.

Wolff believed that the intracranial arteries did not play a major role in the production of the headache. This belief was based on his observation made in six subjects during migraine attacks. He found that raising the intracranial pressure by injecting saline into the spinal canal to achieve pressures of up to 1000 millimeters of water made no difference to the headache. There possibly is a weakness in his argument, since such a level of CSF pressure may not necessarily have been sufficient to significantly diminish the amplitude of the expansile pulsation of intracranial arteries when their intraluminal pressures peaks may be of the order of perhaps 130 millimeters of mercury. Wolff was aware that there could be local areas of edema in the scalp during migraine attacks. He injected saline into these edematous areas and into the corresponding areas on the pain-free side of the scalp, and then aspirated some of the injected fluid from each side. The aspirated fluid from the painful area, but not that from the unaffected side of the head, was found to contain water-soluble materials that seemed capable of producing pain after injection into the scalp. Wolff's attempted identification of these substances led him to believe that the aspirated fluid from the headache site contained both a polypeptide (neurokinin), and a neurokinin-forming enzyme.

Although the final summary of his interpretation of the migraine mechanism (in part cited above) did not make it particularly clear, Wolff elsewhere in his text suggested that any noxious factor within the body that threatened the integrity of cerebral survival tended to lead to a response involving cerebral vasodilatation. If the vasodilatation was of large enough amplitude, extracranial arteries also dilated. Chemicals were then liberated from these extracranial vessels into the surrounding tissue, where they temporarily decreased the pain threshold of the scalp. He thought that the postulated intracranial ischemia of the preheadache phase of migraine that was responsible for the aura, or other noxious events, some of which might be psychological in nature, could initiate the train of circumstances responsible for the headache. This interpretation, of course, still left the instigation of the vasoconstriction that caused the aura inadequately accounted for.

Wolff's ideas were very influential, both at the time and subsequently. They were based on detailed and continuous, largely opportunistic, observation of patients during actual migraine attacks. Moreover, they utilized experimental manipulations to help clarify issues in the understanding of the disordered physiological mechanisms that seemed to be involved in producing the symptoms of the attacks. His studies have sometimes being taken as marking the beginning of the modern reasonably satisfactory understanding of the mechanism of migraine. However, they can also be seen as simply comprising a modification and updating of the Jaccoud, Möllendorf, Eulenburg, and Latham train of thought about migraine pathogenesis. Nevertheless, they differed from the earlier ideas: first, in that Wolff interpreted the aura as one possible cause among others that could produce vasodilatation-mediated headache, though through mechanisms that Wolff could not specify, and, second, in that Wolff recognized the existence of a subsequent tension-type headache that followed the initial vascular headache. As already mentioned, Wolff did not provide a particularly clear view of what initiated the events that led to the migraine aura. By way of contrast, the 19th-century writers had proposed that it arose from cervical sympathetic activity of unspecified cause, and employed the notion of subsequent cervical sympathetic underaction to explain the mechanism of the headache phase, for whose initiation Wolff proposed what seems a vaguely defined pattern of altered cerebral activity. Except in relation to the later-stage tension-type headache element, the 19th-century writers might seem to have produced a more comprehensive interpretation of the migraine mechanism than Wolff had been able to, more than half a century later. However Wolff's interpretation had the advantage that it was based on experimentally verified data obtained from moderate numbers of migraine sufferers. The 19th-century writers' views were based on smaller numbers of subjects, or on individual experience, and they involved unproven assertions of altered sympathetic nervous system activity. It is therefore little wonder that Wolff's contemporaries, better versed in scientific modes of thinking and attitudes than their 19th-century predecessors, gave much greater credence to Wolff's ideas than to the more speculative thinking of an earlier generation. Wolff himself, at no stage in his book, referred to the earlier proponents of the vascular hypothesis of the mechanism of migraine headache.

Even before Wolff had published the final version of his hypothesis on the pathogenesis of migraine, two sets of experimental observations had become available that would prove to have major influences on the way the mechanism of migraine was to be understood in the latter part of the 20th century. Wolff (1963) was aware of the first of these, namely Sicuteri's emerging evidence in the early 1960s that serotonin (5-hydroxytryptamine) might play a significant role in the pathogenesis of migraine. Wolff did not express a view as to the potential importance of this then recent discovery in relation to his own concepts of migraine pathogenesis. If Wolff knew of the second observation, Leão's discovery in 1944 of spreading depression of function in the cerebral cortex, he did not see fit to mention it in his own final comprehensive account of headache mechanisms (Wolff 1963).

Up until Wolff's time, new observations about migraine and new interpretations of its nature had nearly always been made by individuals. From the 1950s onward, the great and sustained proliferation in scientific research and discovery in medicine, the enormously enhanced investigational and analytical capacity of teams of research workers, and the unprecedented proliferation of knowledge make it difficult to refer to all the investigators and investigations that have contributed to the advance in the understanding of migraine mechanisms. From this stage onward in the present account, only the most outstanding individual contributors and the more important or potentially more important findings relevant to the understanding of migraine will be mentioned. Progress in understanding will be traced in relation to the two main schools of thought that emerged from the initial discoveries of Sicuteri and of Leão.

Serotonin-Related Concepts

For some time after Irving Page found serotonin (5-hydroxytryptamine) to be present in biological systems, in the late 1940s (Saxena 1992), the understanding of the physiological role of the substance was rather slow to emerge. The first indications of its possible involvement in the pathogenesis of migraine appeared in the investigations carried out by Federigo Sicuteri (1920–2003; Lance 2004). Sicuteri spent most of his professional career in Florence, where he appears to have followed a continuing interest in pain mechanisms. He had been studying the experimental headache resembling migraine that was evoked by histamine release and found that a drug then code-named UML-491 (and subsequently marketed as methysergide, an antagonist not of histamine but of serotonin) relieved the headache or prevented it from occurring. This led to his measuring the urinary excretion of the main metabolite of serotonin, 5-hydroxyindole acetic acid, which was found in increased quantities during migraine attacks in 15 subjects (Sicuteri et al. 1961). Unfortunately, data on simultaneous urine volumes were not published, leaving the possibility open that diuresis might have contributed to the finding. Nevertheless, the result was consistent with increased serotonin breakdown being present during migraine attacks.

Once the possibility of a biochemical disturbance underlying migraine became apparent, various investigators began to explore the matter. In a series of studies carried out in Sydney, Australia, James Lance and his coworkers confirmed the findings regarding the urinary 5-hydroxyindoleacetic acid excretion (Curran et al. 1965). They also showed that there were reduced plasma serotonin concentrations during migraine attacks. Therefore the increased urinary 5-hydroxyindoleacetic acid excretion during migraine attacks was very reasonably interpreted as a result of increased serotonin breakdown in the body. A substantial part of the body's serotonin content, and virtually all of that in the blood, is contained in the circulating blood platelets. At that time, the action of serotonin on blood vessels was thought to be simply a matter of vasoconstriction. It therefore seemed likely that in migraine attacks, circulating platelets released part of their contained serotonin, resulting in cerebral vasoconstriction, and that this serotonin freed into plasma produced the aura of migraine by causing ischemia of the visual cortex. Once outside the protected environment of the amine storage granules in platelets, the released serotonin would be exposed to the activity of vascular wall monoamine oxidase, resulting in the serotonin being converted to 5-hydroxyindole acetic acid. This inactivation of the released serotonin would lead to a subsequent stage in which there were reduced plasma serotonin concentrations. This would allow the vasodilatation to occur that was thought to account for the headache of migraine. When there was no aura, it was assumed that the initial cerebral vasoconstriction was not severe enough to produce cerebral ischemic manifestations. Thus the series of circulating serotonin changes, of which there was reasonable but not unambiguous scientific evidence, replaced the never proven, and by then almost completely lapsed, notion of altered sympathetic nervous system activity that Latham and his predecessors had invoked to explain the mechanism of migraine.

For a time, it must have seemed that all that remained to be done to have available a reasonably comprehensive interpretation of the mechanism of migraine was to explain the initial circulating serotonin release and the mechanism of the later-stage secondary tension-type headache that might develop in the attacks. Lance et al. (1967) in fact for a time thought they may have obtained evidence that in migraine attacks an unidentified circulating factor was present that caused platelets to release serotonin. Unfortunately, this finding was never substantiated convincingly. On the basis of such serotonin and platelet-centered ideas, Hanington (1978) put forward the idea that migraine was a primary disorder of circulating platelet function. The observation that circulating platelets tended to form aggregates before and during the early phase of migraine attacks was in keeping with this idea (Jones et al. 1981; Nattero et al. 1981). However, by this time, the circulating serotonin hypothesis was beginning to encounter difficulties. Further measurements of plasma serotonin concentrations and urinary excretions of 5-hydroxyindoleacetic acid by various groups of workers failed to produce entirely consistent results, though most tended to be in keeping with the early findings. Very much the greater part of the serotonin in blood is encased within the protected environment of storage granules in platelets and is not able to exert biological effects outside platelets until it has been released into blood plasma. Therefore it came to be appreciated that it would be more relevant to measure serotonin concentrations free in plasma water. Unfortunately, it was never possible to be certain that in separating plasma water from platelets and other plasma components, some platelets did not rupture and release their serotonin. Therefore scientifically convincing plasma water serotonin concentration values do not seem to have become available.

Then, in 1981, Olesen and his colleagues used [133]xenon cerebral blood flow studies to show that there was no measurable alteration in the flow during attacks of migraine without aura. A decrease in flow, though not necessarily sufficient to produce clinically apparent manifestations, had been held by Wolff to initiate the headache phase of migraine, with increased flow during the headache. The finding of Olesen et al. (1981) thus rather undermined the basis of major elements of the vascular hypothesis of the mechanism of production of the most frequently encountered variety of migraine: migraine without aura. It also raised the possibility that migraine with aura and migraine without aura might have different pathophysiologies. Added to the various accumulating difficulties encountered in sustaining the circulating serotonin based concept of migraine pathogenesis, these cerebral blood flow findings seem to have been associated with a declining interest in pursuing the role of circulating serotonin in the disorder. Instead, the interest of those concerned with serotonin in migraine was increasingly transferred to an idea that Sicuteri himself had proposed in 1976. Sicuteri, from an early stage in his investigational work, had apparently been particularly interested in the role of serotonin as an agent that enhanced the pain-producing capabilities of other biological molecules. He had carried out pharmacological studies that tended to suggest that serotonin acted within the brain stem to modulate the activity of the central pain transmission pathway. In the 1960–1970 period, Sicuteri fairly quickly shifted his interest away from hypotheses that envisaged serotonin as acting on the circulation to produce migraine headache. In 1976, he published the idea that migraine headache represented a state of serotonin-mediated central dys-nociception mediated by central receptor hypersensitivity that facilitated the centripetal transmission of trigeminal nociceptive activity (Sicuteri 1972, 1976). Newly developed imaging techniques began to demonstrate an area of increased neuronal activity in the dorsal pons in the region of the locus coeruleus during human migraine attacks (Weiller et al. 1995). A positron-emission tomography study in a small number of migraine sufferers revealed increased brain serotonin synthesis (Chugani et al. 1999). This knowledge, the rapidly increasing understanding of the neurotransmitter anatomy of the brain, and various animal and human pharmacological investigations combined to point toward the major role of serotonin in migraine being that of enhancing the pain of the headache through central mechanisms after the pain itself was initiated by other agencies acting on the trigeminal afferent system. This idea of serotonin-mediated central pain sensitization left the aura of migraine, if one occurred, and the later stage tension headache both unexplained.

Other Neurotransmitters

The evidence for an apparent role of serotonin in migraine pathogenesis inevitably led to the likelihood that the roles of other neurotransmitters, particularly known vasoactive ones, would be explored. Little evidence came to light to suggest that noradrenaline was involved, but there was some evidence obtained that, as was originally suggested by Sicuteri (1977), largely on seemingly rather tenuous pharmacological grounds, dopamine might play a part (Peroutka 1997; Mascia et al. 1998; Gladstone 2007). However, the role of dopamine seems probably to be a minor one that is relevant mainly to the occurrence of nausea and vomiting in the attacks. There also was speculation that substance P might play a part, and quite strong evidence has accumulated that calcitonin gene-related peptide has a significant role (Doods et al. 2007). The latter substance is a very potent vasodilator that is present in trigeminal nerve terminals in proximity to blood vessels in the pia and dura. Calcitonin gene-related peptide also occurs in afferent terminals in the trigeminal nuclei in the brain stem and upper cervical spinal cord. It also possesses pain-producing capabilities. The concentration of calcitonin gene-related peptide has been found to be increased in external, but not in internal, jugular venous blood during migraine attacks (Goadsby et al. 1990). A hypothesis has been developed that increased afferent activity in trigeminal pain fibers from cranial blood vessels leads to calcitonin gene-related peptide release from trigeminal terminals on these vessels. The local presence of the peptide then causes vasodilatation. At the same time, the transmitter's release from trigeminal afferent terminals in the descending spinal nucleus of the nerve plays a part in enhancing the activity in second-level trigeminal sensory pain-transmitting neurons. Among others, Moskowitz made major contributions to this area of knowledge and extended the simplified concept mentioned immediately above by linking the idea with a set of ideas to be touched on later in this chapter (Moskowitz 2007).

There was also speculation about the possible role of nitric oxide in migraine. Some tentative and indirect pharmacological evidence exists that it may play a part (Olesen et al. 1995). Nitric oxide is a potent vasodilator. It appears to mediate the vasodilator effect that serotonin produces on contact with intact endothelium, though serotonin has a constrictor effect on direct contact with vascular smooth muscle, at least in human coronary arteries in vivo (Golino et al. 1991).

As well, markedly raised plasma concentrations of the potent vasoconstrictor endothelin have been found in the early stages of attacks of migraine, whether or not an aura was present (Kallela et al. 1998). This finding was in keeping with the earlier reports of Färkkilä et al. (1992) and Gallai et al. (1994). The ways in which these reported changes in circulating concentrations of vasoactive molecules fit into the overall pathophysiology of migraine remain to be clarified at the time of the present book's writing.

As mentioned earlier, the second major set of ideas that tended to under-mine concepts of the mechanism of migraine derived from Wolff's research arose from a chance observation by a Brazilian PhD student at Harvard, Aristides Leão. In the 1943–1944 period, when Leão was working on experimental models of epilepsy (Leão 1944-a,1944-b; Leão 1947; Leão and Morison 1945), he noted that local stimulation of the cerebral cortex of anesthetized rabbits caused a wave of decreased electrical activity of the cortex. The wave spread from the point of stimulation at a rate of approxi-mately 2 to 3 mm per minute. This wave of depression was accompanied by a spreading local dilatation of the pial arteries. On further investigation, at first carried out by Leão, and subsequently by a number of other workers, it became clear that there was an initial brief phase of spreading excitation that preceded the more prolonged spreading depression of cortical activity. The underlying biochemical mechanisms have been investigated. It appears that the spread of the disturbance is not mediated by neural pathways but by the activity of glia activated by the spread of a high concentration of potassium ions. As mentioned, Leão's initial interest in this phenomenon was related to his work on experimental epileptogenesis. However, a year after his initial publication, he and Morison wrote the following:

> Much has been written about vascular phenomena both in clinical epilepsy and the pre-sumedly related condition of migraine. The latter disease with the marked dilatation of major blood vessels and the slow march of scotomata in the visual and somatic sensory sphere is suggestively similar to the experimental phenomena here described, in spite of the fact that known scotomata are still felt to be vasoconstrictor in nature. (Leão and Morison 1945, p. 44)

Lashley (1941) had earlier mapped the course of his own migraine visual aura, and calculated that its event represented the consequences of a distur-bance which spread over his visual cortex at the rate of about 3 mm a minute. Almost certainly in ignorance of this conclusion, Leão had perceived the possibility that his spreading depression might be the basis of the migraine visual aura. It was left to Milner (1958) to link Lashley's data to that of Leão.

It was some time after its discovery before there was any widespread acceptance that spreading depression might be relevant to human migraine. If it could be shown to occur in humans, it seemed that the phenomenon could explain the aura of migraine, but not the headache. For a long time, there was no evidence forthcoming that the cortical spreading depression phenomenon occurred in humans, even though it was readily elicited in experimental animals. It was only after the serotonin-related vascular hypothesis of migraine genesis began to be regarded as unsatisfactory and the centrally acting serotonin hypothesis in its own right seemed incapable of accounting for the migraine aura, and when more refined methods of measuring human cerebral blood flow and brain activity became available, that it became increasingly accepted that sufficient evidence had been accumulated to sustain the view that cortical spreading depression was the probable basis of the migraine aura.

Thus, in the final decade of the 20th century, reasonable hypotheses with moderately strong degrees of experimental backing began to become available to account individually for the migraine aura (via spreading depression) and the migraine headache (primarily by serotonin-mediated central pain sensitization). The problem remained as to how to explain the frequent but certainly not invariable linkage between the two in a given migraine sufferer. Iadecola (2002) and Bolay et al. (2002) published proposed mechanisms that could achieve such a linkage, and Moskowitz (2007), in a review of his several decades of work into migraine mechanisms, took the possibility a little further. He suggested that high concentrations of ions and possibly neuroactive chemicals resulting from the wave of spreading depression in the cortex might allow some of these ions and molecules to leak into the pia overlying the cortex. There they might activate trigeminal afferent endings around pial blood vessels to produce local vasodilatation (through the agency of local calcitonin gene-related peptide release) and also increase trigeminal afferent pain-conducting activity. This activity might then initiate antidromic activity in trigeminal afferent collaterals from the dural (and presumably the extracranial) arteries, leading to release of calcitonin gene-related peptide at peripheral trigeminal terminals on these vessels. This would produce dilatation of these vessels and cause pain-mediating neural afferent activity to arise from them. The simultaneously increased trigeminal pain input to the descending spinal nucleus of the trigeminal would interact with the serotonin-mediated state of dysnociception in that structure to produce both the headache of migraine and the state of more widespread body surface allodynia that is known to develop as migraine attacks progress (Burstein et al. 2000-a, 2000-b). This whole concept is ingenious, but whether all its individual elements can be demonstrated to occur in human migraine is another matter. There is also the issue of how this mechanism can account for the migraine in those unusual individuals in whom the headache begins before the aura commences.

The above attempts to account for both the aura and the headache of migraine in an all-embracing mechanism have tended to ignore the cranial and cervical myofascial tightness that Wolff had noticed was present in the later stages of migraine headaches. Olesen (1991) had proposed a hypothetical scheme that could link the mechanisms of the processes involved in the earlier and later stage headache of migraine with the supraspinal elements involved in the genesis of migraine attacks. His concept would seem to accommodate the existence of a continuum between migraine and tension-type headache. However, that particular idea does not seem to have been developed further in the literature.

Migraine Genetics

For a very long time, it has been realized that migraine often appears to be inherited. Willis (1672), when writing of headache, was almost certainly referring to migraine when he stated "the Disease is often delivered from the Parents to the Children," while that scrupulous careful observer William Gowers (1888) stated, "Migraine is strongly hereditary; in more than half the cases, inheritance can be traced, and it is usually direct, *i.e.* other members of the family (very often a parent) suffer from paroxysmal headache." With the considerable interest in genetics in the latter half of the 20th century, a good deal of effort went into the attempt to define the genes responsible for the inherited tendency to migraine. Migraine has generally been assumed to have a multigenic basis (Ducros et al. 2002; Wessman et al. 2007), but, apart from detecting three separate genes responsible for the development of particular ion channels that are associated with familial hemiplegic migraine, the efforts of the geneticists had not detected genes related to the more common forms of the disorder until after the end of the first decade of the 21st century, when some additional relevant information began to become available.

Migraine and Epilepsy

An individual may, by virtue of coincidence, experience both epileptic events and migraine at the same or different stages of life. This may have, for instance, been the explanation of the situation in a small group of patients reported by Charles Féré in 1906. Whether the relationship between the two disorders can be more than coincidental is another question, and a more important one.

The Bath physician Caleb Hillier Parry, in his *Elements of Pathology and Therapeutics* (1825-a, 1825-b), drew attention to his perception that an association existed between migraine (sick headache) and epilepsy: "I have known epilepsy occur indiscriminately with sick headach; disappear, as that was cured; and return, several years afterwards, as, from the imprudence of the patient, the sick headach also returned." Parry believed that both the headache and the epilepsy shared the same causal mechanism—namely, excessive determination of blood to the head—a concept that carried the implication that the relationship between the two was more than coincidental. In writing of "sick headach" in his section DCCXII, he had already noted that "this kind of headache not uncommonly occurs as a vicarious affection with epilepsy."

A quarter of a century later, Marshall Hall (1849) also suggested there was a kinship between episodic headache and epilepsy, postulating that both were consequences of obstructed venous outflow from the cranium resulting from the effects of his *trachelismus*, the more severe degree of cerebral venous outflow obstruction being responsible for epilepsy, lesser ones for the headache. Shortly afterward, Edward Sieveking, also in England, wrote the following: "Headache is one of the symptoms that bears so close a relation to the epileptic paroxysm, that it deserves a separate consideration" (1858, p. 45).Sieveking did not explicitly mention either migraine or sick headache in this connection, but he did provide case histories of two instances of a disorder for which he had earlier coined the term *cephalalgia epileptiformis* (Sieveking 1854). His own definition of this condition was that it comprised headache, often quite localized and in that regard resembling the *clavus* of a former day, associated with slight vertiginous attacks, or a solitary seizure in the past, or with "some spasmodic action that alone would not be considered epileptiform." It may be hard to be quite sure from his explanation as to what he meant to include in his concept, though at the time he wrote, *vetriges* was a term applied on the Continent to minor epileptic events. However, one of his case histories provided a reasonably convincing account of hemiplegic migraine. It therefore seems that Sieveking may have been moving a little closer than his predecessors to an idea that epilepsy could cause migraine, though he did not attempt to go into possible pathogenic mechanisms. Nonetheless, he was at pains to make it clear that such an idea did not apply to headache that followed immediately after epileptic seizures, but only to headache that preceded seizures or which recurred habitually. Allbutt (1883) described what would later be called *hemiplegic migraine* under the term *epileptiform migraine*, a designation similar to that which Sieveking had earlier employed for a similar set of clinical phenomena. It reflected a belief that both disorders were of cerebral origin, and paroxysmal in their clinical expression.

In the 1870s, John Hughlings Jackson, having arrived at the realization that epileptic seizures originated in the cerebral cortex, and knowing that accumulating evidence pointed to there being localized representation of function in that part of the cerebrum, began to explore the limits of the range of phenomena that could be embraced by his notion of epilepsy, much as Willis (1670) had done two centuries earlier in relation to the concept of convulsive disease. Jackson speculated as to whether entities such as asthma and chronic cough might be epileptic when he wrote the following:

> I think the sensory symptoms of the paroxysm are owing to a "discharging lesion" of convolutions evolved out of the optic thalamus, i.e. of "sensory middle centres" analogous to the "middle motor area" I believe the headache and vomiting to be post-paroxysmal. (Jackson 1876/1931, p. 153n)

In that same publication, he addressed the matter, from his standpoint, as follows: "However, in some cases of migraine, which in my nomenclature are epilepsies, the development of sensations during discharges of sensory centres is slow and deliberate, and consciousness is not lost" (Jackson 1876/1931, p. 139).

Jackson repeated the notion at other places in his writings and, at a time when no really satisfactory interpretation of the pathogenesis of migraine was available, and when the power of his intellect was becoming increasingly apparent to his medical colleagues, others adopted the idea. James Ross, of Manchester, in the shortened version of his encyclopedic two-volume neurology textbook (1885), extended the concept by proposing that the effects of the discharging lesion might extend to the medulla oblongata and even to the ciliospinal region of the spinal cord at the cervicothoracic junction to produce altered cervical sympathetic activity, thus providing a possible explanation for a vascular-type headache mechanism along the lines suggested a little earlier in the ideas of Du Bois-Reymond, Möllendorf, Jaccoud, Latham, and Eulenburg. Gowers (1888) was cautious about the nature of any relationship between epilepsy and migraine. He reported that he had encountered at least 12 cases of various patterns of association between the two disorders, and concluded that both disorders probably arose from disturbances of function in nerve cells of the brain, but that the disturbances were "of a different kind." As already mentioned, his thinking may have been influenced by Sidney Ringer (1877), his former colleague, who had proposed that both epilepsy and migraine arose not from brain overaction, Liveing's "nerve storm" in the case of migraine, but from loss of "resistance" (i.e., loss of inhibition).

Jackson's idea that migraine was a variety of epilepsy kept recurring in the English-language literature (e.g., Collier 1928), until at least the posthumous appearance of Wilson's magnum opus (1940). It probably was knowledge of the electroencephalographic appearances of human epileptic seizures that finally made the idea untenable. The concept of an epileptic type of basis for migraine did not seem to arouse much enthusiasm among

Continental writers on headache at any stage. Certainly, there were occasional reports of an association between the two disorders (e.g., Féré 1906; Kovalesky 1906), but without attempts being made to interpret it beyond the two disorders having a possible genetic relationship. Lennox (1946) published a small book, seemingly intended for a semipopular readership, titled *Science and Seizures: New Light on Epilepsy and Migraine*. In the book, he attempted to use statistics to bring out affinities between the two disorders, though his statistical approach to the matter might not be considered particularly satisfactory today.

The Precipitation of Migraine Attacks

Among migraine suffers, and to some extent in the wider community, there is a long-standing belief that various circumstances and factors, both endogenous and exogenous, physical and psychical, will bring on migraine attacks in those predisposed to the disorder. Thomas (1889) linked the names of putative attack-provoking factors with the names of prominent figures of the past who had chosen to blame various of these factors for causing their migraine attacks: wine (Haller), chocolate (Lasegue), milk (Armangué), acid drinks (Claude Bernard), and alcohol in general (See, who held that beer, especially English beer, was much worse in this regard than all other forms of alcohol). Numerous other substances and situations have also been nominated for addition to such a list of migraine provocants (Dalessio et al. 1986; Debney and Hedge 1986; Olesen 1986). These particular substances may provoke migraine in certain susceptible individuals, though there seems to have been surprisingly little scientific study of the matter. Where there has been, the outcome has not always been as expected on the basis of clinical impressions.

For instance, on the grounds that tyramine in cheese could cause headache in patients taking monoamine oxidase inhibitors, Hanington (1967) hypothesized that the amine in various items of diet might be a hitherto unrecognized precipitant of migraine in individuals relatively deficient in intestinal monoamine oxidase activity. A very small preliminary study, in four patients with diet-related migraine, suggested that the idea might be valid. However, in a larger subsequent study, Moffett et al. (1972) failed to find any significant relationship between oral tyramine intake and the occurrence of headache attacks in migraine sufferers.

Nevertheless, certain beverages and foods continued to have a reputation among migraine sufferers for bringing on their headaches. Chocolate is notorious in this regard, but a double-blind, placebo (carob)-controlled study failed to obtain evidence for the association, not only in a group of migraine sufferers, but also in those who believed that such an association was present in themselves (Marcus et al. 1997). In an earlier study, Moffett et al. (1974) had found that chocolate rarely precipitated migraine.

Migraine sufferers have sometimes been thought more vulnerable to attacks during the approach, and presence, of particular weather conditions. Overall, the evidence for this belief is not strong, though, for instance, Cooke et al. (2000) were able to show that, in a subset of migraine sufferers in Alberta, Canada, there was a real association between headache attacks and the presence of warm westerly "Chinook" winds.

The tendency for migraine attacks to occur particularly around the time of menstruation in some women of reproductive age has been known for a long time, though the association has at times been somewhat loosely defined (MacGregor 1996). Van der Linden (1666) probably was the first to draw attention to the phenomenon when he described the presence of a consistent association between migraine and menstruation in the then 31-year-old Marchioness of Brandenburg. He described this type of migraine as *hemicrania menstrua*. Later studies have showed that the relationship seems to be determined by the time course of the behavior of circulating female sex hormone concentrations (Somerville 1972).

Migraine with, and without, Aura: The One Disorder?

In the latter part of the 20th century, a number of writers touched on the question of whether migraine with, and migraine without, aura are separate disorders. The question is an important one in relation to the understanding of migraine, and some relevant data have been published.

Russell et al. (1996) compared the clinical characteristics of the two groups in migraine sufferers drawn from the general population and showed that menstruation was a precipitating factor in the attacks only in those whose episodes lacked an aura. There also were differences in patterns of age of onset. The authors concluded that the two types of migraine were separate and distinct entities. A little later, in a study of migraine lifetime prevalence rates in monozygotic and same-sex dizygotic twins, Russell et al. (2002) found no statistically significant difference between observed and expected rates of co-occurrence of the two types of migraine in twins of either sex. They interpreted this finding as also suggesting that the two clinical types of migraine were distinct disorders. Further, Stewart et al. (2000) found that there was a tendency for migraine attacks to be more frequent on the last two premenstrual days and the first two days of menstruation in women whose migraine lacked auras, when compared with women who had migraine with auras.

In the past half-century, a considerable amount of scientific information about aspects of the pathogenesis of migraine has accumulated. However, it has not yet proved possible to develop a securely established and enduring understanding of all aspects of the production of the disorder. Part of the problem may be that investigations appear to have often been carried out, and their findings interpreted, without relating them to the stage of evolution of the individual migraine attack. One consequence of this is that a variety of observations exist whose relevance can neither be taken into consideration with confidence nor confidently and validly discarded. Critchley and Ferguson (1933) wrote three-quarters of a century ago that "migraine has been the happy hunting ground of the theorist." To the category of the theorist may now be added that of the experimentalist. Despite the seekers for a satisfactory explanation for migraine, after a very long pursuit, closing in progressively on the object of their chase from more than one direction, their quarry had so far managed to evade being taken into any well-secured final intellectual captivity.

CHAPTER 6
The Treatment of Migraine

At the present time, migraine treatment is often discussed in terms of (i) the treatment of individual headache attacks and (ii) the prevention of attacks. Attack prevention is then sometimes subdivided into (a) long-term continuing management and (b) strategically timed preventive intervention. In the writings of the past, these various aspects of migraine treatment were usually not so clearly distinguished, though to an extent the probable purposes of various recommended treatments can be deduced from their natures or from the immediate context in which their use has been described. As well, in the earlier literature, the intended durations of use of various preventive treatments is often not made clear, though some contemporary accounts are also vulnerable to this criticism.

Until migraine started to become a generally recognized medical entity in the late 18th century, it seems inevitable that attacks of what would now be accepted as the disorder, unless they were hemicranial in the distribution of the pain, would be included under the designations of *cephalalgia,* or sometimes *cephalaea,* and would have been treated as headache in general was then treated (chapter 3). Such treatment is not considered in the present chapter unless a description of *cephalalgia* or *cephalaea* in the earlier headache literature can be identified with reasonable probability as being that of migraine and where there also is information concerning its treatment. Further, the treatments mentioned in earlier accounts of *hemicrania* have been taken into consideration only when there appear to be reasonable grounds for believing that present-day migraine was recognizable in the accounts.

Until comparatively recent times, the medical profession lacked the intellectual tools that enabled it to distinguish reliably between genuine therapeutic responses and apparent beneficial responses that represented no more than the effects of chance, or of spontaneous recovery that took place with the passing of time. Consequently, the earlier headache literature is replete with reports of proposed migraine treatments, often based on particular theories of headache causation or on small numbers of sufferers, that subsequently did not meet the expectations that they initially engendered. The following account should be read in the light of this knowledge, and also of recognition that relatively little purpose would probably be served by an exhaustive recitation of all the numerous remedies that were recommended in the available early literature.

THE TREATMENT OF MIGRAINE ATTACKS

The Ancient World

The earliest recorded physical treatment of an attack of possible migraine appears in the Ebers papyrus (ca.1500 B.C.), where it was advised that in *hemicrania*, the pain-affected part should be anointed with the skull of a catfish, fried in oil (Nunn 2002). But whether this particular *hemicrania* was migraine is far from certain. The only intimation of treatment aspects in relation to the instance of highly probable migraine with a visual aura that was described in the later Hippocratic writings (Smith 1994) was the terse statement that followed the description of its clinical features. The sufferer was given a draught of hellebore, and the reader was told that "phlebotomy helped." Aretaeus, early second century A.D., treated all headache similarly (see chapter 3), but advised that in *hemicrania*, locally acting remedies should be applied to the affected side of the head. One might anticipate that he and any disciples he had would have treated migraine along those lines. It is difficult to be sure whether Galen was dealing with present-day migraine when he discussed treatment aspects, but in volume 8 of the Kühn edition (1833) there is mention of purgation and venesection in relation to treating *hemicrania*, and in volume 12 there are details of a number of compound preparations for treating the symptom. Whether such measures would have been recommended if Galen had known of present-day migraine is another matter.

In Bussemaker and Daremberg's (1873) translation of the writings of the late ancient–early medieval commentator Oribasius, there is a section on *migraine*, that word being taken as a synonym for *hemicrania*, though the exact equivalence between the two may not be entirely certain. At the outset of treatment, a decision had to be made as to whether the sufferer would be better purged or bled. Before the attack, the forehead was to be rubbed with a cotton rag containing warming materials; once the pain had begun, specifics ("hémicraniques") were used. If the sufferer experienced a great warmth with the pain, cooling materials were applied; if these failed to afford relief, warming substances were substituted, perhaps reinforced by materials with astringent properties. Lukewarm oil with a little euphorbe (the sap of a *Euphorbia* species) could be injected into the ear on the affected side to enhance the sufferer's comfort.

Medieval Times

There appears to have been little conceptual advance regarding the treatment of identifiable migraine attacks in this period. Gonzáles-Hernández and Domínguez-Rodríguez (2008) have made available some material concerning the treatment of hemicranial attacks that was contained in the *Compendium medicinae* of Gilbertus Anglicus (ca. 1180–1240/1250). "Arabic" pills (which contained a mix of liver-colored aloes, brome, mastics, laurel bays, sammony, and cloves mixed with cabbage juice or fennel preserved in honey) were to be swallowed, and aromatic substances (e.g., cumin, anise) in the diet were to be avoided. As well, plasters might be applied to the head. The surgical writings of Albucasis (1106/7–1187) contained the recommendation that if medical treatment failed to afford relief of *hemicrania*, the area of the affected temple should be cauterized by means of an iron heated in the fire. Alternatively, an incision was to be made in the scalp of the pain-affected area and caustic material inserted into the wound (Albucasis 1861).

Avicenna recommended the local application of a mixture of opium, absinthe, and wild cucumber in oil, according to De Villiers (1819).

The Scientific Revolution

Thomas Willis (1672), in writing of "headach" in his *De anima brutorum*, did not indicate the treatment he used in relation to the individual cases of probable migraine whose clinical details he had recorded. However, after describing a particular head pain-producing mechanism that suggested that he was thinking of migraine headache, namely that blood was rushing "by heaps into the Membranes of the Head . . . distending the Vessels above measure," he recommended that blood be removed from the arm, or the jugular vein, and that the following steps be taken:

> Let there be Medicines of Vinegar, Rosecakes and Nutmeg, or some other *Epithems* or Medicines of the same nature applyed to the Head; also give to drink *Juleps, Emulsions* or *Decoctions* which allay the fervour or madness of the Blood. Let the Belly be cooled and kept soluble by the use of clysters. (Willis 1672/1683, p. 114)

All this seems rather similar to what was written a thousand and more years earlier, though the rationales for using the same types of therapeutic measures had changed with the passing of time.

Wepfer, at much the same time as Willis, had no important alternative suggestions, unless one regards applying a Cantharides plaster to the head as a therapeutic advance. Even so, according to Isler (1987-a), Wepfer's therapy was less violent than that of his predecessors and contemporaries. Because Wepfer's *hemicrania* included entities other than migraine, it may be important to note that he managed the subject of his Observation 54, his patient with probably the most unambiguous migraine, by means of clysters, purgatives, and emetics (Wepfer 1727).

The 18th and 19th Centuries

For his own hemicranial migraine, John Fordyce (1758) took large doses of the herb valerian (a sedative) and considered it to be helpful. However, he sometimes had recourse to plunging his head into cold water. He commended the use of emetics and also noted that pressure over the region of the supraorbital nerve would provide a degree of pain relief.

An example of what a well-intentioned and intelligent nonmedical author recommended for relieving *hemicrania*, which would have included instances of migraine, may be found in *Primitive Physic* written by John Wesley, the founder of Methodism. This work first appeared in 1747 and achieved sufficient popularity to be republished in numerous editions over the course of more than a century. In a later edition (Wesley 1858), for a *hemicrania* it recommended cold bathing, or shaving part of the head and making a blister there. If the headache could be ascribed to an overloaded stomach, the book advised taking an emetic powder with warm water, or an aqueous fluid of senna; if the headache appeared related to excessive blood flow to the head, cold applications should be applied to that part, and warm ones to the feet; if the headache appeared to be related to rheumatism longer term therapy with niter or fluid extract of henbane was suggested. In the latter case, the therapy seemed intended for prevention of recurrences rather than for providing more immediate relief. Probably these relatively innocuous recommendations were based on the available medical literature or other sources of medical advice, but they may well reflect the widespread community management of migraine in 18th- and early 19th-century England.

In Diderot's *Encyclopedia* (1765), the author of the article on migraine, probably Jean Jacques Ménuret de Chambaud (Isler et al. 2005), indicated that there was no certain cure for the disorder, and commented that its management should be relegated to the charlatans whose daring equaled their ignorance. He mentioned that some patients obtained great benefit from arteriotomy, but that in others it was useless. The response of the headache to bloodletting was inconsistent. Vomiting sometimes brought attacks to their end. The author recommended that sufferers should endure their pain patiently, though if the pain became too severe, it could be alleviated by the scents of aromatic essences, or of volatile spirits or fetid substances. Repeated enemas could be useful, because constipation was often present during attacks and sometimes caused them. The author believed that one of his own migraine attacks had been cured by taking an emetic. He favored employing stomach bitters, tonics, iron preparations, and, in particular, quinine for longer term migraine management. He also thought some benefit might be derived from applying blistering plasters.

Soon after this material in the *Encyclopedia* became available, Samuel Tissot's account of the disorder appeared. Tissot drew a clear distinction between treatment of the migraine attack itself and the use of measures intended to prevent further attacks. Subsequent authors on the whole preserved this distinction. Therefore, from here on in the present account, treatments for migraine attacks are discussed separately from, and also prior to, the preventive management of migraine. However, many 19th-century authors dealt with these matters in the opposite sequence.

During migraine attacks, Tissot (1780) advised that the sufferer should be placed in quiet surroundings and in darkness. Coffee could be given, or a light infusion of camomile, and opium employed if the pain was excessive. The limbs might be bathed, but local applications placed on patients' foreheads almost never helped. Pressure over the supraorbital nerve at the eyebrow on the affected side might produce benefit. Unfortunately, Tissot did not consider whether the benefit was derived from compressing the nerve itself or its accompanying artery. Bleeding from the temporal artery might be considered, or else bleeding from the jugular vein. He mentioned that one author (Sigaud de la Fond) claimed that he had seen migraine cease on a number of occasions when the patient's face was turned toward the north, and the south pole of a small bar magnet that had been placed on the site of the pain was then moved about. It seems that what Tissot described for treating migraine attacks was based on a mixture of his own practice and recommendations drawn from various sources in the literature.

More or less simultaneously to Tissot, in England John Fothergill commended his own qualifications for commenting on the treatment of sick headache, in other words, migraine:

> Having had some little experience of this complaint myself, and having met with numerous occasions of seeing it in others, in the variety of degrees of force and continuance;

and having likewise attended to the different ideas and modes of treatment, in regard to this distemper, I thought it might be useful to suggest what had occurred to me on the subject. (1784, p. 107)

Fothergill went on to write that it was not difficult to obtain speedy headache relief by using an emetic or a mild cathartic and that an anodyne would for the most part soon restore sufferers to their usual health.

Among the set of French-language authors who took up the topic of migraine in the 19th century, Martin (1829) discussed the treatment of the attacks on the basis of their presumed mechanism. When the attacks were thought due to plethora, he recommended bleeding, or a more gradual removal of blood by the application of leeches, and the use of cold evaporative compresses placed on the head. When the attacks were thought to be related to nervous over excitability, he recommended the application of ether, cologne, or opium to the head. For attacks ascribable to malfunction of other organs, particularly the stomach, the intake of compound pills intended to restore normal function to these organs was, in his view, the desirable course of therapeutic action.

Two years later, Piorry (1831), whose interest lay particularly in the visual aura component of the headache attack, advised placing the patient in darkness, avoiding all use of the eyes. Belladonna was to be rubbed into the affected side of the head after the sufferer had been warned that the pupils would still be dilated the next day. Wine, strong coffee, and alcoholic liquors should be given and the patient's feet placed in hot water.

In Adelon's *Dictionnaire*, Calmeil (1839) provided the type of advice for managing migraine attacks that many subsequent 19th-century French authors advocated. At the onset of the attack, or as it developed, cold infusions of tea, coffee, orange leaves, European veronica, sage, camomile, or similar substances were to be drunk. Cooling and rapidly evaporating lotions containing alcohol, ether, or water of mélisse, should be applied to the head. At times opium might be necessary. Calmeil observed that sometimes doing nothing except providing conditions conducive to complete rest was the best policy. He noted that Paré had opened the temporal artery in recalcitrant migraine and suggested that bleeding from the jugular vein or the veins of the feet should be considered when managing violent attacks of headache in which there was alarming congestion of the head and face.

A decade after Sir Charles Locock (1857-a, 1857-b) first reported the successful use of potassium bromide in the prevention of epileptic seizures, Barudel (1867) described the use of this substance in treating migraine.

Jaccoud (1869) saw a place for undertaking no active measures in managing migraine attacks, but merely ensuring rest and tranquility for the sufferer. If necessary, he seemed to be prepared to go as far as recommending measures such as the intake of an infusion of camomile, or of orange flowers, or simply drinking pure water. His was perhaps the least vigorous of all the published 19th-century active management regimens for migraine attacks. Soon after, in England, Hubert Airy (1870), in his account of the migraine aura, mentioned in passing that for his own migraine, he had tried to induce vomiting and had applied mustard plasters. He confessed that he had obtained no discernable benefit from either measure.

In his monograph *On Megrim*, Edward Liveing (1873) provided a rather extensive review of published material on the treatment of migraine attacks. To this he added some therapeutic views based on his own experience. For the attacks, he advised bed rest in quiet darkened surroundings. Early in the attack, full doses of brandy or other form of alcohol should be given (he regarded brandy as a stimulant). Potassium bromide at this stage sometimes helped, but more often it failed. Potassium bicarbonate could be used, or tincture of valerian or sal volatile. Strong tea or coffee might be helpful, and guarana might be prescribed. Samuel Wilks had introduced guarana into English medical practice, and found that it could help relieve migraine attacks, though unfortunately, from his point of view, not his own (Wilks 1878). Guarana was subsequently proved to be simply a source of caffeine. Emetics were sometimes given to induce vomiting, because it had been noted that the act of vomiting sometimes terminated migraine attacks. Chloroform inhalations gave relief, but the benefit was too transient to be useful in practice. Rubbing belladonna into the affected area of the scalp, compressing the supraorbital nerve, compressing the carotid artery on the headache side, applying mustard plasters to the legs, and galvanic stimulation of the cervical sympathetic trunk had all been used by the time Liveing wrote, but he did not seem particularly impressed by their efficacies. He concluded his account as follows, embodying his appreciation of the situation in his translation of Tissot's words:

> During the attacks there is scarcely anything to be done; moreover the patients are so
> much afraid of all noise, motion, or anything approaching them, that they infinitely prefer
> to be left perfectly quiet than tormented with useless measures. (Liveing 1873, p. 471)

Liveing's contemporary and fellow countryman P. W. Latham (1873) dealt briefly with the treatment of migraine attacks in his monograph on the subject. He advised that the patient should not be bled and should not be given calomel or other laxative. The sufferer should be ensured perfect rest, have cold applications placed on the head, and be given potassium citrate, soda water, potassium bromide, or guarana. Latham commented that Trousseau had not been impressed with the effectiveness of the latter.

In the writings of these 19th-century English authors, one can see the development an increasingly conservative attitude toward the treatment of migraine attacks, the gradual supplanting of a largely botanical-based antimigraine pharmacopoeia with increasing numbers of pure inorganic and organic chemicals, and the appearance of a degree of skepticism concerning the efficacy of any available treatment.

In Germany, Eulenburg (1877) knew of the various treatments mentioned immediately above and added a few further agents to the list of those recommended for the management of migraine attacks. He mentioned that because migraine was a periodic disorder and quinine relieved the periodic fever of malaria, the drug had also been used in migraine prevention. Eulenburg considered it ineffective in this regard, but believed that in big doses, it could shorten individual migraine attacks. He mentioned that some authors claimed it was most effective in the angioparalytic variety of the disorder. Eulenburg stated that the potent vasodilating agent amyl nitrate had been used for Du Bois-Reymond's sympatheticotonic migraine. From the tone of his writing, he did not appear to be overly impressed with its effectiveness, or with that of electrical stimulation of the cervical sympathetic nerve trunk. He accepted the efficacy of carotid compression but knew that the benefit did not outlast the duration of the compression. He expressed a reluctance to use narcotics to relieve migraine pain and mentioned an agent, Ergotin, an aqueous extract of ergot, which was a vasoconstrictor and useful both in angioparalytic migraine and what he termed "non-unilateral *cephalalgia vasomotoria*" (presumably this would be equivalent to migraine with bilateral head pain, as Eulenburg had been writing about the topic of migraine under the designation of *hemicrania*). The fascinating history of Ergotin and other ergot derivatives, a family of chemicals that contains among its members ergotamine, the first specific migraine-relieving agent and one that was to pave the way to the present-day treatment of migraine attacks, will be taken up shortly.

However, the medical literature in the final quarter 19th century and the first two decades of the 20th, before the ergot derivatives became established in human therapeutics, contains some further information on measures employed in those times to treat migraine attacks.

Much of the material in the French- and English-language literature on migraine up to his time was collected in a monograph on the subject written by the librarian Louis Hyacinth Thomas (1887). Thomas was not a clinician, and his account was almost inevitably a reiteration of what others, whom he carefully acknowledged individually, had written and claimed concerning the treatment of the disorder. Thomas did not always distinguish whether particular substances were used only in managing attacks of headache or were taken continuously for headache prevention. Among the agents that he recorded as having been used in treating attacks were several substances not mentioned so far in the present account. These included a powder comprising quinine mixed with either opium or tobacco, sodium salicylate, inhalations of nitroglycerine, or carbon dioxide or, surprisingly, hydrogen sulfide, and also chloroform, chloral, and cannabis indica. He stated that a medicated pomade containing potassium cyanide or belladonna had been applied to the scalp.

Norström (1885), in Paris, reported the presence in migraine sufferers of areas of induration in the cervical muscles, particularly those of the back and sides of the neck. He was able to provide headache relief by massaging these areas. Possibly he achieved his reported success by treating the secondary tension-type headache that develops in the later stage of migraine attacks (see chapter 5).

In his final systematic account of the topic of migraine in volume 2 of the second edition of his *Manual of the Diseases of the Nervous System*, William Gowers (1893) commented on the variable outcome of the immediate treatment of migraine attacks. He repeated the by then familiar advice about organizing rest for the sufferer. Purgation at the onset of migraine headache usually was not useful. By analogy with the response in epilepsy, another periodic disorder, potassium bromide used alone or taken in combination with Ergotin might be helpful. However, Gowers considered that the latter substance merely lessened the degree of throbbing of the head pain and did not render the sufferer pain-free. At the onset of the headache, but only then, nitroglycerine could be beneficial. The analgesics acetanilide, phenacetin, and Indian hemp, taken by mouth, could lessen pain in the attacks, but injected morphine was not particularly effective. Overall, in his view, caffeine and guarana had proved disappointing, but the sedation provided by a dose of chloral could reduce suffering in the attacks. Sedative liniments containing belladonna or aconite, and mustard plasters applied to the nape of the neck, were sometimes employed, and menthol might be rubbed into the skin of the headache-affected area. Gowers discussed the electrical treatment of the attacks, and observed that "the value of the treatment is, to say the least, seldom perceptible."

Several other English-language authors wrote monographs on headache in the latter half of the 19th century but usually did not deal with migraine as a specific entity. As a result, the treatments they advocated for headaches of various types, or for headache in general, cannot easily be equated with what they might have used when they treated migraine itself, had they recognized that entity.

Auerbach (1913), a German author whose account of headache was translated into English, suggested the usual management practices for migraine attacks, namely ensuring absolute rest in a darkened room with cold, wet compresses or an ice bag applied to the head, and the use of analgesics, of which an increased range had become available, for example antipyrine, phenacetin, pyramidal, and aspirin. The use of injected morphine was reserved for very severe head pain.

Critchley and Ferguson (1933) stated that it was useless to try to "fight off an attack" of migraine. Rather, the sufferer should retire to a quiet darkened room as soon as possible and should take the analgesic remedies Veramon or phenacetin with caffeine, or Compral. They did not mention using any ergot derivative, though such substances were by then becoming available and were beginning to provide the mainstay of therapy for the individual headache attack. Admittedly, there was a persisting hesitancy about using them, at least partly because of the long history of toxic manifestations associated with ergot intake.

Ergot Derivatives in Migraine Therapy

Ergot is the sclerotium of the fungus *Claviceps purpurea* that infests rye (figure 6-1) and, to a lesser extent, other grasses that are used as sources of human and animal food, for example wheat (Barger 1931). The fully developed fungal sclerotium is a hard dark gray or purple-black cylindrical structure up to 14 mm long and 6 mm in diameter. It resembles a cock's spur in shape. As it grows, it replaces the grain of the grass. The ripening grass crop, and with it the fungal sclerotia, may be eaten by grazing animals. Alternatively, the ripened crop, containing the *Claviceps* sclerotia, may be harvested, if the sclerotia have not already fallen to the ground, where they form spores. The spores remain in the soil or later become airborne and then infect the following season's grain crop. The spores grow on the newly infected grass, where they form a secretion (honeydew) that hardens into new sclerotia as the crop ripens, thus completing the fungal life cycle.

Woakes

In the latter third of the 19th century, ergot first entered the history of migraine when it began to emerge as the first substance that possessed a specific action that seemed capable of correcting the mechanism of production

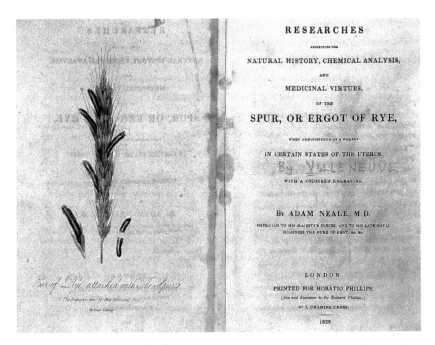

Figure 6-1 Sclerotia of ergot growing on rye. Courtesy of Wellcome Library, London.

of migraine headache. Koehler and Isler (2002) traced the first known record of the use of ergot in treating migraine to an Italian report dated 1862. The first English-language account of its use in migraine appeared in 1868. Then, in the month of August, at Oxford, Edward Woakes (1837–1912), a medical practitioner working in Luton, Bedfordshire, England, who held the qualifications MD (London) and FLS, read a paper with the title *Ergot of Rye in the Treatment of Neuralgia* to the annual meeting of the British Medical Association (Woakes 1868). Woakes later moved to London, where he became senior aural surgeon at London Hospital. In his 1868 paper, Woakes described the use of a liquid extract of ergot in seven patients who suffered what he considered was neuralgic pain. Three had sciatica, only one of whom he thought had benefited from the ergot treatment that he prescribed. However, the ergot treatment did provide relief in an instance of shingles and in two patients whom he had diagnosed as suffering from tic douloureux. Whether the latter diagnoses were correct is arguable, since both sufferers were females in their early twenties, an age group in which idiopathic tic douloureux is unlikely. Koehler and Isler (2002) suggested that these two women may really have suffered from migraine, but the question of diagnosis cannot now be settled. Woakes reported his remaining case, Case IV, as being an instance of *hemicrania,* then often regarded as a form of neuralgia. He described the events as follows:

> John Gray, aged about 35, had been repeatedly under treatment for that form of neural-gia known as brow-ague. His attacks had been cured alike by quinine and sesquioxide of iron. Sometimes they are very severe, and the treatment long continued. He was last seen in May 1868, when he had a very sharp attack of neuralgia of the right temple. He was ordered to take, every four hours, an ounce of a mixture of 2 drachms of liquid extract of ergot in 6 ounces of infusion of ergot. After taking this for two or three days, he was cured more satisfactorily and quickly than in his former attacks. (Woakes 1868, p. 361)

The *Shorter Oxford English Dictionary* indicates that *brow-ague* was a synonym for "megrim." Thus Woakes had probably used ergot to treat migraine at least once, and possibly on three occasions, with apparent success. Admittedly a more skeptical assessment might suspect that the apparent response, at least in the case described immediately above, may have been simply the outcome of spontaneous recovery from a migraine attack.

It might have been expected that at least some of Woakes's audience at Oxford, and some readers of his paper, may have hoped that he had come upon a new method for treating migraine, and would have tried it in their own patients. However, over the following decade or so, there do not appear to have been any subsequent publications in the English language medical literature regarding the use of ergot in migraine treatment. Its possible use, however, was sometimes mentioned in publications from the Continent, for example in the writings of Eulenburg, as will be described shortly. Samuel Wilks, a migraine sufferer who appeared to keep seeking remedies for his own suffering, seems not to have become aware of Woakes's report. Nor did Edward Liveing (1873). If Woakes's contemporary British colleagues tried the drug in migraine treatment, they did not see fit to record the outcomes of their attempts.

Why had Woakes chosen to employ ergot of rye in neuralgic pain? It appears that he had been thinking about the nature of such pain, and began by pondering the nature of the pain associated with herpes zoster. As judged from his account, he had speculated that vasodilatation and exudation of fluid from the vasa nervorum into the peripheral nerves in the sites of the skin lesions of shingles might explain the erythema and fluid-filled vesicle formation that occurred. He hypothesized that the fluid leakage into the underlying peripheral nerves resulted in intraneural swelling and thought that this might be the basis of the associated neuralgia pain. Woakes then proposed that a similar process in peripheral nerves explained other forms of neuralgia pain, including that of migraine. He knew that paralysis of the sympathetic nervous system caused local erythema and fluid exudation. On this basis, he reasoned that if a substance that increased the activity of the sympathetic nervous system was administered, it might relieve neuralgia pain by correcting the pain-producing mechanism that he had envisaged. Woakes was aware that ergot constricted the uterine arteries during childbirth, and he had seen a single instance of ergot administration appear to terminate a hemoptysis. On these grounds, he decided that ergot activated the sympathetic nervous system. Therefore he decided to assess its usefulness in providing relief for various forms of neuralgia pain. Given the state of knowledge of his day, Woakes's chain of argument seems not unreasonable. However, he made rather an intellectual leap by assuming that what applied in one form of peripheral nerve pathology would necessarily apply in others. On the basis of latter-day knowledge, both theoretical and empirical, Woakes's treatment of migraine with ergot might have been expected to have had some chance of success. However, in the one instance of reasonably definite migraine that he treated with the agent, any role that the substance appeared to have in providing benefit may have been more apparent than real.

The next recorded use of ergot of rye in treating migraine seems to be that described by Albert Eulenburg, when he was professor of medicine at the University of Greifswald on the island of Rugen, in the Baltic. In 1875 Tanret, a French chemist, had prepared a crude extract of alkaloids from ergot and this extract, named Ergotin, had become available for therapeutic use (Tanret 1875). Eulenburg (1883), interested in the sympathetic nervous system, compared Ergotin with a German preparation of an ergot citrate, both administered hypodermically. Eulenburg briefly mentioned that a favorable palliative effect had been obtained from the use of these preparations in five cases of migraine, four of which were of Möllendorf's vasoparalytic type. During the final decade of the 19th century, extract of ergot began to be used in treating migraine in United States. W. H. Thompson (1894) provided the first accounts, which Wolff (1963) took to be the initial description of the use of ergot in migraine.

In the early years of the 20th century, the literature continued to mention further use in migraine of various extracts of ergot, without there appearing to be much conspicuous enthusiasm for the therapy. Then, in 1918 a chemist, Arthur Stoll, from the Swiss pharmaceutical firm of Sandoz, was able to isolate the first pure peptide alkaloid, subsequently named ergotamine, from the variety of pharmacologically active substances present in ergot. The pharmacological properties of ergotamine were investigated. Rothlin in 1925 injected it subcutaneously in 2 patients with treatment-resistant migraine and produced relief of their headaches. On this basis, Rothlin later wrote that he had proposed to his Sandoz colleague

Maier that pure ergotamine should receive further study in treating migraine (Rothlin 1955). A year later, Maier (1926) reported using the drug success-fully in relieving migraine headache. The route of administration that he employed is not clear from the original publication. At this time, the ratio-nale for the use of ergotamine was that, contrary to the interpretation that had prevailed in earlier years, migraine headache depended on excessive rather than decreased sympathetic activity, and that ergotamine had a sym-patheticolytic rather than a sympathomimetic effect. Additional reports of the successful use of the pure ergotamine began to appear, first on the Continent, and then, a few years later, in the United States. Most of these favorable reports were based on studies in which the drug was administered by injection, and some authors commented that it was less effective when given by mouth. For instance, Tzanck (1928) achieved a 92 percent success rate in 12 subjects, and 3 years later reported benefit in nearly all of 101 persons in whom the drug was given by mouth or by subcutaneous injec-tion (Tzanck 1931). Logan and Allen (1934) obtained a 94 percent success rate in 71 patients after subcutaneous injection of the drug, Brock et al. (1934) a 78 percent rate in 18 subjects, and Lennox and von Storch (1935) a 90 percent rate in 109 subjects. Such early reports show a much higher effectiveness rates than would be expected from subsequent clinical experi-ence when the drug was more extensively prescribed for intake by mouth.

Probably largely as the result of such reports, by the late 1930s ergot-amine was being administered orally, rectally, by injection, or even by inha-lation, either as the pure substance or in combination with caffeine with or without other agents. It had increasingly become the accepted therapeutic remedy for more severe attacks of migraine. The drug continued in this role over much of the next half century, though it never seemed to achieve the very high success rates that the early publications had demonstrated. Over this time, a great deal of chemical and pharmacological investigation into the various alkaloids contained within ergot had been carried out (Berde and Schild 1978) and another molecule, dihydroergotamine, had found some use as an antimigraine agent.

There seem to have been at least two reasons for the failure of ergotamine to achieve its full potential. One was lack of knowledge of certain aspects of the chemistry and pharmacology of the drug; the other, persisting concerns about the safety of the drug fueled by memories of the history of ergotism.

Pharmacology

In aqueous solution, as used for injection, ergotamine undergoes isomeriza-tion so that, within 24 hours of dissolution, about half the original quantity is in the form of an equilibrium mixture with the biologically inactive ergot-aminine. If the initial studies were carried out with freshly made ergotamine solutions, later use of the same nominal dose of the drug in commercially prepared solutions may have resulted in administration of only half that dose as biologically active substance. Further, it became clear that, after oral administration, the drug underwent extensive metabolic clearance during its absorption and passage through the liver in the portal venous blood. As a result, very little of the dose reached the general circulation as the intact molecule. The actual value of the oral bioavailability of the drug in humans does not seem to have ever been determined accurately, but is estimated to be of the order of 1 percent. Drugs with very low oral bioavailability also tend to show considerable variability in their bioavailability between differ-ent persons. Consequently, to achieve similar therapeutic effects, dosage of such drugs needs to be tailored to individuals. Appreciation of this fact came late in the history of the use of ergotamine in migraine, at a time when it was already being superseded by other agents.

As well as ergotamine, discussed immediately above, the *Claviceps pur-purea* sclerotium, from which ergot is obtained, contains various other pharmacologically active substances. At least 40 of these are other ergot alkaloids (ergolines). Chemically, the biologically active lysergic acid-containing ergot alkaloids are usually divided into amide derivatives (e.g., ergometrine) and peptide derivatives (e.g., ergotamine). The first ergot alkaloid derivative (ergotoxin) isolated from the *Claviceps* sclerotia (in 1906) later proved to be a mixture of the peptide ergot alkaloids ergocris-tine, ergocornine, and ergokryptine. Apart from ergotamine, the first pure alkaloid obtained from ergot, the other ergot alkaloid that found a major therapeutic use was ergometrine (ergonovine), which was isolated by Dudley and Moir in 1935.

Pharmacologically, the lysergic acid derived ergot alkaloids such as ergotamine are (i) serotonin agonists (at $5\text{-HT}_{1B/1D}$ and 5-HT_2 receptors) and therefore arterial constrictors, though ergometrine appears to be a 5-HT_2 antagonist, (ii) dopamine agonists potentially capable of producing dyskinesias and, perhaps, dystonias, hallucinations, and disturbances of mental functioning, (iii) α-noradrenergic antagonists that may increase vasoconstriction (apart from ergometrine) and that may cause contraction of uterine smooth muscle (Berde and Stürmer 1978). These various types of pharmacological effect vary in their degree of development among the different alkaloids. Further, the alkaloid composition of ergots from differ-ent areas, and at different times, may vary, partly depending on the amino acid contents of the soil in which their host plants grow. Knowing some-thing of these pharmacological details is useful in understanding the story of ergotism.

Outbreaks of ergotism, and sporadic instances of the phenomenon, have a long history in medicine, as has been described by a number of authors (e.g., Barger 1931; van Dongen and de Groot 1995; Lee 2009, 2010). Particularly during times of famine, the eating of rye bread contaminated with ergot-containing *Claviceps purpurea* sclerotia caused epidemic ergotism. It was as long ago as 1630 when Tullier recognized the causal role of the fungus (WHO Task Group 1990). Outbreaks of ergotism took place mainly in rye-eating areas and tended to occur after cold, wet winters that were followed by warm spring weather. Rural more than town dwellers usually were affected, particularly at times of hardship when rye formed the main item of community diet. Whole families might be affected, though breast-fed infants of affected mothers were spared. After ergot contamination of rye was recognized as the cause of the problem, public health action, particularly in France, reduced the hazard of acquiring the disorder. Outbreaks of possible ergotism had been reported in ancient times (Hoffmann 1978). In the medieval and early modern literature there were numerous accounts of such outbreaks. Hirsh (1885) tabulated the known record of epidemic ergotism in Europe, and Tissot (1780) reviewed the details of the outbreaks of ergotism in Central and Western Europe up to his time of writing. It was contended by Matossian (1989), mainly on the basis of circumstantial evidence, that ergotism may have been responsible for phenomena attributed in earlier times to witchcraft. Epidemic ergotism usually occurred in either a "gangrenous" or a "convulsive" form. In Europe west of the Rhine, the outbreaks of ergotism were typically of the gangrenous type, whereas in Central and Eastern Europe and in Scandinavia, they were of the convulsive variety. Rarely, both forms occurred in the one outbreak in the one locality (in Lorraine in 1085, and in Russia in 1722, 1824, 1832, 1863, and 1881). Ergotism occurring in local outbreaks and associated either with gangrenous or with what were called convulsive manifestations was reported in various parts of Russia as recently as the earlier part of the 20th century (Barger 1931). Another occurred in Ethiopia in 1979 (Demeke et al. 1979), and a doubtful one was reported from a single location in France in 1951 (Gabbai et al. 1951).

Clinically, gangrenous and convulsive ergotism began similarly. There might be a short period of vaguely ill health and possible gastrointestinal upset, followed by a feeling like ants crawling over the skin of the extremities, particularly the legs. These sensations culminated in local pain. In the gangrenous type, if the disorder progressed further, ischemic manifestations appeared, mainly in the limbs, and ultimately dry gangrene, with a quite substantial mortality, would develop. In the convulsive type, there was distortion of limb and trunk posture with painful involuntary flexion of the fingers and wrists and either flexion or extension at the ankles. Sufferers became drowsy or delirious, and perhaps lethargic, hallucinated, melancholic or manic. There could be double vision, profuse sweating, fever, and muscle stiffness. As the disorder progressed, painful prolonged dystonias of the trunk developed. These involuntary movements could continue for days or weeks. The disorder might recur in subsequent years, often in the same season. There was a 10–20 percent mortality rate.

Sporadic ergotism has usually been the consequence of therapeutic misadventure. Midwives had long been aware that ergot possessed the capacity to accelerate the progress of childbirth, and the substance was formally introduced into medicine for this purpose by Stearns in 1808. Ergot comprised the active component of his "*pulvis parturiens*." But within a few years, the use of ergot for this indication was found to be associated with an increased stillbirth rate (Hosack 1824). The substance thereafter came to be used in obstetrics only for the control of postpartum hemorrhage, until it was replaced in this role by administering a single dose of ergometrine once that became available as the pure substance, though that drug later faded from all obstetric use. Present-day sporadic ergotism is nearly always due to acute or chronic poisoning by ergotamine. It can occur, rarely, after a single oral therapeutic dose of the drug, but is much more likely to be encountered after several therapeutic doses taken reasonably close together. In some instances ergotamine has been taken together with another drug that is an inhibitor of cytochrome $P450_{3A4}$, the isoenzyme that catalyzes ergotamine metabolism. Certain macrolide antibiotics, particularly erythromycin, and certain HIV protease inhibitors, may have this effect (Eadie 2001). Inhibition of the metabolism of the otherwise poorly bioavailable ergot alkaloid is tantamount to providing ergotamine in substantial oral overdosage. The excessive vasoconstriction that may result can produce widespread arterial spasm and associated endothelial injury with local thrombus formation, and possibly gangrene.

Although it has never been proven, it seems likely that different ergot alkaloid compositions of ergots from different geographical regions (mentioned above) account for the two forms of epidemic ergotism. Public health measures should ensure that outbreaks of the disorder do not occur in the future. Nevertheless, continuing medical memories of past events and their sometimes devastating consequences undoubtedly encouraged caution in the use of ergotamine in migraine treatment. The occasional contemporary reports of vasospastic complications from the use of the drug served to enhance that caution, and have perhaps denied ergotamine the place in therapeutics it might have still occupied if it had been subjected to more extensive pharmacological study employing modern analytical methods. Its past ensured that the medical profession was ready to abandon ergotamine once a better alternative appeared, and one did so in the latter part of the 20th century.

Triptan Derivatives

By the 1970s, the relatively indifferent success rate in treating migraine attacks with ergotamine taken by mouth led to the beginnings of a search for other antimigraine drugs. By that time, a good deal of evidence had accumulated indicating that serotonin played a part in the genesis of the migraine attack (see chapter 5). One particularly pertinent observation had been made. Both Kimball et al. (1960) and Anthony et al. (1967) had shown that injected serotonin would relieve migraine headache. Serotonin at that time was believed to act mainly as a vasoconstrictor agent. Further, at least after injection, another known potent vasoconstrictor agent, ergotamine, had well established efficacy in migraine attacks. It was known that orally administered serotonin would be inactivated during absorption from the alimentary tract because of the activity of the enzyme monoamine oxidase in the gut wall. Therefore, in the hope that they might prove useful as antimigraine agents, attempts were made to find molecules with structural resemblances to serotonin but which would not be degraded during absorption from the alimentary tract. During the latter decades of the 20th century, a number of triptan derivatives were synthesized (Humphrey 2007) and underwent testing as treatments for migraine attacks. A considerable amount of work was carried out investigating the molecular pharmacology of sumatriptan, the first triptan derivative shown to be effective in relieving the attacks, and also in studying various of its congeners. Sumatriptan was found to act as a specific agonist at the $5HT_{1B/1D}$ type of serotonin receptor, thereby bringing about vasoconstriction in the cranial vessels. In the light of this knowledge, the mechanism of action of ergotamine was reinvestigated. Ergotamine had long been thought to act as a noradrenaline agonist in producing widespread vasoconstriction. However, there was a structural resemblance between part of its molecule and that of sumatriptan. On reinvestigation, ergotamine also proved to be a highly potent agonist at serotonin $5HT_{1B/1D}$ receptors. On a molecule-for-molecule basis, it was several times more potent than many of the triptans. As well, it had various actions at other types of nonserotonin receptor. By the time this serotonergic mechanism of action of ergotamine was recognized, the drug was long out of patent. With the pharmaceutical industry already actively pursuing the development of new triptan agents, no serious attempt seems to have been made to utilize the accumulating scientific data

and resurrect interest in ergotamine and its therapeutic use. Various triptans, with their much cleaner pharmacological profiles and better safety
records than that of the ergot alkaloid, increasingly became the preferred
treatments for migraine attacks.

Other Agents

Aspirin

Aspirin has often been said to have been synthesized in 1897 by Hoffman,
though his priority in this regard is in some doubt (Sneader 2000). The
substance soon found an ever-growing place in therapeutics as a simple
pain-relieving medication. Its mechanism of action was not determined for
many years until Vane (1971) in London showed that it inhibited prostaglandin synthesis. The drug would almost certainly have been used for
migraine treatment soon after it became available on the market, and it has
been widely self-prescribed since. Thus, for instance, the great early investigator of the cytoarchitectonics of the cerebral cortex, A. W. Campbell, who
spent the latter part of his career practicing clinical neurology in Sydney,
Australia, provided some indication as to the frequency of aspirin use for
headache when he wrote the following concerning the treatment of
migraine:

> To the young woman, however, who carries aspirin tablets in her bag, we offer this
> advice: "your tablets are not as innocuous as sugar. If you are to ease your headache, you
> should take the proper dose and take it in the premonitory stage: also, and this is most
> important, you will help the drug by sitting or lying down for half an hour, in quiet and
> under warm covering." (1933, p. 36)

Vane's work on its mechanism of action stimulated renewed scientific
and clinical interest in aspirin from the 1970s onward. Studies of the drug's
absorption during migraine attacks showed that reduced gastric motility
during and between the attacks in migraineurs (Aurora et al. 2006) delayed
the entry of the drug into the general circulation (Volans 1978).
Consequently the chances of its being effective in providing pain relief in
migraine were decreased. However, in migraine attacks, the simultaneous
administration of dopamine antagonist drugs that enhanced gastric motility (e.g., metoclopramide) increased the rate of absorption of aspirin. As
well, these agents should have diminished any nausea and vomiting that
occurred during the attack. The combination of a sufficient oral dose of
aspirin, usually administered simultaneously with metoclopramide, became

an increasingly used way of dealing with migraine attacks. When formal controlled clinical trials were carried out, the combination generally proved comparable in efficacy to sumatriptan or its congeners taken by mouth in usual dosages (Limmroth et al. 1999; Mett and Tfelt-Hansen 2008). Injectable preparations of lysine aspirin also proved effective in treating migraine attacks. It is salutary to realize that an old, cheap, and seemingly almost trivial drug, when used appropriately, could match the performance of the new, more specific, and more expensive agents in providing migraine relief.

Nonsteroidal Anti-inflammatory Drugs

These drugs have molecular mechanisms of action similar to that of aspirin, though unlike aspirin their action in inhibiting prostaglandin synthesis is reversible. Various members of the class have been used to treat migraine attacks and have achieved a sufficient measure of success to allow them to remain in use for the indication.

Other drugs with analgesic effects (e.g., phenacetin and acetanilide) were recommended for administration during migraine attacks in the earlier part of the 20th century, but had ceased to be used before modern methods had elucidated their mechanisms of action at a molecular level.

Cannabis

Cannabis has a very long record of being used for certain of its pharmacological effects. In the second half of the 19th century, its use was explored in the medical treatment of a number of disorders. Several prominent Victorian era physicians, including Gowers (1888) and Russell Reynolds (1890), recommended it in the management of migraine, and it came to be included in some contemporary pharmacopoeias in Britain and North America for the purpose of headache management. In the first edition of Osler's (1892) *The Principles and Practice of Medicine*, it was stated in connection with the treatment of migraine that "*cannabis indica* is probably the most satisfactory remedy." This statement continued to appear in subsequent editions of the book. However, growing concerns about the abuse properties of the drug saw it disappear from orthodox medical recommendations concerning migraine treatment. Russo (1998) provided a short account of the history of the use of the drug in migraine and raised the possibility that its employment in this disorder might perhaps be reassessed employing modern scientific methods.

The surviving second century A.D. writings of Aretaeus the Cappadocian contained a considerable amount of detail regarding the short-term treatment of *cephalea* before the author proceeded to state that the disorder may become chronic. Further, if an episode settled, it might recur at a later date. He then dealt with measures that seemed intended for long-term effects before going on to indicate that the measures used for *cephalea* can also be used for *heterocrania* (i.e., *hemicrania*). It therefore seems probable that, had Aretaeus recognized the modern entity of migraine in his patients, his preventive measures would have involved shaving the head and cauterizing the scalp down to the muscle, or to the underlying skull bone; the resulting eschar would have then been treated with various applications: for example, rose oil, wine, lentil with honey. Exercise would have been recommended for the benefit of the shoulders and chest, irritant materials (e.g. mustard) rubbed into the head, and a light diet prescribed. Considerable dietary detail was set down. Probably an appropriate selection from this would have been advised. The sufferer would have been left to find his or her own solution to the dictum "Sexual intercourse is a self-inflicted evil to the head and nerves" (p. 463), but sea voyages and living by the sea would have met with approval. Thus the recommendations may have ranged from gentle conservatism to the heroic. Some, if followed, may have proved more onerous than the headaches they were intended to prevent.

Because Galen's *hemicrania* included disorders other than migraine, and migraine probably was present among those who suffered from *cephalalgia* and *cephalea*, it is difficult to know what measures he might have employed if he had known the present-day entity of migraine as a discrete type of headache.

The account of *cephalea* in Oribasius (Bussemaker and Daremberg, 1873) suggested that instances of migraine would have fallen within this headache category, in that the presence of intolerance to noise and light were mentioned in his account of the subject. Oribasius indicated that treatment was difficult, and seemed to recommend mainly the use of measures directed against the presumed underlying humoral disturbance, namely various measures intended to promote removal of the humor that was present in increased proportions. This was to be achieved via evacuation of the contents of the alimentary tract, by promoting nasal discharges or by removing blood from the body.

The medieval Arabian physicians made little contribution of importance to the preventive treatment of headache and, not knowing of the entity as such, did not deal specifically with migraine as a topic. Abulcasis, as he also did in relation to the management of short-term headache, and with the proviso that medical measures should already have been found inadequate to help the patient, was prepared to cauterize the chronic headache sufferer's head with a hot iron or by means of locally applied caustic substances (Abulcasis 1861).

Charles Le Pois (1618), who described what can reasonably confidently be identified as migraine without aura in himself and in one other person, seemed unable to find any satisfactory method for alleviating his own problem. Apparently, at least in 1618, he was unaware of the mixture that Lazarus Riverius (1589–1655) had stated that Fernel claimed he had devised a remedy that had never failed in treating *hemicrania*. The mixture consisted of ½ oz. aloes, 3 grains each of powder of electuary of pearls, the "three Sanders," and red roses, mixed with syrup of wormwood and violets. This was taken in a dose of 1 drachm twice weekly, an hour before supper (Culpeper 1658).

When Thomas Willis (1672/1683) described the almost lifelong saga of the migrainous headaches that afflicted Anne, Countess of Conway (also see chapter 4), he mentioned that by the time she had consulted him, her situation was as follows:

> Some years before, she had endured from an oyntment of Quicksilver, a long and troublesome Salivation, so that she ran the hazards of her life. Afterwards twice a Cure was attempted (though in vain) by a Flux at the Mouth, from a Mercurial Powder, which the noted Emperick *Charles Hues* ordinarily gave: with like success with the rest she tried the Baths, Spaw-waters, almost of every kind and nature: she admitted of frequent Blood-letting, and also once the opening of an Artery; she had also made about her several Issues, sometimes in the hinder part of her head, and sometimes in the forepart, and in other parts. She also took the Air of several Countries beside her own native Air, she went into *Ireland* and into *France*: there was no kind of Medicines both *Cephalicks, Antiscorbutics, Hystericals*, all famous *Specificks*, which she took not, both from the Learned and the unlearned, from quacks, and old Women; and yet notwithstanding, she professed, that she had received from no Remedy, or method of Curing, any thing of Cure or Ease, but that the coutumacious and rebellious Disease, refused to be tamed, being deaf to the charms of every Medicine. (Willis 1672/1683, p. 122)

This statement gives some indication of the way in which recalcitrant migraine may have been managed around the time of the restoration of the monarchy in England, assuming that sufferer had the financial wherewithal to afford the treatments, and the courage or desperation to endure them. Willis appears to have been prudent enough not to indicate what therapeutic measures he advised in the countess's situation, though elsewhere in his account he described the treatments he recommended for such situations.

Between headache attacks, Willis advised that blood might be removed from the veins of the feet by applying leeches. Medicines of vinegar, rose cakes, and nutmeg, or some other *epithems* or medicines of the same nature were to be applied to the head: juleps, emulsions, or decoctions that "allay the fervour or madness of the blood" were to be taken by mouth, and the belly cooled by the use of clysters. For prevention of further episodes, whey or "spaw-waters" and water itself were to be drunk, and a thin and cooling dietary regimen followed. Wine, spiced meats, baths, Venus, violent motions of the mind or body, and all hot things were to be shunned. And he went on to acknowledge that many sufferers tried to find their own solutions to their headache problems:

> There is no need here to add a method or particular form of Medicines, when in this case, almost everybody labouring, is wont to be his own Physician, being taught by frequent experience, from things hurting or helping. (Willis 1672/1683, p. 115)

According to Tissot (1780), Willis's contemporary Johan Jakob Wepfer (1727), in his posthumous *Observationes*, included a variety of advice for the management of migraine. However, Tissot probably considered that Wepfer's *hemicrania* corresponded closely, if not exactly, to the entity of migraine, whereas some of Wepfer's cases of *hemicrania* probably represented examples of unilateral head pain from other causes. Tissot stated that the measures Wepfer advised included maintaining sobriety; avoiding food that is difficult to digest; supping lightly; keeping out of cold and humid air; undertaking daily exercise on foot and weekly horse or carriage riding; reading and writing without lowering the head; shaving the head; applying vesicatories, setons, or the cautery; drinking milk to calm the blood (goat's milk was beneficial in one man with stomach cramps); establishing sweating; repeatedly opening the temporal arteries; douching with a cephalic decoction; bathing the legs; using a cephalic powder with wild valerian root as its base. Such measures seem designed for the longer term management of the disorder, though some might have also been employed during acute episodes, in particular the bleeding and leg bathing. The suggested use of valerian is interesting. The plant has known sedative properties and is included in the present-day *WHO Monographs on Selected Medicinal Plants* (Anonymous 1999) for this purpose. However, among chemical constituents of valerian is isovaleric acid, which has a degree of chemical structural resemblance to the molecule of valproic acid, an antiepileptic drug that in several clinical trials has been shown to prevent migraine (Silberstein 1997). There is some evidence that valerian itself may possess a degree of antiepileptic activity (Eadie 2004). Therefore it may be the case that, as early as the 17th century, a substance with epileptic seizure–preventing properties was being used in migraine prevention. Even if this were the case, it is unlikely that it would have been realized, both because of the inconsistency of response of migraine to preventive drugs and because of the probable variation in the amount of active ingredient that would have been present in different valerian-containing preparations.

Samuel Tissot (1780), in his account of migraine, went into what was essentially the nonpharmacological prevention of the disorder at some length. If plethora was present, he advised regular bleedings and also indicated that anything that increased the quantity of blood should be avoided. Thus nourishment, sweets, warm food, wine, chocolate, liqueurs, violent exercise, warm rooms, and oversleeping should be minimized or avoided altogether. If migraine was believed to depend on stomach disturbance, and Tissot regarded this as a common situation, consuming a light diet and drinking considerable quantities of water were desirable. If the sufferer had only mild and infrequent attacks of headache, and had good health between the attacks, it was often better to leave well alone and simply have the patient follow a prudent diet and avoid overtreatment. In the case of menstrual migraine, if the stomach disturbance was more severe and involved slow emptying of that organ, vomiting should be induced by giving ipecacuanha for some days, possibly together with a bitter laxative. For the latter purpose, Tissot preferred infusions of marsh clover. He claimed that good effects were obtained from kina, conserve of genièvre (jenever), or an herbal tea of orange leaves. If the stomach tended to sourness, he advised the regular use of magnesia, and the drinking of spa water and cold water. Fatty or viscous foods, pastries, sweets, acid substances, warm water, wine, and milk foods should be avoided.

On the whole, Tissot accorded an excessive importance to disturbances of the stomach as a cause of migraine, but the treatments he suggested were in general relatively innocuous, and from a modern standpoint were unlikely to do any great harm even if they provided no genuine physical benefit.

Probably independently of knowledge of Tissot's publication, in 1778 John Fothergill of London also regarded dietary factors as playing a major role in the production of migraine (Fothergill 1784). Consequently he advised mainly measures intended to overcome this presumed cause of the disorder. He wrote,

> We are, perhaps, too ready, in chronic cases, where digestion is concerned, to confide in the *Materia Medica*, and judge it sufficient to select and enjoin such articles in our prescriptions, as are of known use in such cases. But unless the whole plan of diet, both in kind and quantity, are made to conspire with medical prescription, the benefits arising from this are hourly annihilated by neglect or indulgence. (p. 114)

If the bowels tended to be costive, Fothergill recommended the use of gentle laxatives. If there was excess acid bile (he did not indicate how this was to be determined), he advised the use of small doses of stomach bitters and an alkaline salt or chalybeate, mineral or vegetable acids, soap, magnesia, or rhubarb. He advocated the prolonged intake of mineral waters, and commented that, contrary to fairly widespread present-day belief, chocolate did not seem to matter in relation to migraine occurrence, though coffee and sugar both tended to cause attacks.

William Heberden (1802) in his posthumously published *Commentaries*, when writing on the entity *capitis dolores intermittens*, which would appear to be largely equivalent to migraine, provided a skeptical comment that also reflects on the contemporary migraine-preventing treatment practices of his time and country:

> In an attempt to cure this malady, evacuations have proved not only useless, but harmful; and bleeding in particular has been very detrimental. Cataplasms have not been well borne, and have rather added to the misery of patients. The Peruvian bark has very often been tried in vain, so have the root of valerian, the fetid gums, myrrh, musk, camphor, opium, extract of hemlock, sneezing powders, blisters, deep caustic, electrifying, warm pediluvia, epithems of aether, anodyne balsam, sp. vini, linamentum saponaceum, and the oil of amber, opening the temporal artery, and drawing some of the teeth: nor has a supervening of the gout made any alteration in this obstinate ailment. (Heberden 1802, pp. 81–82)

Despite this expression of therapeutic destitution, Heberden then proceeded to suggest that it might be worth trying the bark for one week, or producing a blister behind the ear during the attack, or having the patient drink tartar emetic with opium, or drink extract cicutae to the point of experiencing giddiness, and to employ cold bathing. He seemed to advise continuing these measures for some days after the headache had settled, so that he may have had some prophylactic intention in mind.

Up to the time when the idea that migraine originated in the stomach began to pass from favor, attempts to prevent recurrences of the disorder were often focused on optimizing the function of the alimentary tract. Thus Mearse (1832), in the fifth edition of his monograph *On the Causes, Cure, and Prevention of Sick-Headache*—in other words, nonhemicranial migraine without aura—dealt with the maintenance therapy of the disorder in relation to the diet to be followed, the intake of liquids, the pattern of exercise that was to be undertaken, and the desirability of a change of air. Such approaches to longer term migraine management began to disappear after medical opinion moved in the direction of the disorder being due to altered function of various parts of the nervous system.

In his 1831 paper, Pierre-Adolphe Piorry was in particular concerned with what was later called, particularly in the French literature, *migraine ophthalmique*, in other words, migraine with a visual aura. In considering the prevention of this particular type of migraine, Piorry accorded the first priority to avoiding its provocation. Work that employed the eyes extensively should not be engaged in when digestion of food in the stomach was still going on. Nevertheless, the sufferer need not be afraid to follow occupations involving spiritual activity, as this activity of itself would not produce attacks. Very bright light, and also going from dark places into brightly lit spaces, should be avoided. The sufferer should learn to gradually accustom himself or herself to tolerate the glare of the day. Piorry believed that if potential migraine sufferers had to fix their sight on an object for a long time, eating of a mouthful of bread would prevent the headache that would otherwise probably occur. He admitted that plethora was sometimes the cause of migraine. If this appeared to be the case, bleeding was indicated. If the subject had a sedentary lifestyle and was not in robust health, it was necessary to provide a substantial food intake. If constipation seemed to increase the frequency of occurrence of the attacks of visual disturbance, purgatives were indicated. If there was a pattern of intermittent attacks, quinine sulphate should be employed.

Thus Piorry's approach differed from the usual one up to his time in that he emphasized preventive measures directed against the provocation of the visual aura of migraine. This was an aspect that his predecessors had almost uniformly neglected, as they had either overlooked aura phenomena, or had failed to note their existence. Late in his life, four decades after his earlier account, Piorry returned briefly to the management of this type of migraine. He then indicated that some spoonfuls of good quality wine, in which a biscuit was soaked, could be very useful in preventing the attacks (Piorry 1875).

Henri Labarraque, in his Paris MD thesis (1837), which was quite often cited by contemporary and later writers for its historical material and coverage of the literature, discussed the preventive treatment of migraine. In relation to the latter purpose, he mentioned an array of treatment approaches, many of which continued to be recommended in the subsequent literature on migraine treatment. The preventive treatments were aimed at attacking the cause of the individual patient's migraine and mitigating any predisposition to it. Thus a compound pill of opium and camphor might be prescribed for twice daily intake to reduce any general body hypersensitivity in the migraine sufferer. Any underlying affection of the stomach was managed by trying to induce vomiting, and by having the sufferer take purgatives, bitters, or lavages. If there was gastric pain, an infusion of camomile tea sweetened with syrup of orange flowers was recommended, and for any indigestion, a pill containing extracts of valerian, asafetida, castor, and syrup of amber was to be taken twice daily. If such measures did not suffice, a plaster of theriac (a concoction of multiple herbal and other ingredients) was to be applied to the region of the stomach. If plethora was detected, bleeding was to be carried out, sometimes by applying leeches to the anal area. If there was anemia, iron was to be given. And to enhance bodily secretions, menstrual flow was to be increased by hot cataplasms, and sweating induced by mustard-containing footbaths.

Labarraque provided advice concerning the dietary management of an irritable stomach: eating white meats (chicken, veal, fish), fresh green vegetables, and colored or plain water. Coffee was to be avoided. If there was a tendency to plethora, tight clothing (e.g., cravats and corsets), should not be worn, the feet should be kept cool, the head lightly covered, penetrating smells avoided, moderate exercise undertaken, and strong emotion (love, jealousy, anger, and all strong passions) restrained to deny them the opportunity to provoke attacks. The prescription of such advice, if it did little else, should at least have reassured migraine sufferers that their problems were receiving attention. Although the rationales for the suggested measures were made explicit and are fairly obvious, the whole therapeutic approach was directed at perceived causes of the disorder. There was no understanding of how the presumed causes were translated by sufferer's body into the symptoms of the attacks. Therefore treatment could not be directed toward preventing the intermediate stages in the migraine attack's pathogenesis.

Labarraque also provided some interesting information about the methods that a number of distinguished literary and scientific men of an earlier generation had adopted in the hope of ridding themselves of their migraine. He gave no indication that he had considered the possibility that any improvement in their disorder was coincidental rather than being a consequence of the measures they had employed. In the words of Liveing's translation,

> Marmontél, who was for seven years tormented by paroxysms of migraine of a very painful character, and who had consulted the Queen's physician to no purpose, cured himself by following the prescription of a farrier who advised him to drink water, to eat little, and to take exercise.
>
> Haller, too, was very subject to megrim, and he cured himself by drinking every day a large quantity of fresh water, and exchanging a highly nutritious regimen for a much lighter dietary, which had the effect of not taxing the nervous susceptibility of his stomach so much.
>
> Linnaeus again cured himself by the same means, and by taking exercise every day before dinner. (1873, p. 433)

Mauritz Romberg (1853), in volume 1 of his *Manual*, in the section "*Hemicrania, la Migrène*," commented prudently, in the words of Sieveking's translation, "In our treatment, whether with a view to palliation or to a radical cure, we cannot be sufficiently on our guard against the abuse of medicines" (p. 177). When the migraine did not appear to be secondary to alimentary tract or other bodily disturbance, in other words, when it was regarded as purely "neuralgic" in character, Romberg advised against any violent therapeutic interference as part of an attempted radical cure. The serviceable and noninjurious remedies that he favored included

> prolonged exhibition of an infusion of quassia, of menyanthes combined with valerian, of the waters of Spa or Pyrmont if there be an anaemic constitution . . . ; of bark of quina if there be marked periodicity, or we may have recourse to sea bathing. Arsenic, in the shape of Fowler's solution, in doses of from four to eight drops three times daily, and nitrate of silver, one third to half a grain twice a day, are sometimes of use. (Romberg 1853, p. 178)

The Paris 1870 MD thesis of the Englishwoman Elizabeth Garrett Anderson (Wilkinson and Isler, 1999) contained statements regarding migraine prevention that were generally similar to others in the then recent literature. She emphasized that the nervous system, rather than the digestive one, should be the focus of therapy—to treat the latter was simply to try to relieve one exciting cause of the headaches. She recommended forbidding alcohol intake, following a simple diet, never reheating meat, and ensuring that something was eaten every four to five hours. One new touch was to recommend that, once each fortnight, a pill containing Pil. Hyd, colchicine, and hyoscyamus should be taken. This was intended to prevent congestion in the portal circulation or the accumulation of intestinal mucus that might occur even in the absence of constipation. To act as a tonic, she recommended colchicine, potassium bromide, or digitalis, the latter intended to improve the circulation.

Edward Liveing, in his monograph *On Megrim* (1873), recorded how Robert Bentley Todd, of King's College Hospital in London, had some 15 years earlier mentioned to him that he had found that potassium iodide was "the only remedy productive of any permanent benefit in cases of confirmed Sick-headache, for which he was often consulted." Liveing's own account of the preventive treatment of migraine began with a clear statement of what he considered the intention of this aspect of the therapy of the disorder should be:

> Here our aim must be twofold—First, to lessen the tendency to explosive action in the nervous centres by measures directed to the improvement of the general health, the

removal of accessory causes, and the diversion of nervous energy into natural channels, as well as by pharmaceutical remedies; and, Secondly, to avoid or remove the exciting course of the seizures, and so to reduce as far as possible the number of attacks. (1873, p. 429)

He proceeded to give the then usual advice about improving the sufferer's general level of health, diet modification, lifestyle organization both in relation to work and to domestic activities, and indicated the desirability of attaining emotional tranquility. He mentioned the idea of avoiding excessive brainwork, a notion that tends to appear more often in the English than in the Continental literature.

Liveing addressed preventive drug treatment:

> Good drugs in sufficient doses are indispensable; but even when these are provided there still remains a want of uniformity in their therapeutic effects which has led some practitioners too hastily to discard some remedies of this class as useless, and attribute the benefit which in other hands has undoubtedly followed their exhibition to a mere co-incident improvement. This may be the case with a few of the remedies which at various times have enjoyed an ephemeral reputation for the cure of nervous complaints, the caprice of which is well-known, but the beneficial influence of others is too well attested to be thus explained away, although the nature of their operation is not understood. (p. 437)

Liveing then discussed the employment three classes of drugs: sedatives, tonics, and specifics. The sedatives were intended to quiet the oversensitivity of the migrainous nervous system. The agents he discussed under this category were belladonna, hyoscyamus, and atropine (all centrally acting anticholinergics). As tonics, he discussed the use of iron, strychnine, and quinine. He stated that the latter was useful in (probably malarious) brow ague but not of much use in other forms of migraine. His specifics were potassium iodide, which he considered of uncertain benefit, and potassium bromide, which he had begun to use regularly "after reading Locock's paper." The latter statement is interesting in that Sir Charles Locock himself never published a paper on potassium bromide. The *Lancet* and the *Medical Times and Gazette* had published reports of a discussion that followed Sieveking's paper on epilepsy read to the Royal Medico-Chirurgical Society of London in 1857. These reports contain mention of Locock's statement made to the meeting after the paper was read. In that statement, Locock had described the efficacy of potassium bromide in "hysterical," in other words, catamenial, epilepsy. Liveing also mentioned that Symonds had found that common salt was helpful in the variety of migraine known as bilious headache, though Liveing personally had no experience of its use in this situation. He did mention that valerian and zinc valerinate were useful pharmaceutical agents in migraine prevention.

The Montpellier MD thesis of Auguste Thomas (1889) contained an exhaustive account of the treatments of migraine recorded in the literature of the first nine decades of the 19th century.

In the second edition of his famous and influential *Manual*, William Gowers (1893) did not devote a great deal of text to the prevention of migraine. After mentioning the usual lifestyle and dietary measures recommended in this situation, he stated, "There is much variation in the effect of the intermediate treatment. As already mentioned, the measures that do great good in one case will fail in another, apparently quite similar" (p. 854). By analogy with the effectiveness of bromide in treating epilepsy, he suggested that this chemical might be the first agent to be tried in migraine prevention, though he felt it was of service in this role less often than might have been expected. He stated that ergot might usefully be combined with it. However, in the majority of cases, the drug that had most influence was nitroglycerine, which had "a striking effect in many patients, rendering their attacks far slighter and far less frequent, and often, after a time, stopping them altogether." He stated that nitroglycerine should be taken three times a day after food, and its dose increased cautiously, in stages. He indicated that it was most conveniently administered in a 1 percent solution in alcohol and that it was very usefully combined with tincture of nux vomica and tincture of gelsemium and dilute phosphoric acid, or with lithium citrate and acid syrup of lemon. This combination later became known as Gowers's mixture and continued to be mentioned in connection with migraine prevention in some neurology books for at least the next half century. It seems somewhat paradoxical that Gowers should have thought so highly of an agent that has since been used as an experimental tool for inducing migraine attacks in humans (Iversen and Olesen 1989).

When writing on migraine, the London neurologist Wilfred Harris (1907) commented that an old treatment, the insertion of a seton into the back of the neck where it remained for some time, was beneficial. This was long after one might have imagined that such a therapy would have been consigned to the dust heap of history.

Jellife and White (1923), in their textbook of nervous system disease, with its rather strong psychological orientation, indicated that they felt that medication taken between migraine attacks was largely useless. For preventing attacks of the disorder, they continued to advise measures intended to promote gastrointestinal tract hygiene and enhance health in general before they commented that "migraine is one of the most universal scapegoats for meliorizing psychological conflicts."

Arthur Hurst, physician and neurologist at Guy's Hospital in London, in his 1924 Savill Lecture dealing with migraine, advanced the following proposition in relation to prevention of attacks:

> The most important part of treatment is the prevention of eye-strain. . . . [P]ersonally I have never yet seen a case in which eyestrain was not present, and I have only seen two in which its correction did not either cure the patient or lead to very considerable improvement. (p. 5)

The correction process that Hurst had in mind was one that required pains-taking work by oculists to remedy defects in the balance of the external eye muscles. As to other measures to prevent migraine, he felt that bromides were of minor value, that arsenic was useless, and that the effectiveness of Gowers's mixture was not very impressive. He considered that the only other useful agent was luminal (phenobarbital). He went on:

> Attempts to treat supposed intestinal toxaemia by aperients, other digestive or meta-bolic disorders by freak diet, and endocrine deficiencies by glandular preparations— though happily most of the latter are completely inert—aggravate the patient's general health without influencing his migraine. (p. 5)

Hurst's opinion seems a curious mixture of critical insight about the relative inefficacy of many by then conventional migraine-preventing measures, and unbridled enthusiasm for an approach to prevention in which few others found consistent and sustained merit. As noted above, he did mention the use of phenobarbital, which may have had a degree of genuine effectiveness in migraine prevention, though this was never conclusively demonstrated.

The early part of the 20th century saw not only a number of unsustain-able though ingenious hypotheses of the pathogenesis of the migraine attack (see chapter 5), but also reports of various preventive therapies that failed to meet the expectations initially held of them, and so did not become established in more general use. Thus the London physician Thomas Hunt (1933) reported that regular oral bile salt administration improved migraine in 19 of 22 subjects, but the matter then seemed to disappear from the lit-erature. In the sixth edition of their textbook on medical treatment, Dunlop et al. (1953) suggested the regular intake of urea or, if that failed, nicotinic acid used twice daily, as preventive therapy for migraine. Apart from this, the measures they recommended were the usual ones for their time.

The editions of the book *Headache and Other Head Pain* that Harold Wolff authored were concerned mainly with headache mechanisms.

Nevertheless, Wolff (1963) did discuss the treatment of migraine. As a preventive, he advised the use of daily ergotamine intake for 10 days when a run of migraine attacks was occurring. He discussed measures such as ligation of the temporal artery, histamine desensitization, and the regular intake of potassium thiocyanate, a treatment that does not seem to have hitherto appeared in the antimigraine armamentarium. He also discussed the continuous oral use of endocrine preparations for the prevention of migraine attacks. In particular, he mentioned Leyton (1958; a reference difficult to trace) and his recommended prolonged courses of chorionic gonadotrophin therapy. Wolff tended to give pride of place among migraine preventives to the lysergic acid derivative methysergide, then recently available and to be considered further below.

Wolff's publication stands at a watershed in the history of migraine preventive treatment. Prior to his time, treatment recommendations largely depended on the published views of prominent individual medical figures whose opinions were based on a mixture of the writings of earlier authorities and of their own interpretations of their personal experience, nearly always unassisted by any form of statistical data analysis. From Wolff's time onward, the role of individual authoritative figures in influencing therapeutic practice increasingly lessened, pharmacological knowledge expanded with almost explosive rapidity, experimental design was taken more into account, and statistical methods were more often applied to numerical data. As a result, the assessment of benefit, or lack of benefit, from various agents proposed for use in an antimigraine role was placed on a more secure and objective scientific foundation. From this point in the present account of the story of migraine, preventive therapy is more easily recounted in terms of individual drugs or classes of drugs, dealt with chronologically in relation to their date of introduction into treatment, than considered in relation to the names of prominent medical figures.

Drugs Affecting Serotonin-Related Mechanisms

Several classes of drug have been found that may interfere with mechanisms that involve the various actions of serotonin.

Methysergide

Once the chemical structure of the pharmacologically active ergot alkaloids was deduced, the Swiss pharmaceutical company Sandoz expended a deal of effort in chemical manipulations of the component lysergic acid molecule in the hope of deriving new compounds that might possess important pharmacological activities. Methylation of lysergic acid (Troxler and Hofmann 1957) produced the derivative 1-methyl-D-lysergic acid-L-2-butanolamide, which later received the generic name of methysergide. It was found to be a strong antagonist to the action of serotonin on the isolated rat uterus. Its use was then explored in the treatment of migraine by Sicuteri (1959). The drug appears to be a mixed agonist and antagonist at various types of serotonin receptor. According to Haigler (1982), the drug acts as an agonist at brain $5HT_1$ and $5HT_2$ receptors.

Methysergide was the first migraine-preventing agent for which there was reasonable scientific evidence of efficacy. Unfortunately, with the passage of time and growing experience, it became clear that the drug possessed an array of significant adverse effects. These included a tendency held in common with many other ergot derivatives, that of causing fibrotic reactions in various serous membranes of the body and particularly in the connective tissues surrounding the ureters. The far-from-universal efficacy of the drug in migraine prevention, the potential seriousness of the fibrotic reactions, and their possible medicolegal consequences, have ensured that the drug's use diminished in more recent times once safer, though probably not more effective, agents for preventing migraine became available. Koehler and Tfelt-Hansen (2008) have made available a history of the drug's use in migraine prevention.

For a time, ergotamine itself, in various oral preparations containing a variety of additional components, was used on a regular basis for migraine prevention. The always threatening hazard of tissue damage from excessive drug-induced vasoconstriction and the possibility of producing medication-overuse headache combined to ensure that this pattern of use of the drug progressively disappeared from clinical practice. In the belief that it may be safer than ergotamine, dihydroergotamine sometimes continued to be used for this purpose, especially in North America.

Antiserotonin Agents

Several drugs conventionally classed as antihistamine (H_1 receptor blocking) agents also possess antiserotonin activity and have come into use as migraine preventives. Pizotifen had its efficacy demonstrated in clinical trials of not particularly high quality (Speight and Avery 1972). By virtue of similarity of molecular structure and mechanism of action to pizotifen, both cyproheptadine and methdilazine found their way into therapeutics in attempts to prevent migraine (Lance et al. 1970). In this role, the drugs in this family appear somewhat more effective than placebo. Their efficacy is modest but their adverse effects are not particularly dangerous. For want of better alternatives, they continued to have some use in migraine prevention, at least to the end of the 20th century.

Monoamine Oxidase Inhibitors

At least one monoamine oxidase inhibitor (phenelzine) showed some effectiveness in the prevention of migraine, though only in studies that lacked a placebo control group (Kimball et al. 1960; Anthony and Lance 1969). Presumably the action of the inhibitor would be to raise circulating and cerebral serotonin concentrations, but also the concentrations of other biogenic amines. It may be this combined effect which explains the drug's action in preventing migraine. The use of the drug did not become part of regular medical practice, mainly because of the risk of serious adverse effects from failure to metabolically inactivate various catecholamines as well as serotonin, both in the central nervous system and throughout the remainder of the body, and because of the inconvenience of the dietary precautions that are necessary for safe usage of this class of agent.

Amitriptyline

In clinical trials, the tricyclic antidepressant amitriptyline, which blocks reuptake of serotonin into nerve terminals, was found to have a moderate degree of efficacy in preventing migraine (Gomersall and Stuart 1973; Couch et al. 1976). Most of the subsequently marketed serotonin reuptake-blocking antidepressants do not seem to have produced consistent therapeutic results when used for migraine prevention. Amitriptyline has a metabolite, nortriptyline, which blocks noradrenaline reuptake into nerve terminals, and it may be this additional factor, perhaps plus the anticholinergic effect of the parent substance, that make amitriptyline a more reliable agent for preventing migraine than its more modern therapeutic successors. Again, the efficacy of amitriptyline in preventing migraine recurrences appears to be relatively modest.

Drugs Affecting Catecholamine Mechanisms

Propranolol was the first of the beta-adrenoceptor blocking agents to find a significant and continuing place in human therapeutics. Its initial use was for the treatment of hypertension and anginal chest pain. While it was being used for these conditions, patients reported that their headaches were reduced. As a result, formal placebo-controlled clinical trials of the drug in migraine prevention were carried out. They demonstrated that migraine attacks were less frequent during treatment with the drug as compared with when a placebo was in use (Stensrud and Sjaastad 1976, 1980; Biggs and Milac 1979). Subsequent studies utilizing other beta-blockers for migraine prevention have tended to show that agents of this class, if they lack intrinsic sympathomimetic activity, have some efficacy in preventing migraine (e.g., atenolol and metoprolol). Beta-blockers that possess some sympathomimetic activity as well as a beta-blocking capacity do not seem particularly effective in this role (pindolol, oxprenolol). The relative overall lack of adverse effects in drugs of this class has resulted in their continued use as migraine preventives, even though they do not possess any outstanding effectiveness. Whether their mechanism of action depends on their effect at beta-adreno-ceptors is uncertain. There is evidence that propranolol may interfere with platelet serotonin transport (Rudnick et al. 1981), and it may have as yet unrecognized effects on other serotonin-mediated biological mechanisms.

Nonsteroidal Anti-inflammatory Agents

As mentioned earlier in this chapter, aspirin has been used for many years with reasonable success as a treatment for actual migraine headache attacks. The drug has also been used in a migraine preventive role. In a well-designed, small-scale, double-blind controlled trial O'Neill and Mann (1978) demonstrated that an aspirin dose of 650 mg twice daily did have a migraine-preventing effect. Ryan and Ryan (1982) obtained a similar result in another study, as did Masel et al. (1980). However, the latter authors had used the drug in combination with dipyridamole. Therefore the benefit found in their study cannot necessarily be ascribed purely to the aspirin. Subsequent studies in which attempted aspirin prophylaxis for migraine resulted in evidences of benefit were summarized by Limmroth et al. (1999) and Lampl et al. (2007). The earlier studies mentioned immediately above were carried out at a time when the platelet hypothesis of migraine pathogenesis was in vogue. The mechanism of action of the aspirin as a migraine prophylactic was then seen as being the prevention of platelet adhesion, the preliminary event to platelet release of serotonin. It is uncertain whether this is the real mode of action of aspirin in preventing migraine or whether cyclooxygenase inhibition due to the drug achieves antimigraine effects through disruption of other metabolic pathways and in other tissues.

For some time, continued oral intake of the herb feverfew has had the reputation of being able to reduce the frequency of migraine or prevent the attacks occurring. Some limited clinical trials support this belief (Hylands et al. 1987). The latter authors have provided a deal of scientific information about the plant, including details of its chemistry and possible mechanism of action.

More recently, various other nonsteroidal anti-inflammatory agents have been used on a regular basis with the intention of preventing migraine. They have generally proved to possess some effectiveness in this regard (Peto et al. 1988; Buring et al. 1990).

Antiepileptic Drugs

As mentioned earlier in this chapter, phenobarbital, formerly widely used as a sedative but now employed almost exclusively as an antiepileptic agent, was recommended for migraine prevention in the earlier years of the 20th century, though no controlled trials to prove that the drug was effective were ever carried out. As new antiepileptic agents have appeared, some were tried for migraine prevention. There were a few reports that phenytoin was of use, though the evidence was mainly anecdotal. Swanson and Vick (1978) reported that the drug had some effectiveness in preventing attacks of basilar artery migraine in a relatively small number of subjects. More recently, sodium valproate, or valproic acid itself, has proved moderately effective in preventing most common varieties of migraine when used in doses that are usually tolerated comfortably (Sorenson 1988). Valproate possesses several known mechanisms of antiepileptic action, but the molecular means whereby it can prevent migraine remain uncertain (Cutrer et al. 1997). The antiepileptic drug gabapentin has also shown some effectiveness in trials (Matthew et al. 2001). Lamotrigine was also tried in migraine prevention after it became established as an antiepileptic agent, but the earlier studies did not find proof of effectiveness (Steiner et al. 1997-a). However, Lampl et al. (1999, 2005) found that the drug was effective in preventing migraine with aura, but not migraine without aura. This finding, if substantiated, may raise interesting issues in relation to the possibility that there is a fundamental difference between these two patterns of migraine attack, a matter already considered in chapter 5. Topiramate was also studied with the possibility in mind of its having a migraine-preventing action. The drug proved to possess this capacity (Storey et al. 2001).

There appears to be reasonably convincing evidence that these various antiepileptic drugs, with their rather disparate mechanisms of action, do possess real migraine-preventing activity. The biochemical basis of their actions in this regard is unclear.

Calcium Channel Antagonists

Two calcium channel antagonists, verapamil and flunarizine, have been studied sufficiently often and for long enough to make it likely that they do possess some genuine migraine preventing capacity. Their exact mechanisms of producing this effect await clarification.

Dopamine Antagonists

Two dopamine antagonists, metoclopramide and domperidone, have been used to overcome the nausea that often accompanies migraine attacks, and to prevent vomiting in the attacks. One study had shown a dose-related effect of the latter when used in migraine prevention (MacGregor et al. 1993).

Endocrine Therapies

Nevil Leyton, a London medical practitioner who had an interest in migraine, wrote a small book that appeared in 1954, with a second edition two years later. In his preface, he described how, three hours after injecting stilboestrol, a synthetic estrogenic compound, into a young woman, she developed a typical attack of her migraine. An oral dose of a natural estrogen produced a similar response. On this basis, Layton reasoned that blocking the production of endogenous estrogen should protect against migraine. He began to inject migraine sufferers of either gender with 11-month courses of "anterior-pituitary-like hormone prepared from pregnancy urine" with the intention of modifying estrogen production while causing little interference with the menstrual cycle in females. Later he managed more severe migraine with intensive in-patient therapy using histamine desensitization and adrenocorticotrophic hormone. By 1953, he had treated almost 2000 patients and reported the following:

> Eighty percent of the patients seen have been either relieved entirely of their migraine or the attacks shortened and the interval between them so prolonged that only a minor degree of discomfort and interference with normal life remains. (Leyton 1953, p. 39)

Half of the second edition of his book comprised a series of "typical" case reports, but no more detailed statistical analysis of the overall outcome of therapy was provided apart from the numbers cited earlier in this paragraph. Despite the impressive results that he described, Layton's approach did not come into more general use.

There have been a number of attempts to achieve the prevention of menstrual migraine by administering progesterone, or to defer the headaches to more convenient times by administering estrogen derivatives when the premenstrual fall in circulating concentrations of this hormone is anticipated. Some success may be achieved (Somerville et al. 1972), but with the disadvantage that, as time passes, unacceptable patterns of disturbance may develop in female reproductive organ function.

Miscellaneous Migraine-Preventing Agents

Reasonable-quality studies have shown that a number of drugs with no obvious mechanism of action in common have degrees of migraine-preventing capacities. How these drugs act in migraine in terms of their known mechanisms of action is also often obscure. One good-quality study showed that the vitamin riboflavin was effective in some instances in preventing otherwise recalcitrant migraine (Schoenen et al. 1998). The antispasticity agent baclofen, which has some capacity to diminish other varieties of pain such as that of trigeminal neuralgia, has a proven degree of effectiveness in migraine prevention (Hering-Hanit 1999). Two trials have shown that the antihypertensive agent lisinopril, an angiotensin-converting enzyme inhibitor, can achieve a measure of migraine prevention (Schrader et al. 2001), as can the angiotensin-receptor blocking agent candesarten (Tronvik et al. 2003). Botulinum toxin injected every few months also seems capable of a degree of migraine prevention (Evers et al. 2004; Dodick et al. 2005). As well, high oral magnesium dicitrate dosage was found to achieve some degree of migraine prevention in a study of adequate quality (Peikert et al. 1996; Pfaffenrath et al. 1996).

In the present state of knowledge, it does not seem possible to discern any single mechanism of molecular action by which these various substances achieve migraine prevention. Possibly most of the individual substances, or the members of each pharmacological group, may act by preventing the effects of certain factors that provoke migraine attacks in particular sufferers, or by interrupting various chemical stages in the production of the disorder's manifestations. If so, the prevention that they achieve would not be due to any interruption of the final common pathway of the migraine mechanism. Rather, it may involve interference with mechanisms that vary from individual to individual sufferer. In this regard, it would be interesting to know the extent to which migraine sufferers who have failed to achieve headache prevention with one type of prophylactic agent may benefit from receiving another agent with a different probable mechanism of action.

Spinal Manipulation

At least in some countries, migraine sufferers often seem to seek chiropractic advice and receive chiropractic treatment (General Chiropractic Council 2004). Until the early years of the 21st century, and subsequent to the time period that the present book is intended to cover, little quality scientific work had been published assessing the efficacy of chiropractic treatment in the disorder, and no persuasive evidence of its effectiveness had become available (Posadzki and Ernst 2011).

Acupuncture

Acupuncture became a fairly extensively used means of preventing migraine in the latter part of the 20th century, particularly in Europe (Diener 2008). However, a meta-analysis of published data failed to find convincing evidence for the efficacy of the procedure (Melchart et al. 1999). A more recent, large-scale, randomized controlled clinical trial resulted in a similar conclusion (Diener et al. 2006).

Ligation of Arteries

For a time, various scalp arteries and the middle meningeal artery itself were occasionally ligated to try to treat medically intractable migraine. The longer term results did not seem to justify the procedures, and they appear to have been abandoned.

Closure of a Patent Foramen Ovale

It has been known for some time that there is a statistical association between suffering from migraine and the presence of a patent foramen ovale (Del Sette et al. 1998; Anzola et al. 1999). In one study, some 38 percent of patients with refractory migraine had a patent foramen ovale (Tepper et al. 2007). Although a number of studies have been carried out, as yet it has not been established that surgical closure of the foramen is of unequivocal benefit in preventing migraine. There have been suggestions that the procedure may benefit patients who have migraine with auras. The association between a potential right-to-left shunt within the heart and migraine, and the possible benefit from preventing such blood shunting, have raised the possibility that some circulating chemical substance exists that can pro-voke migraine and is formed elsewhere in the body and is normally inacti-vated during the passage of venous blood through the lungs. If there was a right-to-left shunt of blood so that it bypassed the lungs, such a postulated substance could reach the cerebral circulation and the brain without being inactivated. This possibility remains a matter for speculation at the time of writing.

Electrical Therapy

During the 19th century, there was a good deal of exploration of the possi-bility of using electricity to treat various disorders, including migraine. Several authors recommended its use, for example Garrett Anderson in 1870 (Wilkinson and Isler 1999), Russell Reynolds (1874, 1876) and Eulenburg (1877), but Gowers (1888) and Osler (1892) were skeptical. In this case, the skeptics appear to have been correct.

There is considerable further interesting material on various earlier non-pharmacological treatments of migraine in a recent paper authored by Koehler and Boes (2010).

CHAPTER 7

The Trigeminal Autonomic Cephalalgias

The term *trigeminal autonomic cephalalgia* did not appear in the medical literature until quite recently. Goadsby and Lipton (1997) seem to have coined it to take in a group of unilateral headache disorders with a significant number of features in common, yet with sufficient differences between them to appear to be separate entities. All have affinities to migraine, but their clinical features allow them to be plainly distinguished from it. Nevertheless, as more instances are recorded of the relatively uncommon painful hemicranial entities that comprise the trigeminal autonomic cephalalgias, it seems possible that enough instances of intermediate forms may be described to result in the currently recognized individual varieties becoming merged into a diagnostic continuum. However, that situation certainly has not been reached at the time of writing.

The individual disorders originally embraced by the concept of trigeminal autonomic cephalalgia were (i) cluster headache, (ii) chronic paroxysmal hemicrania, (iii) SUNCT/SUNA (short-lasting unilateral neuralgiform headache attacks with conjunctival injection and tearing/short-lasting unilateral neuralgiform headache attacks with cranial autonomic features) syndrome, and (iv) hemicrania continua. However, the International Headache Society subsequently decided to exclude the latter entity from the trigeminal autonomic cephalalgia category. If all these entities, including hemicrania continua, had been recognized in earlier times, they would have almost certainly been included in the ancient headache category of *hemicrania*. That is another reason why the *hemicrania* of the past cannot be equated precisely with present-day migraine. In fact, the modern trigeminal autonomic cephalalgia headache category to a considerable extent corresponds to the group of head pain conditions that Wilfred Harris (1926), in his book *Neuritis and Neuralgia*, dealt with under the designation *migrainous neuralgia*. In relation to this particular head pain category Harris seems to have described, both then and also later (Harris 1936), what would now be identified as cluster headache, dealing with it under the name *ciliary neuralgia*. He also gave an account of a probable instance of chronic paroxysmal hemicrania. However, within his migrainous neuralgia category, he also included certain other patterns of headache. Some of these probably were instances of migraine itself, and there are others that may have proved to be cluster headache if additional diagnostic information had been recorded.

A further problem of terminology exists because Edwin Bickerstaff (1959), when writing exclusively, but with great clarity, on cluster headache, titled his influential *Lancet* paper "The Periodic Migrainous Neuralgia of Wilfred Harris." In so doing, he partly sacrificed nosological accuracy to pay tribute to a great English authority on neuralgic types of head pain, one who in 1959 was nearing the end of his long life (1869–1960; Boes et al. 2002).

In what is to follow, the trigeminal autonomic cephalalgias will be considered individually. There is much more information available about cluster headache than about the other, even more recently recognized, varieties of this headache category.

CLUSTER HEADACHE

The Clinical Manifestations

Kunkle et al. (1952, 1954) first applied the term *cluster headache* to the one-sided headache disorder here being considered. The name acknowledged the peculiar time pattern of the occurrence of the pain attacks that were the disorder's most characteristic feature. At the time, these authors considered that cluster headache was not a discrete nosological entity but simply a migraine variant. The name cluster headache was both apt and avoided the uncertainties engendered by the shifting and never closely defined meaning of *migrainous neuralgia*, the term by which the disorder had often been known earlier in the 20th century. Almost inevitably, cluster headache increasingly became the preferred name for the condition. The 1988 version of the International Headache Society's Classification of Headache defined cluster headache in terms of (i) attacks of severe, strictly unilateral, pain in the orbit, the supraorbital region, and/or the temple, lasting 15 to 180 minutes and occurring between once every two days and eight times a day, and associated with (ii) one or more of unilateral conjunctival injection, lacrimation, nasal congestion, rhinorrhea, sweating of the forehead or face, miosis, ptosis, eyelid edema, and with, in the great majority, (iii) the attacks occurring in a series lasting for weeks or months, in other words, in clusters, with months or years of freedom from such headaches between the clusters, but much less commonly with attacks showing no periods of remission. The diagnostic criteria have remained essentially unaltered since, and had actually been recognized in practice in earlier times, though on the whole, less weight was previously placed on the associated features such as the red eye and the unilateral lacrimation. In a few of the cases he described under the designation of migrainous neuralgia, Harris (1926) had noted the presence of such features, though he seemed to regard them almost as irrelevant or inconvenient curiosities. Only when the full clinical picture of the disorder and also its agreed name emerged in the mid-20th century did the entity become more widely known. As a result, identifying earlier reports of the condition in the literature usually involves a degree of uncertainty. This is so because past authors may neither have sought nor, if they knew of it, appreciated the significance of the time pattern of the attacks, or their associated features. They may have therefore described instances of cluster headache under other diagnostic designations.

The earliest known report of possible, though perhaps not probable, cluster headache may well be that of Nicolas Tulp (Koehler 1993, 1996; Mendizabal 1999; Gordon 2004). Tulp (1593–1674), born Nicolas Pieterszoon, physician and anatomist, of Amsterdam, in his *Observationes medicae*, published in 1641, described the case of Isaac van Halmaal, who, in the words of Koehler's translation,

> in the beginning of the summer season, was afflicted with a very severe headache, occurring and disappearing daily on fixed hours, with such an intensity that he often assured me that he could not bear the pain anymore or he would succumb shortly. For rarely it lasted longer than two hours. And the rest of the day there was no fever, nor indisposition of the urine, nor any infirmity of the pulse. But this recurring pain lasted until the fourteenth day. (1993, p. 19)

The timing and duration of the pain are consistent with cluster headache, but there is no indication that it was experienced unilaterally, and no mention of any other of the typical associated features of the entity.

Thomas Willis (1672) followed soon after Tulp, though his report of possible cluster headache could scarcely be regarded as more convincing than that of the latter. In *De Anima Brutorum*, Willis described it as follows:

> A venerable Matron of about forty five years of Age, of a lean habit of Body, and indeed with a Cholerick Temper, after she had lived for a long time obnoxious to Headaches, wont to be caused occasionally, she began about the beginning of Autumn to be troubled by a periodical pain of the Head: This Distemper invading her about four of the

Clock in the Afternoon, was wont to continue until midnight, when being wearied with the pain and watching, she was compelled to sleep; then afterwards awakening from out of a profound sleep, she found herself well again. She being sick after this manner for three weeks, suffered the daily fits of this Disease, and forebode to take any Medicine, which she greatly abhorr'd; but at length her Appetite being lost, and her strength worn out, being forced to seek for Care; after letting blood and a gentle Purge, she took twice a day for a week or two, the quantity of a Chestnut of the following *Electuary*, and grew perfectly well. (1672/1683, p. 124)

The formula of the electuary scarcely matters at this point—in terms of modern knowledge, it could scarcely be expected to have had any specific efficacy, though it may have had an effect on the taste buds. Willis's account did not specify the headache site, and the duration of the attacks was rather long for cluster headache, but the occurrence of the headache at a consistent time of day, the pain severity, the duration of the apparent cluster, and its probable spontaneous resolution might be seen as suggestive of the disorder, even in the absence of any mention of associated autonomic phenomena.

Arkink et al. (2010) have suggested that a probable instance of cluster headache was reported to the Royal Society of London in 1702 by one of the society's fellows, the Reverend Mr. Abraham de la Pryme (1671–1704). That reverend gentleman had written to the secretary of the society concerning two matters: subterranean trees and the poison of rabies (de la Pryme 1702). In Pryme's letter, there was incidental mention of the following matter. A few years earlier, Pryme's brother had lost a greyhound bitch and her litter of whelps to rabies, and two of the brother's servants had put their fingers in the mouth of the last surviving whelp a day or two before the animal died, presumably to see if the swallowing difficulty was due to some local source of obstruction. Pryme's letter went on, initially referring to the dogs:

They being dead were soon forgot, until that about 3 weeks after, my Brother's Servant, a most strong laborious Man, that had frequently put his Fingers into the Whelps mouth, began to be troubled now and then with an exceeding pain in the Head, sometimes once, sometimes twice a day, so very vehement that he was forc'd to hold his Head with both his hands, to hinder it from riving in two, which fits commonly held him about an hour at a time, in which his Throat would contract, as he said, and his Pulse tremble, and his Eyes behold every thing of a fiery red colour. Thus was he tormented for a whole week together, but being of a strong constitution, and returning to his labour in every interval, he sweat and wrought it off, without any Physic.

But it went worse with one of his fellow Servants, a young Apprentice of about 14 years of age, who had made much of the Whelp as he, but was not of so strong a Constitution, he was seiz'd also with a pain in his Head, was somewhat Feverish, sometimes better, sometimes worse, cough'd much, had a good stomach, eat heartily, but could drink nothing. (de la Pryme 1702, pp. 1075–1076)

The apprentice died a few days later. Perhaps there is enough detail in the account to allow the reader to decide whether a retrospective diagnosis of cluster headache would be warranted in the first subject described.

A report of a rather more persuasive early example of cluster headache was recognized by Isler (1993). His translation of the original Latin, though omitting several sentences, is reproduced below. The case history was originally published in 1745, in the *Commentaria* of Gerard van Swieten, of Vienna, who had previously been one of Boerhaave's pupils.

A healthy, robust man of middle age (was suffering from) troublesome pain which came on every day at the same hour at the same spot above the orbit of the left eye, where the nerve emerges from the opening of the frontal bone; after a short time the left eye began to redden, and to overflow with tears; then he felt as if his eye was slowly forced out of its orbit with so much pain, that he nearly went mad. After a few hours all these evils ceased, and nothing in the eye appeared at all changed. . . . I objectively perceived, how that artery in the angle of the eye was pulsating more rapidly, and stronger than it usually and naturally does. I therefore believed that there was a fever, but a local one; and I gave Peruvian bark (quinine) and cured it with good luck. (Isler 1993, p. 73)

In this account, there is mention not only of the headache being unilateral and situated in the frontal part of the head, but also of the timing of attacks and of the occurrence of some autonomic manifestations, and also the probable spontaneous resolution of the cluster. Only evidence that the attack clusters were recurrent is not available.

Not long afterward, another of Boerhaave's former pupils, Robert Whytt, professor of the theory of medicine in the University of Edinburgh, in his 1768 posthumously published *Observations on the Nature, Causes, and Cure of Those Disorders which Are Commonly Called Nervous, Hypochondriac or Hysteric*, discussed "periodic headache":

These either affect almost the whole head, especially in the forepart, or only one side of it; sometimes no more than one of the eyes, with part of the fore-head and temple on the same side. They generally return once a day, nearly at the same hour, and as regularly as the fit of a quotidian ague. In some cases they are attended with a visible swelling, not only of the eye affected, but also of that side of the forehead. Sometimes the eye seems to sink within its orbit; at other times, nothing can be observed but that the eyes want their usual lustre, and look as if the person had watched long, or drunk too much. (Whytt 1768, p. 620)

In that description, there is contained more or less the same items of information that van Swieten had recorded, though the evidence of autonomic disturbance may not be so definite.

At much the same time as Whytt, in the latter half of the 18th century, Morgagni described the suffering of an associate of his youth, one Lawrence Bagattrini. Giovanni Battista Morgagni (1682–1771) had followed in the distinguished lineage of his great predecessors Versalius and Fallopius in the chair of anatomy at Padua, which he occupied for the last 56 years of his long life. His *De sedibus et causis morborum per anatomen indagatis* appeared posthumously in 1779. In it, the account of Bagattrini's illness, in translation, read as follows:

> I remember when I was a young man, I had a patient among my compatriots, by name Lawrence Bagattrini, who had been seized long before with an external, but very violent hemicrania, which returned every day at the eleventh hour, according to the method of reckoning the hours among the Italians. Whatever I did, had either no effect at all, or at least only that of shortening and alleviating the pain, for it still returned at the same hour, and if any little error, or irregularity, was committed, it returned with its formed vehemence. Having for many days used all other remedies in vain, I at length got the better of the disorder, by means of a slight decoction of the woods; which gently agitating and impelling the circulating juices, threw the patient into sweats, and relieved him of his disorder. And Balonius testifies that the same method succeeded with him also, in intolerable hemicranias, that returned every day, at a certain hour. (Kelly 1971, p. 336)

This particular account may seem less persuasive than those of van Swieten and Whytt, in that the headache was not stated to be frontal in its site though it was one-sided. Further, no autonomic features of the attacks were described. Nonetheless, cluster headache still seems the most probable diagnosis.

In 1777, probably shortly after Whytt and Morgagni had their encounters with probable cluster headache sufferers, a medical student named Johan Müller experienced what was almost certainly an attack of cluster headache. He described it years later, though details of the time pattern and whether there was a cluster of attacks are not available. Isler, as so often has been the case in relation to aspects of headache history, provided a translation of the account:

> 1777, the 28th of April, 8 o'clock in the morning [I received] at the right orbit, just above the arcus superciliaries, at a place which can be covered by a three-penny piece, a quite peculiar pressing perception. . . . Increased from minute to minute [and] finally transformed itself into a painful feeling that mounted up to an insupportable degree.

The pain was tearing, gnawing, boring, throbbing. . . . [T]he eye became so sensitive that it could not support the light, it became inflamed, spasmodically contracted and tearing, the temporal vessels pulsated uncommonly strongly. (Isler 1987-b, reproduced in Mendizabal 1999, p. 1414)

The attack lasted four hours and then resolved. While it was present, Müller could not find a position of comfort for his body. However, one could question whether this particular account provides sufficient information to permit recognition of cluster headache.

Marshall Hall, famous for his recognition of the reflex arc, may have been referring to cluster headache among other entities, when he wrote the following, in what was basically note form, concerning augmented action of the sentient nerves:

735. The *hemicrania intermittens*, or *brow ague*, is apt to recur in spring or autumn, from exposure to the north-east wind: it prevails in damp and marshy districts, and is frequently observed to accompany the epidemic influenza. It frequently exists as a complication of intermittent [here a word seems to have been omitted from the printing in the available account].

736. The ague pain occupies the brow, the temple, the forehead, the occiput, &c; it is often excruciating, occasionally producing delirium, and, still more frequently, redness of the conjunctiva. It may recur once or twice in the course of the day. (Hall 1836, p. 169)

There is no indication that Hall thought he may have been considering more that one distinct entity in this section of his book. There also is no explicit indication of the characteristic short-term periodicity of the headache, though "brow-ague" was considered of malarious origin at Hall's time of writing, and malaria was regarded as a paradigm of disorders with periodic recurrences. However, the account contains mention of the red eye and the seasonal pattern of recurrence of the painful disorder.

Mauritz Romberg, in his Manual of the Nervous Diseases of Man, wrote of ciliary neuralgia:

Painful sensations in the eye, which are generally confined to one side, and are excited or increased by rays of light and by visual effort, are the characteristic symptoms of this affection. In the higher degrees photophobia is present; this is therefore the term generally applied to the affection. The patient avoids solar and artificial light, as the bulb of the eye becomes painful when exposed to their influence, and the eyelids contract painfully. The pupil is contracted. The pain not unfrequently extends over the head and face. The eye generally weeps and becomes red. These symptoms occur in paroxysms, of a uniform or irregular character, and isolated or combined with facial neuralgia or hemi-crania. (1853 [Sieveking's translation], p. 56)

It has been inferred that this description may refer to cluster headache (Mendizabal 1999), though the characteristic time pattern of the disorder is not particularly obvious from the account. Both the wording itself and the material that follows the paragraph cited suggest that Romberg was dealing mainly with local eye disorders and was fitting the material described into his concept of nervous system disease at a time when neurology was beginning to emerge as a particular area of medical interest.

Francis Anstie (1866) wrote of two cases of periodically recurring neuralgias of the fifth cranial nerve: "In both of these cases there was unilateral flushing of the face and congestion of the conjunctivae, to a slight degree, during the painful attack." There was no indication that Anstie thought he had come across a new form of trigeminal pain syndrome. Conceivably, he may have encountered instances of cluster headache, but there is not sufficient detail to be sure.

Möllendorf (1867) had described what was sometimes called "red migraine," and Rudolph Bing, beginning in 1913 (Bing 1952), had written on "erythroprosopalgia," both entities sometimes taken to be cluster headache. However, Möllendorf referred to a red face, rather than a red eye, which occurred in otherwise ordinary migraine, and Bing also had described facial rather than conjunctival redness.

Until this point, in the light of knowledge of the characteristic features of the headache syndrome, one can go back in the literature to find reports of instances of possible or even probable cluster headache. However, the old accounts provide no sense that their authors envisaged that they were dealing with a new and perhaps important headache entity. It was rather that they had noted an unusual set of headache-related phenomena that seemed worth recording. That situation came to its end with the writings of the London neurologist Wilfred Harris (figure 7-1), in the period between the two world wars of the 20th century. Harris collected sufficient material relevant to the disorder of cluster headache to allow the concept of a new and characteristic headache entity to begin to emerge.

Harris

In his monograph *Neuritis and Neuralgia*, Wilfred Harris (1926) covered the topic of what was to later be named cluster headache in part of his chapter "Migraine and Allied Neuralgias." There he dealt very briefly with migraine itself before going into the subject of migrainous neuralgia in

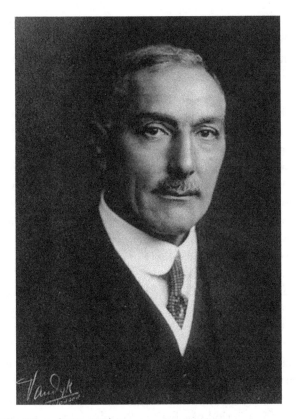

Figure 7-1 Wilfred Harris (1869–1960). Courtesy of Sage Publications.

greater detail. He subdivided that particular subject into (i) migrainous supraorbital neuralgia and (ii) periodic migrainous neuralgia, with a subset of the latter being designated *ciliary neuralgia*. Harris's account of these disorders has been very carefully analyzed by Boes et al. (2002). To present-day interpretations, some of the migrainous neuralgia case histories that Harris provided appear to describe instances of migraine. In others, it is difficult to be sure what type of headache was present. However, there are a few accounts that would meet modern-day criteria for cluster headache. Writing of his migrainous neuralgia, before dealing with its periodic subset, Harris noted the following:

> Sometimes the attacks are as frequent as three or four in the week, the patient being hardly ever free from pain, and in a few cases that I have met with excruciating pain at the temple at side of the head or in the cheek might last for an hour or even less, but would be repeated three or four times a day, the daily paroxysms continuing for years. (1926, p. 295)

One can see that present-day chronic (i.e., nonperiodic) cluster headache could be accommodated within that time pattern of headache, but so could other conditions causing head pain. For instance, Harris recounted this case history:

> A New Zealand sheep farmer, *aet.* 26, when staying in this country, noticed one night when getting into bed a sharp, heavy pain in his right temple as if he had been struck, the pain keeping him awake for hours.
>
> Next morning the pain had gone, but every day of his life since the same pain returned between 4.30 and 5 in the afternoon. There was occasional nausea, but never vomiting. No treatment had ever done him any good, though exposure to cold always made it worse. This he noticed especially during the winter months when in the trenches during the War. His father had for years suffered from some form of pain in his head, which caused him to commit suicide at the age of 60. (1926, p. 300)

This head pain, as described, had the regular time of occurrence that is very suggestive of cluster headache, but it is arguable whether enough additional features were recorded to permit the confident retrospective diagnosis of that entity.

When Harris turned to his category of periodic migrainous neuralgia, he emphasized the long-term periodicity of its occurrence: "In other cases the migrainous neuralgia may occur daily at about the same time and last for several hours for a period of a few weeks only in the year, and may recur annually at about the same time." And among his examples, he included this description:

> A young man of 25, when aged 19 began to suffer from daily attacks, for three or four weeks every year, of severe pain in the back of the right eyeball and forehead, with lachrymation and reddening of the eye; would last for an hour or two, no nausea, but voracious appetite accompanying the neuralgia. (Harris 1926, p. 305)

In this particular instance, the autonomic disturbance of cluster headache was present, and there was enough information available to infer that the attacks occurred in clusters, with headache-free intervals. But when Harris proceeded to consider his entity of ciliary neuralgia, he began by stating this:

> Under this heading I include those cases of migrainous neuralgia in which pain is referred locally to the eyeball alone or to the back of the eyeball, and I label them as ciliary more for descriptive purposes than with any certainty of their pathology.
>
> Indeed I am convinced that these cases are a form of substituted migrainous neuralgia. (1926, p. 307)

He then proceeded to describe an illustrative case, in which the diagnosis of cluster headache appears readily sustainable:

> A man, *aet.* 47, had his first attack of neuralgia in January 1917, when in the trenches in front of Beaumont Hamel. The pain struck him suddenly across the left temple and fore-head, and lasted three-quarters of an hour, like an "electric battery," while his face became flushed and he felt faint. The neuralgia recurred thrice daily, at about eight hour inter-vals, for six weeks, and then disappeared entirely for two years. Ever since his first attack he had a left cervical sympathetic paralysis, there being slight ptosis, with a small pupil. In subsequent attacks the neuralgia began on the left side of the top of the head, the eyeball being very painful, and red, and the pain spreading down the nose into the left side of the cheek. The second attack lasted for six weeks, while his third attack did not occur till three years later, the pain awakening him shortly before 5 a.m. (pp. 307–308)

While Harris in his 1926 monograph had clearly described the clinical phenomena of cluster headache, particularly in relation to his account of ciliary neuralgia, the possible recognition of a characteristic new headache entity was obscured by its being described mixed in among examples of probably related headache disorders. His acknowledged expertise in inject-ing alcohol into various cranial nerves and into parts of the Gasserian gan-glion itself ensured that Harris had a considerable consultant practice among head pain sufferers. He continued to accumulate additional cases, and he came to realize that he had encountered a possible new headache disorder. In 1936, he wrote of "ciliary (migrainous) neuralgia" in the *British Medical Journal*:

> In 1926 I described under the heading "ciliary neuralgia" a form of migrainous neuralgia in which the pain is especially located in, behind, or around the eyeball. I did not wish by using the term "ciliary" to suggest that the pathology of the condition was necessarily associated with either the ciliary ganglion or the ciliary body within the eyeball, but rather to define a variety of migrainous neuralgia in which the eye is clearly affected, not only by the reference of pain within or behind it, but also in many cases by extreme con-gestion and reddening of the conjunctiva, with lachyrimation. (Harris 1936, p. 457)

He went on to define the essential natures of his migrainous and ciliary neuralgias:

> It is essentially a paroxysmal recurrent neuralgia, usually strictly unilateral, though occa-sionally, like some migraines, spreading at the end of an attack to the opposite side, though the pain is almost invariably more severe on one and the same side.... When the eyeball itself is prominently affected by the pain I speak of this variety of migrainous neuralgia as ciliary neuralgia. (p. 458)

By the time he wrote this, Harris had collected a total of 26 instances of his ciliary neuralgia, and noted that the ocular autonomic abnormalities were present in 10 of them. Although his account did not bring out the details of the periodicity of the recurrences of the disorder as clearly as it might have, there appear to be reasonable grounds for regarding Wilfred Harris as the first to recognize the existence of the discrete type of head pain that was later to become known as cluster headache.

Horton

In a series of papers commencing in 1939, and at that time apparently unaware of Harris's writings, Bayard Horton (1895–1980; figure 7-2) of the Mayo Clinic described what he and others considered was a novel type of headache. In 1939 he and his colleagues set down the origins of the concept in the *Journal of the American Medical Association*:

> This new syndrome of vascular headache, which MacLean, Craig and I tentatively called "erythromelalgia of the head" and which I shall call "histaminic cephalgia" hereafter, was first encountered and recognized at the Mayo Clinic in September 1937. At that time the syndrome had not been described adequately in the literature. The observations which have been made with reference to this specific type of headache warrant its establishment as a distinct clinical entity, classic in its symptomatology and unique in its response to histamine therapy. (Horton et al. 1939, p. 377)

With the passage of time, his awareness of the manifestations of the syndrome broadened, as evidenced by his description of it:

> Histaminic cephalgia (Horton's headache) is an unusual kind of headache with typical symptomatology. The brevity and severity of the pain, its tendency to awaken the patient an hour or so after he has gone to sleep at night, and the accompanying localized vasomotor phenomena are its outstanding characteristics. The pain is unilateral and may involve any region of the head and neck. Attacks of histaminic cephalgia do not shift from side to side, as is so often observed in migraine. During a given series, attacks always occur on the same side, with but rare exceptions.
>
> Attacks may occur frequently, and they usually last less than an hour....
>
> In the typical full-blown attack, the pain is associated with profuse congestion and watering of the eye, stuffiness of the nostril or unilateral rhinorrhea. Frequently, sweating, orbital edema, and swelling of the temporal vessels occur on the affected side. The affected region may be sore to the touch for a while after an attack has ceased ... Horner's syndrome, which is common, may disappear after a given series of attacks have ceased, or it may persist indefinitely.

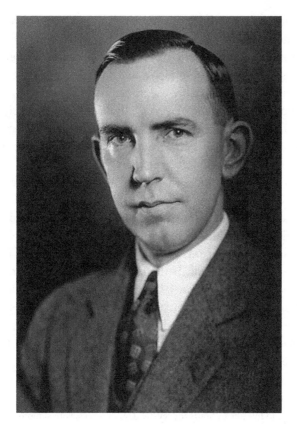

Figure 7-2 Bayard Horton (1895–1980). Courtesy of Sage Publications.

> Remissions and exacerbations occur spontaneously. Succeeding series of attacks
> seem to last longer, to be more severe, and, frequently, to be more difficult to treat. Most
> patients experience remissions which may last for many months or years, but eventually
> remissions may cease to occur and attacks become continuous. (Horton 1964, p. 228)

In many ways, this account of the individual headache episode reads very
much like a description of the features of an attack of cluster headache,
although the pain distribution may have been more extensive than is typical
of the latter disorder. The features of altered autonomic function were made
quite clear, but the peculiar timing pattern of the disorder was perhaps not
as obvious as it might have been. Horton had shown that when the disorder
in the sufferer was in a phase of activity, subcutaneous injection of histamine could provoke attacks (Horton 1941). Stemming from this observation, he administered courses of histamine desensitization and believed
that these were beneficial, or even curative. However, he probably had not
given enough attention to the possibility that spontaneous remission of

clusters of attacks during the desensitization process might have accounted for the apparent benefit.

There seems little doubt that Horton had described cluster headache under his designation of histaminic cephalgia. His account of the clinical features of the disorder probably was more adequate than that of Harris, but his opinion that histamine played a causal rather than merely a provoking role diverted medical knowledge along a false trail for a time. In addition, the fact that Horton was able to collect some 72 cases between 1937 and 1941, and could record that "from 1937 to January, 1958, I saw 1402 patients with histaminic cephalgia—1226 men and 176 women," whereas Harris, a senior London neurological consultant with a considerable reputation for managing head pain, could collect no more than 26 cases over more than a decade (up until 1936), does require explanation. Nonetheless, it seems to have been Horton's writings, more than those of Harris, that made the disorder substantially better known to the medical profession.

Kunkle and his colleagues in 1952 presented to the American Neurological Association a paper in which they described the features of 30 cases of an unusual form of periodic headache. All of the characteristic features of cluster headache were described, and more weight was given to the time pattern of the disorder:

> A peculiar feature in 24 of the group was the occurrence of the headaches in recurrent clusters of one to five per 24 hours for several days or weeks, with symptom-free intermissions lasting two months to two years, or occasionally longer. A regular periodicity in the occurrence of the individual headaches or the clusters was noted in only a few patients. (Kunkle et al. 1952, p. 241)

After making this statement, in the course of the article, the authors repeatedly referred to the condition they discussed as "cluster headache." As already mentioned, in so doing, they introduced a term that medicine has found advantageous to employ ever since.

In 1956, the British neurological clinician Sir Charles Symonds published in the journal *Brain* a paper titled "A Particular Variety of Headache," based on his experience of 17 cluster headache sufferers. The account was well organized, and though it contained nothing that was novel, it described the time pattern of the occurrence of individual attacks, and of the clusters, more clearly that the earlier writings had. Edwin Bickerstaff, a Birmingham neurologist, shortly afterward chose to deal with the disorder in the pages of the *Lancet* (1959). He produced a well organized and comprehensive account that probably reached a much wider readership than the more restricted neurological journal, however prestigious.

By the 1960s, the clinical phenomenology of cluster headache (or migrainous neuralgia as it was sometimes still termed) had become reasonably well known among those interested in headache. The disorder, unlike migraine, was usually considered not to be inherited until evidence surfaced (Russell et al. 1995; Russell 1997) that, in certain families, it appeared to have been transmitted in an autosomal dominant fashion. During the latter part of the 20th century, little more of importance was added to its spectrum of clinical manifestations, and interest shifted to matters more germane to its mechanism of production and its management. It was increasingly recognized that in a minority of instances, the disorder might not undergo spontaneous remissions from its outset, or that after several remissions, the disorder might fail to remit after becoming active again. Hence it sometimes became necessary to qualify the diagnosis of cluster headache with the prefixed word episodic or chronic. Over the years, various designations not already mentioned had been applied to cluster headache. They are listed in some accounts of the disorder, though some refer to other disturbances, for example, Möllendorf's "red migraine" (Möllendorf 1867) and Raeder's "paratrigeminal syndrome" (Raeder 1924); the remainder have disappeared from use.

The Mechanism of Cluster Headache

The early instances of probable cluster headache recorded in the literature were regarded merely as examples of unusual headaches or as migraine peculiarities. Their mechanism, if it was considered at all, was probably seen in the same light as that of the headache disorder category to which they were thought to belong. Wilfred Harris (1926, 1936) provided his interpretation of the mechanism of migrainous neuralgia after pointing out that his views of its pathogenesis were "necessarily mainly speculative." Because of the resemblance of the disorder to migraine, in which Harris thought the fundamental process was "a vasomotor spasm of the cortical and possibly meningeal vessels," he considered that in migrainous neuralgia there perhaps was

> vasomotor spasm in these cases affecting the more anterior regions of the meninges, and thus causing referred pain over areas of the trigeminal nerve through recurrent meningeal branches of the three divisions of this nerve. Possibly on account of this anterior area of the meninges being involved in migrainous neuralgias, we have an explanation of the practically invariable absence in them of visual spectra, which are associated with the posterior occipital vascular supply. (1926, p. 306)

His ciliary neuralgia was, he thought, simply "a form of substituted migrainous neuralgia," whatever precisely he meant by that. He made no attempt to account for the associated autonomic features, which he had noted in a minority of his cases, or for the tendency to a periodic pattern of occurrence of the disorder.

Horton's proposed mechanism of the disorder was somewhat different. It needed to account for the existence of a peculiar temporal pattern of sensitivity to histamine that he had detected. As well, Horton placed more emphasis on the extracranial arterial circulation as the site of pain origin. He had noted that compression of the common carotid and sometimes the temporal artery on the affected side, and also the intravenous injection of adrenaline (epinephrine), could relieve the pain of the attacks. Further, histamine and alcohol could provoke attacks, though only when the disorder was in an active phase (Horton 1941). He therefore argued that the pain arose from dilated cranial arteries, in keeping with what Wolff had shown was the probable mechanism and site of origin of migraine headache pain. Again, Horton's was an incomplete interpretation of the mechanism of cluster headache. It left unexplained the autonomic features and the periodicity, and Horton was well aware of both of these. His concept of histamine sensitivity as the cause of the disorder continued to be of interest for some time. However, later, he found it necessary to acknowledge that "in spite of abundant and sometimes plausible speculation, evidence that histamine is a causative agent is not yet convincing" (Horton 1959).

Completely unambiguous evidence regarding the role of histamine in the production of cluster headache never became available, though Sjaastad (1970) found increased urinary histamine excretion during cluster attacks in 3 of 6 sufferers, and Anthony and Lance (1971) measured increases in blood histamine concentrations during the headaches in 19 of 22 attacks experienced by 20 patients. However, Anthony et al. (1978) and Graham et al. (Kudrow 1987) later found that histamine receptor blocking agents (for H_1 and H_2 receptors) failed to prevent cluster attacks. It became increasingly accepted that histamine was merely a headache-provoking agent, and was not involved in the essential mechanism of cluster headache genesis.

Gardner et al. (1947) took the autonomic features of cluster headache into account and hypothesized that the pathological basis of the condition was a neuralgia of the greater superficial petrosal nerve. On this basis, they proceeded to divide the nerve and achieved immediate or delayed headache relief in some three-quarters of the cases on whom they had operated. Unfortunately, within the next three years, the attacks recurred in three of those who had obtained immediate relief from the surgery. The immediate and subsequent experience of the outcome of the operation was essentially similar when carried out by Stowell (1970). The suggestion of greater superficial petrosal neuralgia brings to mind the entity that Sluder had been describing from 1908 onward (Sluder 1918). In this condition, Sluder postulated that nasal infection led to involvement of the area of the sphenopalatine ganglion. The existence of such infection in Sluder's neuralgia was never proven. Nor was it proven that events in the sphenopalatine ganglion were responsible for pain in the middle part of the face, extending from the side of the nose to the mastoid region and ear on the same side. In the disorder that Sluder had described, there also was some reddening of the ipsilateral eyeball and pupillary dilatation (not constriction), as well as nasal stuffiness and discharge. The pain occurred in episodes lasting between a few hours and several days. Application of cocaine to the lateral wall of the nose near the sphenopalatine ganglion yielded relief. Thus what Sluder described in some respects resembled cluster headache, but there were sufficient differences to indicate that it was not the same disorder, whatever its real nature may have been.

Kunkle et al. (1952) carried out intrathecal injections of saline during cluster headache attacks in two subjects with the intention of raising their intracranial pressures and thus diminishing the amplitude of pulsation of intracranial arteries. They found that no headache relief occurred. Having noted that temporal artery compression produced relief in several patients with cluster headache, and that head jolting did not increase the headache, they concluded that the pain of cluster headache arose from the extracranial branches of the carotid artery. However, they then went on to state that in other patients, head jolting did increase the pain, which to them implied that in these persons, the pain of cluster headache arose intracranially. Neither Symonds (1956) nor Bickerstaff (1959) put forward any ideas about the cluster headache mechanism, though Bickerstaff argued for an affinity between the disorder and migraine, partly on the grounds that family history of migraine and past history of that disorder were a good deal more frequent in his cluster headache patients than the published experience of earlier authors would have suggested. Wolff (1963) was more concerned with persuading his readers that cluster headache was a migraine variant, and not a separate type of headache, than in explaining issues relating to its mechanism, particularly those issues that concerned the autonomic features and the periodicity.

Beginning in the seventh and eighth decades of the 20th century, some biochemical and cerebral blood flow data potentially relevant to human cluster headache appeared in print. Kudrow (1976) showed that there was reduction in plasma testosterone and luteinizing hormone levels during headache clusters, though subsequent investigations suggested that the reduction in testosterone levels might be a nonspecific response to pain (Nelson 1978; Klimek 1982). D'Andrea et al. (1992) demonstrated reduced platelet contents of noradrenaline and adrenaline in cluster headache sufferers, and increased platelet tyrosine concentrations during the headache attacks. They interpreted these findings as suggesting the presence of decreased sympathetic nervous system activity (which would correlate with the ocular sympathetic palsy encountered in some cluster headache sufferers). Chazot et al. (1984) found decreased plasma melatonin levels and a disturbed circadian melatonin rhythm in cluster headache sufferers. The early cerebral blood flow studies carried out during cluster headache attacks (Broch et al. 1970; Sjaastad et al. 1974) did not produce any easily interpretable conclusions, though an angiogram carried out during an attack demonstrated narrowing of a segment of the ipsilateral internal carotid artery in the carotid canal (Ekbom and Greitz 1970). Consistent with this observation, Kudrow (1979) and Nattero et al. (1980) obtained Doppler evidence of decreased blood flow in the supraorbital artery on the headache-affected side. This finding correlated with the earlier thermographic data of Lance and Anthony (1971).

Clinical and biochemical data consistent with decreased sympathetic nervous system activity and evidence of an altered internal carotid artery caliber had been published by Ekbon and Greitz (1970). This material provided a background for Hardebo's (1994) hypothesis that cluster headache was due to a chronic inflammatory process that was present in the cavernous sinus. Hardebo suggested that such a process, during periods when its activity was increased, would cause decreased venous outflow from the sinus and also ocular sympathetic disturbance (as can also occur in cavernous sinus thrombosis). There also would be irritation of the ophthalmic division of the trigeminal within the cavernous sinus, and this could cause unilateral anterior head pain. The local venous congestion from the obstructed sinus could produce what might be interpreted as the effects of parasympathetic overactivity in the affected trigeminal territory. No additional evidence to support this hypothesis appears to have become available. Remahl et al. (2000) could obtain no clinical or laboratory evidence to support the presence of inflammation anywhere in the body when cluster headache was active. However, the idea that the ocular sympathetic pathway may be affected at the level of the cavernous sinus continues to be held, though its mechanism remains unproven.

Goadsby and Edvinsson (1994) collected external jugular venous blood from the headache-affected side during cluster headache attacks, and found that it contained increased concentrations of the highly potent vasodilator calcitonin gene-related peptide (CGRP) and also vasoactive intestinal peptide. There was no change in the venous plasma concentrations of neuropeptide Y or substance P. Calcitonin gene-related peptide is released from trigeminal nerve terminals when they are activated. Soon afterward, May et al. (1998) described evidence obtained from brain imaging showing that there was activation of the hypothalamus in the region of the suprachiasmatic nucleus in the floor of the third ventricle during cluster headache attacks. This hypothalamic nucleus appears to exercise a timing function in the nervous system. This knowledge, taken in conjunction with the ipsilateral calcitonin gene-related peptide changes in jugular venous blood and an awareness of the increasingly well understood trigeminovascular reflex loop, paved the way to new (and at the time of writing, still current) concepts of the probable mechanism of cluster headache. Further studies have generally been supportive of these concepts, but the newer information is too recent to have yet found a definitive place in the corpus of established medical understandings.

In essence, the most recent concept of the cluster headache mechanism is that various factors, many as yet not identified, may activate the suprachiasmatic nuclear area of the hypothalamus and/or the trigeminal afferent side of the trigeminovascular reflex arc. The afferent limb of this arc begins in trigeminal afferents terminals in the periphery or in afferent terminals around extracranial or meningeal blood vessels. The cell bodies of the afferent neurons are in the Gasserian ganglion, and the incoming trigeminal axons terminate in the descending spinal nucleus of the trigeminal (the nucleus caudalis). Afferents from the forehead and scalp synapse in the lowermost part of the nucleus, at the second cervical level. The second neuron in the reflex arc terminates in the superior salivatory nucleus of the medulla oblongata. Parasympathetic efferent axons from neurons in this nucleus leave the brain stem in the nervus intermedius of Wrisberg, then join with and run in the facial nerve, leave it via the greater superficial petrosal nerve, synapse in the greater superficial petrosal ganglion, and then terminate around cranial blood vessels and on cells of the lachrymal glands. Activation anywhere in the afferent limb of this arc is thought to result in pain, particularly in the upper part of the head, and a parasympathetic discharge will occur. Further, trigeminal afferent activation will result in the peripheral release of calcitonin gene-related peptide, leading to consequent vasodilatation. Thus, in the last years of the 20th century, an explanation of the mechanism of cluster headache seems to have been developing that is capable of accounting for not only the pain and the associated vasodilatation of cluster headache, but also for the autonomic (parasympathetic only) features and the periodicity. Time will tell whether the set of ideas will prove correct in the longer term.

The Treatment of Cluster Headache

Because individual attacks of cluster headache are relatively short-lived, compared with typical migraine episodes, it is often difficult to be sure whether any treatment taken at the onset of the pain has really provided relief, rather than simply having been present in the body when the pain resolved spontaneously. Further, the attacks may occur several times a day. Consequently, the literature dealing with treatment of cluster headache has been concerned mainly with the prevention of attacks. It has more or less been accepted that available analgesic agents will be used in an attempt to relieve the pain of individual attacks. However, a few agents have become available that, if administered appropriately, seem capable of providing specific relief of individual cluster headache attacks. With the exception of inhaled oxygen in relatively high concentration, these agents can also serve as attack preventives.

Earlier Therapies

There is little concerning apparently successful treatment of cluster headache recorded in the writings of the earlier authors who described probable instances of the disorder. As mentioned earlier in this chapter, Willis's "venerable matron" "grew perfectly well" after bloodletting and drinking an "electuary." His prescription for the latter was as follows:

> Take of the Conserve of the Flowers of Succory and Fumitory, each three ounces; of the Powder of the Root of Aron compound two drams and a half, of Ivory one dram and a half, of yellow Sanders, and of Lignum Aloes, each half a dram of the Salt of Wormwood one dram and a half, of Vitriol of Steel one dram, of the Syrup of the Five Roots what will suffice to make an Electuary. (1672/1683, p. 124)

Van Swieten (1745) prescribed nothing so elegant or so complicated—he simply employed the Peruvian bark whose quinine content may have rendered it effective against periodic fevers of malarial origin. In earlier times, its known effectiveness in this particular situation caused it to be used indiscriminately, and hopefully, for many other periodically recurring conditions. In the absence of knowledge of the natural history of cluster headache in past centuries, it is understandable that if any prescribed remedy happened to be taken at the time when a cluster of the headache attacks in a sufferer resolved spontaneously, that remedy might be credited with possessing curative properties.

Wilfred Harris (1926), in comparatively modern times, occasionally allowed sufferers to try to obtain pain relief by administering injections of morphia and hyoscine in anticipation of attacks, though this was a course that he did not recommend. In his writings on migrainous neuralgia, and in particular those on his ciliary neuralgia subset, Harris observed that "some cases will benefit notably from luminal," in other words, phenobarbital. He seemed to employ this drug, in conjunction with aspirin, as his medical treatment of first choice, with phenazone and butyl chloral hydrate as less favored alternatives—basically he used simple analgesics and sedatives. He then proceeded to record the following:

> In many sufferers all drugs are useless, though in them some relief may be obtained by a mustard leaf on the back of the neck, by painting Frozoclone on the forehead, or by inhaling the vapour of Chlorylen, twenty or thirty drops on a handkerchief.
>
> Others in which the pain is located over the supra-orbital distribution, in the eyeball or in one fixed spot in the temple may occasionally show brilliant results with alcohol injections of the supra-orbital nerve, of the infra-orbital nerve or the tender spot in the temple itself. (Harris 1926, p. 313)

Harris went on to confess that, on anatomical grounds, it was difficult to explain how injecting the infraorbital nerve could instantly relieve pain in the eyeball, and then suggested that:

> Probably the alcohol injection acts in a reflex manner inhibiting the attacks of vasomotor spasm, and acting in this way it might not matter very much which branch of the fifth nerve is injected, though it is only natural to suppose that reflex inhibition of the vaso-motor meningeal spasm causing the pain is most likely to be successful when that nerve is injected over whose territory the neuralgic pain is referred. (p. 313)

In such an idea, one can see some elements of the present-day theories of cluster headache and migraine pathogenesis: that activity in one part of the trigeminovascular reflex mechanism may produce consequences in other parts.

By the time of his later writing on the disorder, and with increased experience of it, Harris stated the following:

> Since 1909 I have treated a considerable number of migrainous neuralgias with alcohol injections, of either the supra-orbital or the infra-orbital nerves, being guided by the principal location of the pain. Of late years I have, instead, in several cases injected the inner portion of the Gasserian ganglion so as to obtain a permanent anaesthesia and a lasting cure. (1936, p. 458)

Whether Harris's cure really proved lasting is more problematical—Harris (1940-a) indicated that of the 29 cases he had treated with his alcohol injections since 1931, 5 of the 10 who initially showed a good response had subsequently relapsed, though the remaining 19 appeared cured (at least at the time of his reporting).

Horton, from 1939 onward, was chiefly concerned from the therapeutic standpoint with the use of histamine desensitization as a remedy for his "histaminic headache" (Horton et al. 1939). His failure, and that of others, to recognize the existence of spontaneous remission in the disorder, took some time to become apparent. A little more than a decade after Horton's original description, Kunkle et al. wrote the following:

> Improvement in the headaches after an elaborate program of histamine injections has not been shown, by controlled experiments, to be due to a desensitizing effect of this agent. The characteristic tendency of the headache to occur in clusters of unpredictable length, followed by short or long spontaneous remissions, represents a major obstacle in the evaluation of any prophylactic regimen. (1952, p. 242)

While Horton's histamine desensitization approach has long since been abandoned, in one of the case histories in his 1941 paper, there was mention that before being referred to Horton, an attack in this patient had been relieved by injected dihydroergotamine. This was an observation that Horton (1941) did not pursue and that seemingly went unnoticed by others for a time.

Current Therapies

Ergotamine and Dihydroergotamine

As long ago as 1878, a Dr. Schumacher published in the *Lancet* an account of a right-sided headache that woke the sufferer nightly at 2:00 to 2:30 a.m. and that appeared to be controlled by the administration of Ergotin. During the attacks, the arteries in the sufferer's right temple pulsated forcibly. In the morning after the attacks, the sclera of her right eye was injected. This appearance cleared during the day but returned overnight. Whether the available details are sufficient to permit cluster headache to be recognized in retrospect is problematic, but this account may represent the first recorded description of the response of cluster headache to an ergot derivative.

It is usually accepted that Ekbom, in 1943, and again in 1945 (Ekbom 1947), was the first to write of orally administered ergotamine as a successful preventive for cluster headache. However, Harris (1940-b) had mentioned in one of his case histories that a compound tablet containing ergotamine had failed to prevent attacks. Ekbom used the drug in an oral dosage of between 2 and 3 mg a day, and obtained improvement in 13 of

16 sufferers. Kunkle et al. (1952) then found that intravenous ergotamine rapidly terminated individual attacks in 4 of their subjects, and Symonds (1956) reported treating 8 patients successfully with regular, strategically timed, daily or more frequent injections of ergotamine tartrate administered until headache attacks ceased. No therapeutic mishaps occurred. Symonds's higher success rate from injected ergotamine may have resulted from the fact that the consequences of the very low oral bioavailability of the drug (see chapter 6) were not then appreciated. Bickerstaff (1959) followed Symonds's practice in using the drug by regular injection several times a day in his 16 patients. There was only 1 failure, and 12 obtained complete relief from the time of their first injection. Schiller (1962) produced what he considered satisfactory outcomes in 33 of 41 cluster headache sufferers, employing either orally administered or injected ergotamine. Following these reports, regular ergotamine administration came into increasing use as a preventive for cluster headache attacks. It was always appreciated that the drug could be administered orally with success if an adequate but nontoxic dose could be found in the individual sufferer. However, there remained a continuing concern regarding the potential toxicity of the drug, particularly when it was employed in such a pattern of regular use. Consequently, as other agents became available, they gradually took over the role of the preferred cluster headache preventive.

Triptans

When another 5-hydroxytryptamine$_{1B/1D}$ receptor agonist, sumatriptan, became available some years later, it also proved effective in providing relief when injected during individual attacks of cluster headache. Rapidity of absorption issues and an incomplete oral bioavailability made it, like ergotamine, not particularly easy to use orally in relieving existing cluster headaches. As well, sumatriptan's relatively brief elimination half-life of around two hours made the drug inconvenient to employ as an attack preventive, and its use in regular oral administration, perhaps several times a day, proved unduly expensive. The same limitations have applied to many subsequently available triptan derivatives such as zolmitriptan. None of these seems to have achieved any widespread use for cluster headache prevention.

Methysergide

This lysergic acid derivative, later shown to be a 5-HT$_2$ receptor antagonist, was tried with benefit by Sicuteri (1959) in two cases of cluster headache soon after the molecule was synthesized. Other early publications demonstrating its effectiveness included those of Lance et al. (1963) and Lance and Anthony (1971). The history of methysergide use in migraine and cluster headache was recorded by Koehler and Tfelt-Hansen (2008). As experience with methysergide grew, the drug continued to prove reasonably effective in a headache prophylactic role. Unfortunately, its adverse effect profile and subsequent litigation issues (which also surfaced when it was used for migraine management) limited its use and ensured that newer and apparently safer agents, when they became available, would be preferred.

Verapamil

In these recent litigious times, at least in Western society, the calcium channel antagonist verapamil, with a relatively good safety profile, has increasingly taken on the role of the preferred prophylactic against attacks of cluster headache. Evidence of its effectiveness in this regard was provided by authors such as Gabai and Spierings (1989), Bussone et al. (1990), and Leone et al. (2000), particularly after it was realized that higher than conventional oral doses might be needed to achieve optimal effects. The molecular mechanisms whereby verapamil produces its benefit in cluster headache prevention do not appear to have yet been established.

Glucocorticoids

Horton (1964) reported that he had stopped cluster headache attacks occurring in one patient by giving a course of adrenocorticotrophic hormone injections. This report may have stimulated trials of oral corticosteroid administration in cluster headache, but possibly these agents were tried simply because other treatments had not proved adequate. Oral steroids, particularly prednisone or prednisolone, in moderate dosage, have come into reasonably frequent and successful use in the attempt to prevent cluster headache attacks recurring.

There have also been several reports that corticosteroids, usually injected into the suboccipital region near the greater occipital nerve, will prevent headache attacks during a cluster. In one trial, the injected steroid, betamethasone, provided in a short- or a long-acting preparation, proved significantly more effective than a placebo injection in cluster headache treatment (Ambrosini et al. 2005). Whether the injection site, the mode of administration, or the steroid dose, or combinations of these, determines the beneficial response does not seem to have been clarified.

Lithium

On the basis that lithium provided benefit in one periodically recurring disorder, manic-depressive psychosis, Ekbom in 1974 (Ekbom 1977) considered that it might also be useful in the prevention of cluster headache. He (Ekbom 1977) and also Kudrow (1977) published data that were in keeping with this expectation when they were managing the treatment of chronic cluster headache sufferers. Lithium has had some further use in the disorder, despite the necessity of monitoring its plasma concentrations to reduce the risk of toxicity due to overdosage. It has been pointed out that the onset of benefit from lithium in cluster headache sufferers can be delayed for several weeks. As a result, the drug has been employed particularly in managing chronic cluster headache that was refractory to other agents. The apparent delay in the preventive effect of lithium raises the possibility that spontaneous remission of a headache cluster may at times have been mistakenly considered a genuine therapeutic response to the drug. Moreover, Steiner et al. (1997-b) failed to demonstrate benefit from lithium therapy in episodic cluster headache in a placebo-controlled study. If the drug does have a cluster headache–preventing effect, its mode of achieving this, and the drug's apparent success in chronic but not in episodic cluster headache, remains to be explained.

Oxygen

In a significant proportion of cluster headache sufferers, inhalation of 100 percent oxygen during the headache seems to abort the attack. Kudrow (1981) reported pain relief in 75 percent of those so treated. This was a response rate slightly greater than that achieved with sublingual ergotamine, though the limitations of the latter mode of administration of the drug (Sutherland et al. 1974) were not appreciated at the time of Kudrow's report. Fogan (1985) found inhaled oxygen more effective than inhaled air. The oxygen might be expected to produce a vasoconstrictive effect, though it is not clear whether that is the mechanism through which its benefit is achieved in cluster headache.

Melatonin

Leone et al. (1996) showed that melatonin could prevent cluster headache attacks, an interesting finding in the light of the reported altered circadian melatonin rhythms in sufferers (see above).

Wilfred Harris's selective partial destruction of the Gasserian ganglion or of particular trigeminal, greater occipital, and parasympathetic peripheral nerve branches by means of alcohol injection, and direct surgical severance of such nervous structures, have all tended to fall from favor as time has passed. Nevertheless, as recently as 1993, Kirkpatrick et al. described the relative effectiveness of trigeminal root section in medically intractable chronic migrainous neuralgia. Once evidence was obtained that there was activation of a localized part of the hypothalamus during cluster headache attacks, the possibility of electrical deactivation of this region was explored. Stereotaxic placement of electrodes in the requisite site, with subsequent electrical stimulation of the region via these, was reported to be successful in two subjects (Leone et al. 2001). There were subsequent reports of benefit from the procedure.

In comparatively recent years, a considerable amount of information has been amassed concerning the pathogenic mechanism of cluster headache, and this has resulted in some new treatment approaches being devised for sufferers who do not respond to the more customary therapeutic measures. At the time of writing, it is uncertain how much of the accumulating recent data will find a lasting place in the understanding of this type of headache, and how much will gradually fade from memory because it will have led nowhere or will have been deemed flawed.

CHRONIC PAROXYSMAL HEMICRANIA

This entity is appreciably less common than cluster headache and, unlike the latter, is more often encountered in women. Simplistically, its clinical features are similar to those of cluster headache but the attacks are shorter and more frequent. However, the disorder has a different pattern of therapeutic responsiveness, with indomethacin providing specific headache prevention. Chronic paroxysmal hemicrania as an entity was first described by Sjaastad and Dale (1974). Many of the earlier subsequent publications concerning the disorder emanated from Sjaastad's and other Nordic sources. In retrospect, the disorder may have been described long ago by Oppermann (1747) under the designation *hemicrania horologica*. He gave an account of a 35-year-old woman who had bouts of hemicranial pain that lasted for 15 minutes and recurred regularly every hour. In reporting a very similar instance a quarter of a millennium later, Granella and D'Andrea (2003) advanced the view that neither case was really an instance of chronic paroxysmal hemicrania because the timing of the recurrent attacks was too regular, and because no features of autonomic disturbance were mentioned in either report. It seems unlikely that the issue of diagnosis in Oppermann's case so long ago can ever be settled definitively.

The individual attacks of chronic paroxysmal hemicrania last from 2 to 45 minutes, and occur from 1 to 40 times a day. The pain distribution, in the upper anterior part of the head, is similar to that which applies in cluster headache, and the attacks are accompanied by the same pattern of autonomic disturbance, though the features of this disturbance may often be incomplete. In a significant minority of cases, sudden neck movement seems to induce the attacks (Sjaastad 1987). Oral dosage of indomethacin, up to 150 mg per day, is effective in suppressing the attacks within a few days of commencement of intake. The disorder seems to exist in both episodic and chronic forms (Sjaastad 1987). Details of the disorder were documented in reviews such as those of Russell (1984), Sjaastad (1987), and Goadsby and Lipton (1997).

Although chronic paroxysmal hemicrania might be regarded merely as a cluster headache variant, just as cluster headache itself was for a time often considered a migraine variant, there are grounds for regarding chronic paroxysmal hemicrania as an independent headache disorder of currently unexplained origin. The main sources of clinical distinction between it and cluster headache are the different gender distributions of the two disorders, the shorter duration and more frequent occurrence of the individual attacks, the different responsiveness to indomethacin, and the provocation of chronic paroxysmal hemicrania attacks by neck movement. Further, Sjaastad (1987) reported that heating of the sufferer's body induced increased sweating on the pain-affected side of the forehead in chronic paroxysmal hemicrania attacks, but caused decreased sweating on the affected side in cluster headache attacks. This was an opposite pattern of response to that produced by injected pilocarpine.

It seems reasonable to speculate that both chronic paroxysmal hemicrania and cluster headache may involve a similar disturbance in a final common pathway mechanism in the trigeminovascular reflex arc, and in the interplay of the suprachiasmatic nucleus with the arc. However, the underlying genetic background and attack initiating mechanisms of the two entities appear to differ, though neither seems to have yet been clarified adequately.

There is another apparently time-determined headache syndrome that was first reported by Raskin in 1988: hypnic headache. In this disorder, episodes of variably located headache, more often bilateral than unilateral, wake older adults from sleep at fixed hours. The disorder itself appears to be benign. No features of cranial autonomic disturbance are discernable, but the nocturnal occurrence of the headache might allow these, if they were present, to go unnoticed. The time pattern of attack recurrence suggests affinities to the disorders discussed immediately above. It is currently unclear where the syndrome will find its definitive place in headache classifications.

SUNCT AND SUNA

Sjaastad and his school (Sjaastad et al. 1989) provided the initial description of the SUNCT syndrome (short-lasting unilateral neuralgiform headache attacks with conjunctival injection and tearing), as well as that of chronic paroxysmal hemicrania. The pain of SUNCT is even more short-lived than that of chronic paroxysmal hemicrania. Each episode lasts for no more than four minutes, and episodes recur at least 20 times a day. The pain may be throbbing or stabbing in character, and is moderately severe. According to Cohen et al. (2006), the International Headache Society considered that SUNCT might be part of a similar disorder with a wider spectrum of autonomic manifestations that was designated as SUNA (short-lasting unilateral neuralgiform headache attacks with cranial autonomic features). These are rare and comparatively newly recognized entities, and much of the literature concerning them originates in the 21st century. At the time of writing, they have been recognized too recently to have accumulated much burden of history, or for their mechanisms of production to have been investigated to any considerable extent.

HEMICRANIA CONTINUA

As mentioned at the beginning of this chapter, when Goadsby and Lipton (1997) enunciated the idea of trigeminal autonomic cephalalgia, they included within the concept an entity, hemicrania continua, which the International Headache Society later decided should not remain within the new headache category, and should be classified otherwise. As described (Sjaastad and Spierings 1984), hemicrania continua is uncommon and comprises continuous unilateral headache with temporary exacerbations and the presence of some autonomic features, though these are not as prominent as those that occur in the accepted trigeminal autonomic cephalalgias. Hemicrania continua is often responsive to indomethacin. However, Warner (1997) reported an instance of the disorder that recovered only after analgesic intake, including that of indomethacin, was ceased. Until the status of the condition is clarified as more data become available, it is difficult to consider the history of its medical understanding in any useful way.

Relationships between the recognized entities within a category as recently designated as that of the trigeminal autonomic cephalalgias may not yet be finally settled. It is likely that the overall category itself will prove valid, but the story of the understanding of the individual entities that are contained within the category may need rethinking if increasing knowledge suggests that the current categorization of the disorders has unacceptable shortcomings.

CHAPTER 8
Tension-Type Headache

At first sight, it may seem rather surprising that relatively little has been published concerning the history of tension-type headache when it is generally considered the most frequent variety of headache that occurs in the community (Kunkle 1959). The character of this type of headache was described in the First International Classification of Headache as follows:

> The pain is typically pressing/tightening in quality, of mild or moderate intensity, bilateral in location and does not worsen with routine physical activity. Nausea is absent, but photophobia or phonophobia may be present. (Headache Classification Committee 1988, p. 29)

Tension-type headache was further subdivided in the 1988 Headache Classification into episodic and chronic varieties, and additional diagnostic criteria for each were provided. The subdivision of tension headache was taken further in the Second International Classification of Headache (Headache Classification Committee 2004). There, some concern was expressed that the earlier definition may have allowed instances of milder migraine without aura to be included in the tension headache category. Nonetheless, the 1988 definition is likely to have been the one that the contemporary generation of clinicians who wrote about headache before 2000 would have employed when applying diagnostic criteria to their patients' headaches. The lay view of tension headache seems to be even broader than the medical one, and may take in almost any headache that is not particularly severe and cannot otherwise be readily explained.

When the 1988 International Headache Society criteria were applied by Rasmussen et al. (1991) to a randomly selected population of Danish adults aged between 25 and 64 years, some 74 percent were found to have experienced tension-type headache, as compared with 10 percent who had suffered migraine. Further, 87 percent of those with migraine also had tension-type headache. Only 1 percent of the tension-type headache sufferers considered that their headaches were severe. The pain was considered moderate in severity in 58 percent and mild in the remainder. By way of contrast, 85 percent of the migraine sufferers considered that their pain was severe. This difference in perceived severity between the two types of headache may have something to do with the comparative neglect in the earlier medical literature of scientific aspects of tension-type headache. It may also go some way toward explaining the relative dearth of material that deals with the history of this particular headache disorder. On the whole, persons with tension-type headache might be expected to be less likely than migraine sufferers to seek medical help for their discomfort. Further, those to whom they went for such help, if they did, may have been less likely to give priority to thinking about comparatively mild headaches when at much the same time they were being called on to deal with more serious and more obtrusive health problems. It is also possible that our comparatively recent ancestors were prepared to cope without the aid of medical ministrations when experiencing degrees of cranial discomfort for which more recent generations have come to expect prompt relief through medical means.

HISTORY OF TENSION-TYPE HEADACHE PHENOMENA

If an Internet search is carried out in the earlier medical literature for the term "tension headache" (the earlier of the two terminological predecessors to the current version "tension-type headache"), instances of the use of the words may be found both in later 19th-century writings and subsequently. However, in most of these instances the juxtaposed words are separated by a comma. In that case, the word pair has not been employed as the name for a single headache entity. Instead, the word *tension* in the combination has referred to the arterial blood pressure, to the intracranial pressure or, occasionally, to the intraocular pressure, and the word *headache* has referred to an associated painful head state. The word pair *tension headache* without an intervening comma did, however, appear in two consecutive papers that were published in the *California State Medical Journal* of 1909 (Franklin 1909; Shiels 1909). There the pair of words did represent a single headache entity, which was further divided into *plus* and *minus* tension varieties. In these two papers, *tension* referred to the tension of the arterial pulse. It is obvious that what was referred to was not present-day tension-type headache but something akin to the older concept of plethoric and anemic headaches (chapter 1). In 1921, Hughson provided an indication of what he meant by the term: "Increased intracranial pressure has long been recognized as a cause of headache; to this type the term 'tension headache' has been applied" (p. 1859).

The term *tension* or *tension-type headache*, used in its present-day sense, or in something close to it, seems to have first appeared in the medical literature around the end of the World War II (1945). It was then used in such a way that it seems to have been expected that readers would already be familiar with it, or at least would not be perplexed by it. At that time, the word *tension* was usually taken to refer to psychological tension rather than to any actual physical pressure, or feeling of physical pressure, experienced in or on some part of the body surface. Friedman and von Storch set out their view of the matter, one that seems to have become fairly generally accepted at the time, at least in the North American literature:

> We believe that the term "tension headache" should be limited to headache occurring in relation to constant or periodic emotional conflicts of which the patients are usually partially aware. Such an emotional state may induce headache by producing changes in the caliber of the cranial vessels and concomitant spasm of the skeletal muscles of the head and neck. The background and pathophysiological mechanism for this headache is similar in many ways to the migraine syndrome. However, tension headaches have no prodromata, are usually bilateral occipital or frontal, and may be accompanied by a variety of associated signs including anxiety, nausea and vomiting. Frequency and duration are variable.
>
> Tension headaches may be differentiated from migraine in that the latter are paroxysmal, unilateral, throbbing, frequently associated with gastrointestinal symptoms and often preceded by an aura. A family history of such headache is prevalent. These factors are infrequent in tension headache. (1953, p. 1128)

At much the same time, Leslie and Dunsworth wrote the following:

> The simple psychoneurotic headache is typically a "tension headache," and may be explained on the basis of hypertonic musculature of the scalp, particularly the temporals. It is felt as a dull chronic superficial discomfort, poorly localized; the tension is obvious too in generalized symptoms throughout the body. (1947, p. 509)

Butler and Thomas also considered tension headaches to be of psychological origin, stating of them, "Basically they are psychosomatic in origin and respond only to psychiatric therapy" (1947, p. 970). In 1956 Drake reviewed the topic of tension headache, and described the features of the headache as follows:

> It occurs in relation to constant or periodic emotional conflict which may be conscious or unconscious. Tension headaches have no prodromata, are usually bilateral, occipital, or frontal, and may be accompanied by anxiety (free-floating or somatized) and such symptoms as nausea and vomiting, dizziness, weakness, irritability, and constipation.

The frequency and duration are variable, but an attack may last for weeks. The discomfort has been described by various authors as "constant, and boring, unlike the throbbing quality of the migraine headache," "bizarre, rarely interfering with sleep, a tight feeling as of a band around the head," "vague and dull, or a sensation of pressure in the head"; "a dull aching tenseness in the neck"; "head caught in a vise, or scalp on too tight, or top of my head blowing off"; "tends to be worse toward evening when the patient is nervous or tired"; "the pain begins in the occipital zone, extends into the forehead and may center there or in the vertex"; and "poorly defined, with a complete lack of any features characterizing them as another type of headache." The patient tends to have a worried and unhappy facial expression but otherwise may present the picture of robust health. (p. 105)

It seems scarcely conceivable that humans had not been subject to emotional stresses before the mid-20th century, and did not sometimes experience headache in relation to such situations. The question therefore arises as to whether tension headache was recognized under some other name prior to the recent half century. Aring (1959), when dealing with the topic of tension headache, provided Wolff's mid-20th-century answer to this question: that what was at that time called *tension headache* had previously been termed indurative, myalgic, nodular, or rheumatic headache. However, Weatherhead's (1835) account of rheumatic headache does not correlate particularly well with the descriptions of mid-20th-century tension headache, though Weatherhead held that the site of his rheumatic headache was "the aponeurosis covering either the temporal or the occipito-frontalis muscle." Weatherhead stated that rheumatic headache was invariably due to exposure of the head to cold. The pain was severe, aching, and heavy, and could be hemicranial in distribution, though it was not pulsatile in character. It was associated with the presence of rheumatism and rheumatic ophthalmia. There were other accounts of rheumatic headache of a rather similar character to that of Weatherhead (e.g., Copland 1858; Corning 1888). Auerbach's (1913) account of what he termed "nodular or rheumatic" headache suggests that this disorder may have overlapped, and perhaps even coincided with, the later accepted category of tension-type headache, though a reader really cannot be sure. Campbell was rather scathing about the entity of rheumatic headache, as it had been described up to his time of writing: "The terms 'rheumatic' and 'arthritic' headache have been used very obscurely, and it is generally quite impossible to identify these headaches from the descriptions given" (1894, p. 208).

Silas Weir Mitchell had earlier perceived an attitudinal difference between North American and British writers on the matter:

As concerns headache, its causes and cures, if we leave out migraine, I do not know a subject in medicine so unsatisfactory in its literature. In England, when all other possible causes fail it is said to be gouty. Gout being there an easy and credible answer to all medical riddles. Indeed; it is curious to see how much it figures as a cause in English medical books, while with us it is, in truth, a disease so rare that probably many country practitioners have never seen a case of acute gout. I myself have seen, in three years, one instance of really acute gout. In fact gout went out when Madeira became a possible wine to the very rich alone.

In place of gout as a hidden cause of headaches, I find the American physician apt to fall back upon neuralgia or rheumatism, and no doubt neuralgic headaches are common enough in all their forms, and are often to be dealt with, I think, as neuralgias of the meningeal branches of the fifth nerve. As to rheumatic headaches, they at least are rare, very rare; that is, occasional fits of pain in the head distinctly to be traced to rheumatism. (1874/1963, p. 70)

No doubt, there had been other accounts of what would pass for tension headache prior to mid-20th century under designations other than the unsatisfactory ones mentioned by Aring (see above). For instance, in the following account, Mitchell provides a description of a headache that he attributed to brain overuse, but which a century later would probably have been considered an example of tension-type headache:

A lad, aged seventeen, worked very hard in a printing-office for two years, during which time he prepared himself for college, where he studied with unusual success and patience. He had a good memory, and acquired readily, but gave himself little rest or sleep, and scarce any physical exercise. Disturbance of that physiological balance which is to be kept by functional alternations of rest and work, told on him after a year, and, without warning, or sense of failing power, late, one night, while preparing for an examination, he began for the first time to have an uneasy sense of pain and distress at the vertex. Next day it was gone, but it began anew when he went to recitation, and thence forward was the inevitable result of severe or long use of the brain. By degrees it grew more common, until any, even the least, intellection, or even steady attention, reading, writing, or calculating, brought it on. By this time it was found that with it came a certain tenderness of the scalp, not always over the seat of pain, but often occipital. Finally, there was added a feeling of distress high up in the cervical region, but no other disturbance of health in any other organ. He had also, for a time, insomnia; but this is much better, and troubles him but little. (1874/1963, p. 73)

It seems to have been only from the mid-20th century onward that the clinical picture of the set of phenomena embraced by the idea of tension-type headache became settled in medical thought, but interpretations of the headache mechanism and its causation continued to range rather widely. As a consequence of this uncertainty as to pathogenesis, the name of tension headache soon became altered to that of *contraction headache* and then, in the 1980s, to the present version of *tension-type headache*. The reasons for these changes are more easily followed in relation to the evolution of the understanding of what is thought to be the tension-type headache mechanism.

MECHANISM OF TENSION-TYPE HEADACHE

Psychological and Muscle Tension Aspects

If it is accepted that before mid-20th century, tension-type headache was recognized under other designations such as that of rheumatic headache, then it seems probable that disorders such as rheumatism or rheumatic fever were believed to be responsible for producing this type of headache. However, the earlier literature did not make clear how these disease processes led to the head pain. From what has been discussed thus far in this chapter, it seems far from clear that any of the earlier described types of headache really corresponded at all closely to present-day tension-type headache. Therefore one really can take up the story of the understanding of the mechanism of tension-type headache no earlier than the period around the middle of the 20th century, when the term *tension headache* began to be used with its present-day meaning.

In the earlier stages of the use of the term *tension headache*, as illustrated by the various material from the literature cited so far in this chapter, it is clear that the word *tension* referred primarily to emotional tension or emotional stress. There were suggestions as to how the emotional state produced headache. For instance, Moench presented one theory:

> The role played by emotional tension cannot be overstressed. . . . Higher animals and primitive man were constantly beset by physical dangers, by larger and more ferocious animals, storms, hunger and the importunate urgings of the testicles. The senses of smell, hearing and sight were a principal defense mechanisms on guard at all times and doubly alerted in times of threat. Raising the nose, eyes and ears as high as possible by lifting the face was accomplished by the contraction of the posterior nuchal muscles. In modern society the physical dangers have been replaced by abstract dangers, the grizzly bears by stock market bears, the thunderstorm by the evangelist, the tribal chieftain by the policeman or the tax collector. Despite the intellectualization of our stresses, many people react in the primitive pattern and face them with head-up alertness, suffering a residual tension in the neck muscles. (1947, pp. 115–116)

Drake (1956) explained that persisting emotional tension caused sustained contraction of the skeletal muscles of the head and neck, and that this resulted in pain perhaps produced by the muscle spasm causing ischemia of the muscles that were involved.

It was the human experimental research carried out by Harold Wolff, more than anything else, that seemed to provide a moderately satisfactory explanation for the way in which the emotional state of the sufferer could bring about headache. The pain in the head was interpreted as being mediated by excessive degrees of contraction in the muscles of the back of the neck and the occipital-frontalis muscles. On the basis of his experimental studies, Wolff described his interpretation of the tension headache mechanism:

> The exceedingly common "tension headache" found in emotionally tense, aggressive, frustrated and anxious people was also associated with electromyographic evidence of prolonged contraction of the muscles of the head and neck. Vasoconstriction of the nutrient arteries and arterioles during such periods of duress and sustained contraction, by furthering the ischemia of the skeletal muscles, may be an additional factor in the resultant headache. Injection with physiologic saline solution of especially tender areas caused an increase in head sensations and pain, whereas injection of 1 percent procaine solution into such areas eliminated untoward head sensations. Furthermore, reduction or elimination of tension by changing the subject's emotions and attitudes by modification of the life situation, and by administration of phenobarbital reduced or eliminated muscle contraction, pressure or tight sensations, and headache. (1963, pp. 692–693)

Wolff's extensive series of investigations into headache mechanisms had also shown the following:

> "Pain and tightness in the back of the head and neck are frequent complaints. The sensations are variously described as: a stiff cap, vise-like, a weight, pressure, a tight band, a cramp, drawing, aching, sore, etc. Tenderness throughout the trapezius muscle is commonly associated with these complaints and is most intense along the top of the shoulders and in the upper neck. Another common complaint is that of pain, pressure, or paresthesia over the vertex of the head. Here, tension in the neck is less obvious, but pain can usually be elicited by palpation of the trapezius muscles. . . . . . .
>
> Observations were made in patients with pain in the occiput and neck associated with inflammation or other dysfunction about the head (pan-sinusitis, migraine headache, and cap-like, vise, or pressure sensations). It was found that in these subjects there was sustained contraction of the neck and head muscles. The intensity of the pain in the neck and over the back of the head could be modified by changing the muscle state." (Wolff 1963, pp. 691–692)

Wolff's account made it clear that he believed that he had demonstrated that sustained contraction in the extracranial muscles and the posterior neck muscles that resulted from emotional tension and personality traits was the explanation of the entity originally described as tension headache. He also believed that the same headache-producing mechanism could be activated by other causes and could result in a descriptively similar pattern of headache, one that was also brought about by heightened tension in the muscles of the scalp and the back of the neck. Thus an ambiguity existed in that the word *tension* could refer to the emotional state or to the state of head and neck muscle contraction present in the headache sufferer, or to both. Further, by the mid-20th century, the laity had become increasingly aware of psychological issues and attuned to the idea of psychologically caused illness. They therefore found it increasingly easy to accept the idea that the word *tension* used in relation to headache referred to a psychological cause of the headache, and perhaps to all headache. This interpretation led to the implication that the tension headache sufferer was deficient in the capacity to cope with the ordinary pressures of life, lacking in moral fiber, even when he or she might in reality be suffering from physical illness. It was probably partly to resolve this difficulty that the 1962 Classification of Headache (Ad Hoc Committee 1962) replaced the term *tension* in the categorization of types of headache with the word *contraction*. In doing this, what had begun its existence as a type of headache with a presumed cause instead became a type of headache with a presumed mechanism. The 1962 definition read as follows:

> Muscle-Contraction Headache. Ache or sensations of tightness, pressure, or constriction, widely varied in intensity, frequency, and duration, sometimes long-lasting, and commonly sub-occipital. It is associated with sustained contraction of skeletal muscles in the absence of permanent structural change, usually as part of the individual's reaction during life stress. The ambiguous and unsatisfactory terms "tension," "psychogenic," and "nervous" headache refer largely to this group. (Ad Hoc Committee 1962, pp. 174–175)

In the years between the 1962 and 1988 headache classifications, problems arose in relation to the diagnosis of contraction headache in individual sufferers. Studies employing electromyography did not consistently show electric evidence of increased muscle activity in the presumably abnormally contracted head and neck muscles in such persons during, and in the intervals between, their headaches. Various explanations for this inconsistency were suggested—for example, sampling of inappropriate muscles or inappropriate parts of muscles that were assumed to have been in a state of heightened contraction. By the time of the 1988 International Headache Classification, it appeared that electromyography had proven no more satisfactory than palpation of the assumed abnormally contracted muscle in detecting states of excessive muscle contraction or tightness. It also appeared that typical contraction headache was sometimes present without there being detectable degrees of abnormal muscle tightness. Biochemical investigations measuring lactate concentrations within tender muscle areas failed to obtain evidence to support Wolff's idea that excessive muscle contraction produced muscle ischemia (Ashina et al. 2002). *Contraction headache* as a term then disappeared from the 1988 Classification of Headache, replaced by *tension-type headache*. This solved one difficulty, but at the price of leaving the headache entity bereft of a name that conveyed much sense of either its cause or its mechanism. Time will show whether this change in nomenclature will prove satisfactory, though one suspects that, except among the headache cognoscenti, usage will gradually lapse back to *tension headache*. Then the old ambiguities may resurface in some form or other.

In the late 20th century, while these difficulties in terminology and understanding were becoming obvious and their solution was being sought, a further difficulty in relation to the concept of contraction headache existed. This difficulty may have led to a number of unresolved problems regarding the interpretation of the mechanism and outcome of treatment of tension-type headache. In the quotation from Wolff's work (cited a few lines above), the association of neck muscle contraction headache with migraine was mentioned. The association was also noted in the Danish study of headache epidemiology (Rasmussen et al. 1991). When he summarized his ideas on the pathophysiology of migraine itself, Wolff wrote, after describing the vascular changes of the migraine headache,

> Secondary to such prolonged pain and distension of cranial arteries, skeletal muscles of the head and neck contract. Prolonged muscle contraction in itself becomes painful, and adds a component to the migraine headache which may outlast the vascular pain. (1963, p. 682)

That is, the postulated contraction or tension-type headache mechanism could come into play in the later stages of migraine attacks. Therefore if a patient experienced, for instance, a not particularly severe attack of migraine without aura, that headache might be interpreted as having been an episodic contraction or tension-type one from the outset, particularly if the sufferer was not assessed until late in the episode. There then might have been two different established types of headache actually present in what would be perceived as a single headache episode. The 2004 International Classification of Headaches acknowledged this possibility (as mentioned above), but it does not always seem to have been taken into account, at least in pre-2004 investigations into the mechanism of tension-type headache, when sufferers from migraine were sometimes used as control subjects.

The 1988 International Headache Classification resolved the difficulty arising from the inconsistent recognition of excessive head muscle contraction in tension-type headache in that it designated varieties with, and without, recognizable excessive muscle contraction. This, however, raised the issue of the mechanism of headache production in those with tension-type headache without detectable excessive muscle contraction. Some investigators pursued more sensitive and more reliable investigative methods for recognizing muscle overcontraction (e.g., Sakai et al. 1995; Ashina et al. 1999-b). These studies demonstrated that increased tightness was present in the trapezii and posterior neck muscles of tension-type headache sufferers. Others sought an explanation in different possible headache-producing mechanisms. The latter investigations of tension-type headache mechanisms have fallen into three main groups: genetic, biochemical, and pain pathway studies.

Genetic Investigations

The study of Ostergaard et al. (1997) showed that the risk of tension-type headache in first-degree relatives of chronic tension-type headache sufferers was increased threefold, suggesting that a genetic predisposition to the disorder existed, its inheritance probably being multifactorial. A twin pair study, in which one twin had frequent episodic tension-type headache, has suggested that an additive genetic effect existed in this population (Ulrich et al. 2004). The possibility may need to be kept in mind that these outcomes could have been influenced if instances of migraine-initiated tension-type headache, with the well-established inheritability of migraine, had inadvertently been included in the populations of tension-type headache sufferers that were studied. Inevitably, headache diagnosis is heavily dependent on information provided by sufferers, and the reliability of such data, even when obtained firsthand, may not always be as great as could be wished, particularly when the matter that is of concern did not occur recently.

Biochemical Studies

In the past two decades, concentrations of various biological molecules have been measured in the body fluids of tension-type headache sufferers, both during the presence of headache and, in episodic varieties of the disorder, in the intervals between headaches. No clear and consistent picture has emerged, and in particular no persuasive biochemical evidence has been obtained that would permit a satisfactory sharp distinction between tension-type headache and migraine. Indeed, Ashina et al. (2000-b) found interictal plasma concentrations of calcitonin gene-related peptide were increased in patients with migraine and in those with episodic tension-type headache in whom the pain had a throbbing character, which would suggest affinities in pathophysiology between the two disorders. Again, in the various investigations, the possibility of contamination of the tension-type headache population studied by unrecognized migraine may have existed, particularly in studies carried out when headache was absent.

Serotonin

Probably because changes in plasma and platelet serotonin levels had been reported in migraine sufferers, circulatory concentrations of this indolealkylamine were measured in persons with tension-type headaches. The interpretation of the values obtained suffers from the same uncertainties and limitations that apply when this substance is measured in migraine, as was mentioned earlier in this book (chapter 5). The values that have been reported have not been entirely consistent between the published studies, the serotonin concentrations sometimes being raised, sometimes normal, and sometimes reduced (Ferrari 1993).

The first study to attract attention to the area appears to have been that of Shulka et al. (1987), who showed that platelets from tension-type headache sufferers took up significantly more serotonin than platelets from migraine sufferers and normal subjects. It was not made clear whether the platelets were collected while headache was present. In later and often better designed studies, platelet serotonin concentration has either been normal or has been reduced (Ferrari et al. 1989; Shimomura and Takahashi 1990; Bendtsen et al. 1997), but platelet serotonin is essentially in storage rather than being readily available for biological activity. Also, platelet serotonin concentrations have been found to be reduced in migraine sufferers during their attacks (Ferrari and Saxena 1993). It is not clear whether the reported changes in serotonin concentration in plasma, and platelets, in tension-type headache are genuine, and if genuine, have any causal role in headache production, or are merely secondary, to perhaps the existence of head pain.

Catecholamines

Castillo et al. (1994) noted reduced concentrations of plasma adrenaline, noradrenaline, and dopamine during attacks of episodic tension-type headache, and Takeshima et al. (1989) recorded reduced plasma noradrenaline levels in persons diagnosed with contraction headache. Dopamine-β-hydroxylase levels were reduced in tension-type headache, but also in migraine (Gallai et al. 1992). Although such findings are consistent with reduced catecholaminergic function, they do not appear to be specific to tension-type headache and may represent, for instance, a reactive change in response to the presence of head pain.

Melatonin

A single study (Claustrat et al. 1989) found reduced nocturnal plasma melatonin concentrations in females with tension-type headache. The relevance of this finding is unclear.

Peptides

Concentrations of various opioid and other endogenous peptides have been measured in the CSF of relatively small numbers of tension-type headache sufferers. The changes that have been found appear to be neither easily interpreted nor useful in distinguishing between such headaches and migraine. Mazzotta et al. (1997) found reduced levels of β-endorphin and substance P in blood mononuclear cells in tension-type headache sufferers. The interpretations of these various findings concerning biological peptides were not made particularly clear when the findings were reported.

So far, it appears that ethically acceptable biochemical studies carried out on accessible human biological materials have not produced unambiguous information concerning the mechanism of headache production in tension-type headache.

Pain Pathway Studies

There is recent evidence consistent with cervical muscle pain being related to increased concentrations of various pain-producing endogenous chemicals (e.g., bradykinin, calcitonin gene-related peptide, substance P, noradrenaline, and serotonin) at myofascial trigger points in these muscles (Fernandez-de-las-Peñas et al. 2007). As well, there are data consistent with continued nociceptive impulses arising from such muscle sites producing a state of central facilitation of pain impulse transmission, possibly mediated through the agency of nitric oxide (Ashina et al. 1999-a; 1999-c; 2000-a).

For instance, nitric oxide synthase inhibition led to relief of the pain of tension-type headache. The central facilitation, or loss of suppression, of nociceptive transmission occurs at the level of the dorsal horn of the spinal cord and the analogous descending spinal nucleus of the trigeminal nerve. The facilitation leads to an augmented perception of pain. The central physiological suppressive process appears to be mediated mainly by serotonergic neurotransmission. A similar loss of suppression in the central pain pathway from the head appears to develop during migraine attacks.

Such a pain facilitatory process could explain an exaggeration of preexisting pain, but whether it could also be the primary initiating process responsible for the syndrome of tension-type headache in the absence of detectable head and neck muscle overcontraction or excessive tightness is more doubtful, though it is not inconceivable (Goadsby 1999). Possibly emotionally driven head and neck muscle overcontraction could sometimes be the instigating event, with reduced central nociceptive suppression providing a secondary pain-reinforcing and -perpetuating mechanism. If the latter were true, other causes of neck and head muscle pain might also be expected to result in pain resembling that of tension-type headache, something that half a century ago Wolff (1963) had suggested was the case in relation to migraine attacks. There is some epidemiological evidence in favor of this view (Goadsby 1999).

TREATMENT OF TENSION-TYPE HEADACHE

As a recognized entity, tension-type headache, under its various guises, is little more that a half century old, so that its therapeutics have had relatively little time to accumulate any considerable burden of history. Further, the content of what has accumulated has usually been determined in awareness of present-day criteria of therapeutic efficacy, so that no substantial pharmacopoeia of dubious or ineffective antiheadache agents has come into existence, unlike the situation that applies for a more venerable headache disorder such as migraine.

For episodic tension-type headache, particularly when infrequent, management has often involved little more than providing relief with simple, readily available analgesics or, later, nonsteroidal anti-inflammatory agents while waiting for the spontaneous resolution of the headache. Some placebo-controlled trials have been carried out showing that at least some of these simple analgesic agents possess some demonstrable degree of therapeutic efficacy in this situation (Bendtsen et al. 2010).

When frequent episodic or chronic tension-type headache first became recognizable in its present character in the medical literature, the disorder was believed to be of emotional origin. As mentioned earlier in this chapter, once the headache had been present for an appreciable period of time, the appropriate treatment was thought to be along psychological lines, for example psychotherapy, relaxation training, EMG feedback, cognition-behavioral therapy, and hypnotherapy (Melis et al. 1991). Such psychological, or perhaps formal psychiatric, management often required a considerable deal of time. Therefore, almost inevitably, remedies that might produce results more speedily tended to be employed first.

Physical therapy has a long record of use in treating chronic and frequent episodic tension-type headache, without a great deal of published evidence on its efficacy. The measures used have included those that have sometimes overlapped with psychological approaches (e.g., EMG feedback), but also manipulation, massage, and the local application of heat or cold to tender, tight head and neck muscles. In the mid-20th century, sedative drugs such as phenobarbital were used, presumably to dampen any emotional element involved in the pathogenesis of the headache. As additional, and more specific, psychotropic drugs became available, these also were tried. Several studies showed reasonably persuasive evidence that the tricyclic antidepressant agent amitriptyline was effective in reducing the severity of the headache in this situation (Lance and Curran 1964; Diamond and Baltes 1971; Göbel et al. 1994). There is some evidence that other antidepressants may also be effective, though not the rather widely used serotonin reuptake inhibitors sertraline (Singh and Misra 2002) and citralopram (Bendtsen et al. 1996). The failure of two relatively specific serotonin reuptake inhibitors in a situation in which drugs that impair reuptake of both serotonin and catecholamines are effective might be thought to provide some clue to the pathogenesis of tension-type headache. However, amitriptyline is also effective in migraine prophylaxis, and in that disorder it has been suggested that its benefit is derived from enhancing central suppression of nociceptive impulses in the descending spinal nucleus of the trigeminal. Drugs that produce muscle relaxation—for example, diazepam, tizanidine, and botulinum toxin—have also been employed, though the latter does not seem to have found an established place in the treatment of the disorder and failed to provide convincing evidence of benefit in a reasonably well designed clinical trial (Rollnik et al. 2000).

The approach that medicine has adopted to the management of tension-type headache over the past half century has been predicated on concepts of the pathogenesis of the disorder, and these concepts do not seem to have been entirely satisfactory. There is evidence that some of the treatment methods employed have been of genuine benefit in some instances. However, many tension-type headache sufferers seem to require relatively little in the way of formal medical measures after they find their way to sources of medical advice and then come to accept that they do not suffer from a disorder that threatens physical well-being or life. The history of tension-type headache and its management leaves a sense of disquiet that the whole situation at the end of the 20th century was still not adequately understood, though new insights were then becoming available (Goadsby 1999).

CERVICOGENIC HEADACHE

The entity termed *cervicogenic headache* was not placed among the primary headaches in the International Headache Classification of 2004, because the disorder is believed to originate from pathological conditions present in the neck. It therefore was regarded as a symptomatic headache. Cervicogenic headache, as the term is currently understood, came to medical notice comparatively recently following a paper written by Sjaastad et al. (1983). It has not yet had time to acquire a history of any great length, or even for its diagnostic criteria to be firmly settled. However, one of Sjaastad's pupils, Torbjørn Fredriksen (1989), in a dissertation has traced reports of what seem to have been the condition back to Bärtschi-Rochaix (1948), who thought that there may have had been an even earlier account given by Schützenberger in 1853. Barré (1926) may have described the same condition under the designation of the "syndrome sympathetique cervical posterior." The clinical features of cervicogenic headache appear to resemble rather closely those of tension-type headache, except that the former is one-sided and the latter bilateral, at least in typical instances. Cervicogenic headache seems to warrant further brief mention in the present context.

Sjaastad et al. (1983), following their identification of the disorder of chronic paroxysmal hemicrania (Sjaastad and Dale 1974), seem to have recognized that among their headache patients there was a group of persons with unilateral headache that did not conform to the clinical pattern of migraine, cluster headache, or chronic paroxysmal hemicrania. Over a two-year period, they identified 22 sufferers from the new disorder (19 of them new headache cases), compared with 10 new instances of cluster headache. Thus the new disorder was not especially rare in the headache population that was studied by Sjaastad et al. (1983). Some two-thirds of the cases of the new disorder, which they termed "cervicogenic headache," were female. They suffered from persistently unilateral head pain that never changed sides. It tended to be maximal toward the front of the head and in the temple, but could extend to the shoulder and arm on the same side. The severity of the pain varied from time to time. It might be present intermittently or continuously, though with fluctuations in severity that lasted from minutes to days. Accompanying the pain there could be slight lachrymation, redness of the eyeball, running of the nose, and blurring of the vision of the eye on the affected side. In severe episodes, nausea was sometimes experienced. The pain could be brought on, or increased, by neck movement, coughing, sneezing, or the effort to defecate. The neck tended to feel stiff, and its mobility might be restricted. Pressure applied over the second cervical nerve root on the affected side, on the greater occipital nerve or over the fourth and fifth cervical transverse processes, evoked pain similar to the sufferer's spontaneous headache. Blocking the second and third cervical nerve roots on the painful side with local anesthetic gave complete but temporary relief in 9 of 11 subjects in whom the procedure was carried out. The authors considered that if neck pathology was present on both sides, there could be a similar but double one-sided unilateral headache. This would appear to be difficult to distinguish clinically from tension-type headache.

Later Sjaastad et al. (1990) published proposed (and implicitly provisional) criteria for the diagnosis of the disorder. The obligatory features were unilaterality of the head pain, without change in side, and the presence of ipsilateral symptoms and signs of neck involvement, together with either (i) pain, seemingly of a similar nature, being triggered by neck movement and/or sustained awkward head positioning, or (ii) pain similar in distribution and character to the spontaneously occurring pain being elicited by external pressure over the ipsilateral upper, posterior neck region, or occipital region. The pain itself should occur in "nonclustering episodes" of varying duration or else be a fluctuating but continuously present one. It should be of moderate, nonexcruciating severity, usually not be throbbing in character, and should begin in the neck, and eventually spread to oculo-fronto-temporal areas, where the maximum pain would often be located. There were additional manifestations that might be present but that were not regarded as essential to the diagnosis, though if they were present, they added support to it.

The topic was subsequently reviewed in some detail by Pöllman et al. (1997), who concluded that the disorder should be understood as "a homogeneous but also unspecific pattern of reaction."

The relationship between the entity, if it proves to be a genuine one, and other types of headache remains to be elucidated satisfactorily (Goadsby 2009).

CHAPTER 9
Cranial Neuralgias

Over the years, a number of neuralgias that occur in the territories of supply of cranial sensory nerves have been described. Some are clearly secondary to various established structural pathologies or mechanical injuries and therefore fall outside the scope of the present book, dealing as it does with the primary headaches. The existence of others as idiopathic entities, for example greater occipital neuralgia, has been questioned in recent times. There remain some that, in the present state of knowledge, can reasonably be regarded as primary and akin to the present-day primary headaches that one expects probably will ultimately prove due to as yet inadequately established pathological processes. The main such primary cranial neuralgias that could be regarded as headaches because of their sites of occurrence are trigeminal neuralgia and the analogous, but more uncommon, glossopharyngeal neuralgia. However, both of these entities at times can also be due to demonstrable structural pathologies. It might be argued that the pain of glossopharyngeal neuralgia is usually experienced too low in the head to warrant being considered a headache, but glossopharyngeal neuralgia is included in the International Headache Society's Classifications of Headache.

TRIGEMINAL NEURALGIA (TIC DOULOUREUX)

Credit for providing the medical literature with the initial influential account of trigeminal neuralgia is often accorded to the Quaker physician John Fothergill (1712–1780), of London, and the disorder is occasionally still referred to as "Fothergill's neuralgia." Fothergill, in 1773, presented to a meeting of the members of the Medical Society of London a paper titled

"Of a Painful Affection of the Face." In it, Fothergill described some 14 instances of a painful disorder affecting the face that was

> nearly akin in appearance to the toothach, and that kind of disorder of the jaw which is sometimes called the rheumatism, sometimes the "ague in the head." . . . This affection seems to be peculiar to people of advancing years, and to women more than to men. I never met with it in any one much under forty, but after this period no age is exempt from it. . . .
>
> The case does not occur very frequently. I can recollect but about fourteen instances in the course of my business. . . .
>
> From imperceptible beginnings, a pain attacks some part or other of the face, or the side of the head: sometimes about the orbit of the eye, sometimes the *ossa malarum*, sometimes the temporal bones, are the parts complained of. The pain comes suddenly, and is excruciating. It lasts but a short time, perhaps a quarter or half a minute, and then goes off; it returns at irregular intervals, sometimes in half an hour, sometimes there are two or three repetitions in a few minutes. The kind of pain is described differently by different persons, as may reasonably be expected; but one sees enough to excite one's compassion, if present during the paroxysm. It returns full as often in the day as in the night. Eating will bring it in on some persons. Talking, or the least motion of the muscles of the face, affects others; the gentlest touch of a hand or a handkerchief will sometimes bring on the pain, whilst a strong pressure on the part has no effect. (Fothergill 1773/1783, pp. 179–181)

After distinguishing between the painful affection he had described and both toothache and rheumatism, Fothergill added further details:

> The disease which is the subject of this essay is seldom observed till between forty and fifty and through the later stages of life. Contrary to what happens in the preceding complaints, the affection I am treating of is more commonly severer in the day than in the night. Sometimes, indeed, it is excited to an extreme degree of violence by the lightest touch of the bed-clothes, which can scarcely be avoided in turning or any other motion in bed. (p. 182)

While Fothergill's paper seems to have been the first formal description of a series of cases of trigeminal neuralgia, there had been earlier recorded accounts of single instances of what very probably was the same condition. Indeed, it has been suggested that Aretaeus's *heterocrania*, in the second century A.D., may have included instances of the disorder (Stookey and Ransohoff 1959). There is little unambiguous evidence to support this view, though it was again mentioned by Rose (1999-b). For a time, it was considered that Avicenna (980–1036) had described the neuralgia under the designation of "Levket," but Lewy (1938), and others since him, have rejected this interpretation. They have argued that this idea arose from a mistranslation and that what had been described in Avicenna's *Canon* was actually facial palsy and hemifacial spasm. However, Ameli (1965) retranslated the original Arabic of the *Canon* into English and then pointed out that, in spasmodic *Leqvet*, it was stated there was not much change in power or sensation, but that "the other sign of the disease is pain." Hence it is possible that medieval Arabian medicine really had encountered and recorded the phenomenon of trigeminal neuralgia, though the scanty available details of the character of the pain must result in an element of uncertainty about the matter.

Wilfred Harris (1926) put forward the interesting suggestion that the disorder was known in England perhaps as early as the 13th century. He based this possibility on the fact that, on two stone pillars in Wells Cathedral in Somerset, there are carved figures illustrating persons behaving as if suffering violent facial pain. One is quite suggestive of the facial grimacing that may occur during a spasm of tic douloureux. Sufferers from toothache and similar pains were reputed to come to the tomb of Bishop Button, the second occupant of the see of Bath and Wells, who died in 1274 and was later canonized. They hoped to be cured of their suffering in the saintly atmosphere of that ecclesiastic environment, and left offerings there that were used to furnish the cathedral. Harris stated that when the bishop's coffin was opened in 1848, his skeleton was noted to possess a perfect set of teeth. Whether these details constitute adequate evidence to sustain Harris's suggestion regarding trigeminal neuralgia is a matter for the reader to judge.

However, there are two accounts, each dating from the latter half of the 17th century, that probably do constitute very early, if not the earliest, reasonably convincing written records of instances of the neuralgia, though one cannot be sure that it was necessarily idiopathic in either case.

The earlier of the two, to which attention was drawn in 1938 by Frederick Lewy (of Lewy body fame), originally appeared in print in 1671 (Lewy 1938). It involved the founder of the Imperial Leopoldian Academy for Natural Sciences, Johannes Laurentius Bausch (1605–1665). The original account appeared in the academy's journal, as part of Bausch's eulogy, which had been written by the two secretaries of the society, Johannes Michael Fehr and Elias Schmidt. The relevant passage, in Lewy's translation of the original Latin, reads as follows:

Joh. Laurent. Bausch had suffered for four years [i.e., since 1660] from a harassing, sharp, shooting pain in his right maxilla. The pain varied in intensity. It was less at times; at other times it retreated deep into the tissues or even completely disappeared. However, on the fifth of November, 1664 the pain grew so intense that our beloved master became bedridden. Suddenly, like a lightning-flash, the pain penetrated his jaws and his brain. He was almost unable to speak and was incapable of taking any solid food. Scurvy complicated the neuralgia. He struggled manfully against this new ailment but could never overcome it completely. During June, 1865 he could again leave his home and enjoy the fresh air. New hope of recovery seemed to appear with the beginning of the fall. However, the pain returned and became worse and worse. Emaciation gradually occurred. On the 15th of December, 1665 he experienced a slight stroke, involving the left side of his body, and at two o'clock in the afternoon of this day he expired, faithful to his Lord. (p. 249)

The second account, describing an event only a few years later, is of particular interest, partly because of the elevated social and intellectual status of some of the persons involved. On a winter evening in early December 1677, John Locke, an Englishman temporarily resident in Paris and possessed of an MB degree from Oxford, and who at some stages of his life chose to practice as a physician, received a request from Margaret Blomer, wife of the chaplain to the household of Ralph Montague, the English ambassador to the Court of France. Locke was asked to come to the aid of the ambassador's wife, Countess of Northumberland in her own right, whom he had known previously in London. He was asked to bring with him "the best blistering plaster you can . . . she is not willing to try any more French experiments" (Woolhouse 2007, p. 140). The countess was suffering from "a violent rheume in her teeth which put her to a very great torment." Details of the subsequent events were recorded by Locke in a journal, which was archived after his death and came to light again only some years ago. Its contents were subsequently published by Dewhurst (1963, pp. 93–99).

The initial relevant entry in the journal read as follows:

Thurs. Dec. 2. About 6 or 7 a clock I was cald to my Lady Ambassadricks whom I found crying out in one of her fits. I had not stayd long but after a little intervall an other began wherein she gave many shreeks. At every shreek her mouth being drawn towards the right eare, and when the fit was over she told me that the pain shot itself all at once like a flash of fire over that side of her tongue, into which she complained there was immediately, when the pain came, as if it were scalding liquor thrown. Her tongue on that side, as I afterward found was also in these fits convulsed, the contracting where of she tooke for swelling, it indeed making it thicker, but as soon as the violent pain ceased it returned to its naturall state.

The severe pain had begun on the previous day, but for three or four days before that she had experienced what she took to be ordinary toothache. Between the episodes of severe pain she suffered pain of varying, but lesser, severity in her teeth. Just prior to her fits of pain she felt a throbbing "in her lower jaw where a tooth hath been drawn in the like fits the last sommer, and a throbbing like wise in the upper jaw just over against it." The episode of similar severe pain the previous summer had lasted some eight to ten days. The tooth that had been removed was said to be "sound." There had been no immediate pain relief following its removal.

No local abnormalities were found to explain the countess's pain. More vigorous measures such as bleeding and applying blistering plasters, though considered, were not employed. Instead, topical laudanum was applied to the affected areas, producing relief. Oil of turpentine was then applied to the gum in the area from which tooth had been removed, but this reactivated the pain. Various means of emptying the countess's bowels were prescribed, and a blistering plaster was applied when her attacks persisted.

Four days after Locke was called in, his journal recorded the following:

> I observed all day that whether it were in the time when her fits were great or litle talkeing was apt to bring them on. Sometimes touching her teeth also of that side presently gave her twitches and fits, but a litle while after she could touch them freely without the least accident.... Opening also her mouth to take in any thing and the motion of eating were apt to putt her into fits.

By two weeks after the onset of symptoms, the exacerbations of pain had ceased. By January 24, 1678, the countess was free from symptoms, though she was still receiving medicines.

Locke recorded his thoughts about the diagnosis in his journal. He inclined to the view that the problem may have arisen from an "impostume" or a "sharp humour" which might "offend" (i.e., injure) a little nerve at the place where the tooth had been removed some months previously. Apparently a small abscess had formed at the site of the tooth removal soon after the earlier dental extraction procedure had been carried out. Whether out of diagnostic uncertainty, prudence in view of the elevated social status of the patient, or from genuine concern for her (there is an impression from the tone of the journal that the latter may have been the case), Locke wrote to London seeking advice from a Dr. Mapletoft, professor of physic at Gresham College and an eminent physician in London. Locke's letter to Mapleton was then shown to Dr. Micklethwaite, recently appointed president of the Royal College of Physicians, to Sir Charles Scarburgh and to a Dr. Dickinson. A separate copy of the letter went secretly from Paris to the former Roundhead soldier Dr. Thomas Sydenham, who had not then achieved his subsequent great reputation and who at the time was unpopular with the London medical establishment. All responded individually. The correspondence was published by Dewhurst (1957). In his reply, Mapletoft totally avoided the issue of diagnosis while committing to paper a plethora of social trivia. Micklethwaite invoked "some pungent vapour which affects ye nerve to quality wch. is a great Business" before proceeding to provide therapeutic counsel. Dickinson also took the view that the problem was of neural origin. It "does depend partly on the weakness of the Nerves traversing to the left side of her Face and partly on the pravity of the Nerval juices." Scarburgh was a little more expansive in his interpretation, again recognizing that the problem involved peripheral nerves:

> Undoubtedly some peculiar disaffection of the nerves of that part from whence the tooth was drawn is a great cause of those sharp and scalding pains, though not the only one, for that Her Honour was before much vexed with the toothache. So that the main original is seated in the Blood and Nerval juices. (Dewhurst 1957, pp. 31–32)

Sydenham evinced a greater awareness of possible psychological factors:

> Distemper I doe not judge to be any ulcer or any venemat quality else upon the gum (whaere it may be supposed some laceration of a nerve was made by that operation) but to be a hystericall quality in the bloud discharging its selfe entirely upon that place and side, where occasion was given by the drawing of the tooth, together with the payne of the operation and the apprehension thereof. (p. 33)

By the time these responses were received in Paris, the countess's problem had probably already resolved itself, at least temporarily. Locke was spared the task of deciding on further management measures, and received for his ministrations "a pair of silver candlesticks, and a silver standish with ink box and sand box and a silver bell" (Woolhouse 2007, p. 141). The countess knew her man, and his interests.

The consensus of consultant medical opinion at the time regarding the countess's problem seems to have been that a local nerve injury resulting from the earlier tooth removal was responsible for the episodes of pain, though some of the sources of advice recognized that this interpretation could scarcely account for the earlier episode of similar pain. In the light of latter-day knowledge, it is easy to see in the features of the countess's pain and its provoking factors a reasonably typical story of tic douloureux. But there is one rather uncharacteristic feature in the account and, unfortunately, what happened subsequently to the countess's pain is not known.

Elizabeth Wriothesley (figure 9-1) was born in 1646, the only child of the great magnate Thomas Wriothesley, fourth Earl of Southampton, who after the restoration of the monarchy in 1660 became lord treasurer of England. At the age of 16, his daughter was married to Joceline Percy, eleventh Earl of Northumberland, who died in 1670, the last of the male Percy line that had come to England with William the Conqueror. The earl's

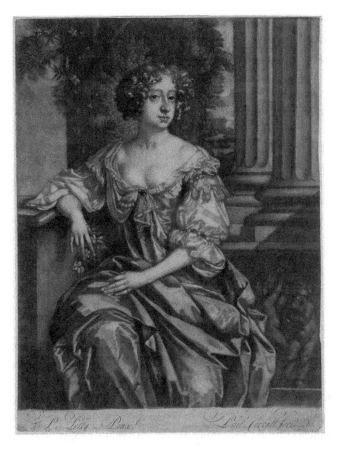

Figure 9-1 Elizabeth, *née* Wriothesley, when Countess of Northumberland, who experienced probable trigeminal neuralgia in 1677. Courtesy of the National Portrait Gallery, London.

eight-year-marriage with Elizabeth Wriothesley had produced no male heir, but only a daughter. After some three years of widowhood, in 1673 the countess married Ralph Montagu, a player in politics and something of a ladies' man, later to become successively Baron, Earl, and finally Duke of Montagu. The countess of Northumberland, by then Duchess of Montagu, died at age 44, in 1690. She was only 30 years old at the time of her first episode of probable trigeminal neuralgia, rather young for the idiopathic variety of the disorder. Her age therefore raises the possibility of underlying neurological disease, perhaps multiple sclerosis, but at that time that disorder was not a known disease entity.

The physician concerned, John Locke (1632–1704), who recorded the events of the countess's illness, had at Oxford been part of the circle that gathered around Thomas Willis, the Sedelian professor of natural philosophy. Together with Richard Lower, Locke had recorded Willis's course of

Oxford lectures (Dewhurst 1980). Locke later became the personal physician and confidant of Lord Ashley (later Earl of Shaftesbury), who was related to the Percy family. Locke's subsequent career, as a civil servant rather than a physician, was linked to that of Shaftesbury for many years, though after the latter's death Locke held senior civil service appointments apparently based on his own merits. He lived out a seemingly solitary life in the shadow of the great personages whose interests he served diligently, yet after death his memory has continued to be preserved while theirs have faded, for this John Locke was also the author of one of the great documents in the history of philosophy, *An Essay Concerning Human Understanding*.

Occasionally in the literature, there has been mention of a possible instance of tic douloureux described by Wepfer (1727) in his *Observationes*. The subject of his Observation 50, seen in 1692, was a woman approximately 60 years old who for eight years had experienced a "*hemicrania.*" In this, the pain began in the right cheek and lower eyelid region, and extended to the right temple, upper lip and side of nose, and to behind the right eye. It was severe, tugging, lancinating, and nearly intolerable in severity, but also brief and momentary, and recurred several to numerous times a day. With it, the lip trembled and the side of the nose retracted. The account does suggest the possibility of trigeminal neuralgia.

A little earlier than Fothergill and his case series, Nicolas André in 1756 recorded three probable instances of the disorder in the somewhat unlikely setting of a section on *Remarques sur certains mouvmens convulsifs* within his *Observatios pratiques sur les maladies de l'urèthre et sur plusiers faits convulsives*. Cole et al. (2005) stated that André had described two instances of the condition, but Brown et al. (1999) provided the details of the three case histories contained in André's work. André was the first to apply the term *tic douloureux* to the disorder, in preference to its earlier description as "spasme cynique" (i.e., cynical spasm). The earlier term, according to Brown et al.,

> borrows its name from its likeness to the one made by angry dogs about to bite.... I will hasten to conclude that the convulsive movements could not be named cynical spasm and that the name tic douloureux fits them much better, because these two words describe contortions and grimaces accompanied by acute and almost unbearable pain. (1999, p. 978)

The condition André described was, again in the words of Brown et al.'s translation,

> a cruel and obscure illness, which causes . . . in the face, some violent motions, some hideous grimaces which are an insurmountable obstacle to the reception of food, which

put off sleep . . . make speech choppy or slurred . . motions, vague and intermittent . . .
nevertheless so frequent as to be felt several times in a day, in an hour, and give sometimes no respite but are renewed every minute. Finally when those who are attacked by
this illness want to articulate a few words, or to move the affected part of the body, the
morbid nerve contracts and removes the ability to act freely. (1999, p. 977)

Thouret (1776) described an instance of facial pain that could pass for
trigeminal neuralgia, though the fact that it was reported to be cured by the
application of a magnet must leave the diagnosis in some doubt.

Eboli et al. (2009) credited the English surgeon and anatomist John
Hunter in 1778 with an early recognition of the phenomena of trigeminal
neuralgia. These authors may well be correct, but the quotation from
Hunter's writings that they cited had more to do with the failure of tooth
extraction to relieve dental pain than to provide persuasive evidence that
the pain represented true trigeminal neuralgia.

Comparatively recently, Govoni et al. (1996) published an account of
the 20-year course of the disorder, and its treatment from 1803 onward, as
it was recorded in the diary of an Italian lawyer, Ruggero Ragazzi (1746–
1824). The account began with the statement from the diary, pathetic in its
tone of resignation, deciphered and translated into English by Govoni and
his colleagues:

The history of tic douloureux, described by me, since I unfortunately suffer from it, is
getting more and more ferocious and nearly always torments me with shooting pains. It
began in 1803 and has continued to the present day, April 1821, and unfortunately will
not leave me for as long as I live. (p. 170)

Rowland (1838) mentioned some other early possible reported instances
of the disorder in his monograph on neuritis.

Fothergill's series of trigeminal neuralgia cases was fairly soon followed
by the publication of further case series (e.g., Méglin 1816), and also individual case records, some of considerable interest because of the wealth of
detail that they contained. All the main clinical features of the disorder were
to be found in the literature by the early 19th century, and relatively little of
major importance concerning clinical phenomenology has been added
since. It is worth mentioning that, in 1868, Armand Trousseau, the great
Parisian clinician, in his *Clinical Lectures*, gave a very detailed account of
some of his experience of patients with the disorder. He considered it under
the designation of "epileptiform neuralgia," and stated that it could present
in either of two varieties. The more common form was manifested as neuralgic facial pain, unaccompanied by convulsive twitching. The other variety, to which he applied the name *tic douloureux*, or *convulsive epileptiform*

neuralgia, involved rapid convulsive action of all the muscles of the half of the face in which the momentary pain was being experienced at the same time. Subsequent authors usually have not observed this distinction into two forms of the disorder, but Trousseau's term *epileptiform neuralgia* continues to be mentioned occasionally.

In later years, some very large case series of the disorder were published, notably that of Wilfred Harris (1940-b), who became a very great authority on the disorder and its management.

Cause and Mechanism

If Wilfred Harris (1926) was correct in his suggestion that trigeminal neuralgia sufferers in the later Middle Ages sought out Bishop Button's tomb in Wells Cathedral, hoping that their presence there, and probably their prayers in sanctified surrounds, would lead to pain relief, there may have been a community perception in those days that some supernatural factor was responsible for the disorder. Govoni et al. (1996), in discussing the pathogenesis of trigeminal neuralgia in their report of the disorder as it affected Ruggero Ragazzi, mentioned that the first hypothesis of the cause of the disorder was that produced by Massa in 1550. He had proposed that the pain was due to tooth decay. Locke's medical contemporaries in the 17th century seem to have regarded the cause of the pain in the Countess of Northumberland either as originating in the former site of the tooth that had been removed or in the nerve that innervated this site. It is impossible to know whether they would have continued to hold this view if they had been able to consider the histories of a series of cases of the neuralgia.

Wepfer (1727) ascribed the possible trigeminal neuralgia in his 60-year-old woman to the effects of a sharp serum and twitching nerves, and pointed out that even after eight years of the episodes of pain, no detectable pathological changes were present that could explain it. André in 1756 recognized that the pain of trigeminal neuralgia originated in peripheral nerves (Brown et al. 1999). He interpreted its pathogenesis in terms of the hollow nerve doctrine that was then extant, the idea that movement of "nervous fluid" within the nerve played the role now attributed to the nerve impulse. André apparently suggested the pain was due to an impedance or obstruction of the flow of this nervous fluid within the lumen of the relevant nerve, possibly as the result of extrinsic compression of the nerve from various pathologies. Fothergill, in 1773, was the first to attempt to explain the origin of the symptoms as they existed in a sizable group of sufferers. He gave thought to the matter and indicated his suspicion that the disorder probably arose from an as yet undetected metastatic malignancy, or was a remote effect of malignancy elsewhere in the body, in some instances possibly in a breast:

On reviewing the cases I have seen of this disorder, I recollected the subjects were mostly women. That they were for the most part, if not all, past the time of menstruation. That they were generally of a firm and somewhat robust habit, generally with black hair, and not subject to any particular diseases. Most of them had borne children and nothing remarkable had occurred about the cessation of the *menses*; in general, rather of a costive habit, and in the middling situations of life. In two of these cares, a small hard tumour in the breast had occasioned some suspicion of a schirrhus, but had never proceeded to give trouble.

These appearances, however, excited my attention, and induced me to suspect that the cause of these extreme pains in the face might possibly be of a cancerous nature. The method of cure and other circumstances seem to corroborate the suspicion. The sex, the time of life, two cases where a tendency to this was obvious, as well as the kind of pain, which was sudden, frequent, and severe, and as suddenly remitting, were to me further confirmation.

In tracing the history of persons afflicted with cancers not apparently proceeding from external causes, we shall find for the most part they have been afflicted with erratic pains in the limbs, often about the loins, sometimes in the thighs, and other muscular parts. These have commonly been considered by the patients as merely rheumatic but if we enquire more particularly, we shall find they are very different. They are not always worse in the night than the day. They are not a dull, heavy, aching pain, and continual, but sharp, lancinating, and remittent. They are not much affected by the weather, nor by any obvious causes; and they frequently disappear for some time; at least, there is a considerable abatement in their violence.

These pains do not always cease when the cancer becomes obvious; they are sometimes severe when the disease is making great progress externally: and experienced surgeons well know how little benefit the unhappy patients have to expect from removing the breast or other diseased part, if the patients have been long subjected to such complaints.

It seems not improbable, but that a sharp corrosive cancerous acrimony may long be pervading, like electrical matter, certain series of vessels, and when collected in a certain quantity, may create these pains; Yet without seizing upon any part with such violence as to destroy its functions. But if a part that favours its operations is once injured, those we call glandular especially, as the breasts, and the subcutaneous glands in the face; and other parts; if these become incapable of resisting or subduing the cancerous matter that may be thrown upon them, the mischief then becomes evident, and advances in proportion to the combination of those causes which favour its progress. An original disposition to form such acrimony, bad health; anxiety, external injury, and extreme sensibility of pain and danger, seem to constitute a part of these causes. (Fothergill 1773/1883, pp. 186–187)

Not long after Fothergill (1773) wrote, Pujol (1787) again made use of the hollow nerve and nervous fluid concept to explain the pain. In a letter to Ruggero Ragazzi written in 1814, Tommasini indicated to the former that his pain was due to an infection of the relevant peripheral nerve (Govoni et al. 1996). A French writer, Méglin (1816), considered the neuralgia a chronic idiopathic or essential nerve malady due to excessive irritation of the nerve of the face. Clearly by this time, the apparent association of some cases of the pain with recognizable local pathology in the region of trigeminal nerve branches was persuading medical opinion to settle on the view that the pain was of peripheral nerve origin, even though a causative abnormality might not always be found. Halford (1833) noted an association of the disorder with various bone abnormalities affecting the skull, for example bone growing where it should not be present, an unusually thick frontal bone pressing on the brain and local nerves, and the presence of diseased bone or bone that had grown preternaturally thick. When such pathologies could not be found, he ascribed the neuralgia to the ever convenient and easily invoked notion of "sympathy."

Almost as soon as the entity of trigeminal neuralgia was recognized, various attempts were made to interrupt the continuity, or otherwise interfere with the function of peripheral trigeminal branches that appeared to be the site of origin of the severe neuralgic pain. Harris (1951) provided a detailed account of the various surgical procedures that had been employed in treating the disorder up to his time of writing. Treatment based on such approaches will be considered in more detail later. In general, the earlier treatment attempts led to temporary pain relief that was not sustained in the longer term. As a result, the site of the physical interference with the function or the continuity of the trigeminal nerve progressively moved centrally in an endeavor to provide sustained pain relief. Coincidentally, these attempts produced evidence of the probable site where the trigeminal dysfunction arose, when no apparently relevant anatomical lesion was visible. The situation culminated in a recognition that the site of origin of apparently idiopathic trigeminal neuralgia usually was in the nerve root between the Gasserian ganglion and the brain stem. However, evidence from macroscopic pathology indicated that disease processes within the adjacent brain stem, for example multiple sclerosis plaques, could also be responsible. The American neurosurgeon Walter Dandy (1934) wrote the following concerning the cause of trigeminal neuralgia: "In a previous communication the writer has come to the conclusion that whatever the cause of trigeminal neuralgia may be, it must be located in the sensory root" (p. 455). Also,

in 10.7 percent of the cases there can be no question whatever about the relationship of the gross lesion to the production of the trigeminal neuralgia. If to these were added the arterial findings, the congenital findings and the case of multiple sclerosis, there would be 42 percent of gross lesions. The addition of the venous branches lying upon the nerve would raise the total to 56 percent, and if also the adherent nerves are included, to 60 percent, leaving forty percent without evidence of a gross lesion. (p. 454)

By way of explanation, elsewhere in the same paper Dandy had indicated that the indisputable gross lesions were mostly acoustic neuromas and cholesteatomas, the arterial findings were basilar artery aneurysms, tortuous or looping basilar artery branches that made contact with the nerve, and arteriovenous malformations, and the congenital findings were abnormal developments of the skull base.

At more or less the same time as the conclusions drawn from these anatomical observations became available, some writers, mostly of a lesser surgical bent, gave thought to the question of the mechanism that was capable of producing pain with the characteristics and distribution of that of trigeminal neuralgia.

In the 19th century, Armand Trousseau, in his then widely read and often quoted *Clinical Lectures* (Bazire translation 1868), evaded the question of the pathogenesis of the disorder when he considered the topic of epileptiform neuralgia, except insofar as the name he applied to it carried etiological connotations. He mentioned that he saw analogies between trigeminal neuralgia and epileptic phenomena, focal epileptic seizures, and angina pectoris. He also recognized that the neuralgia was a phenomenon whose occurrence was peculiar to the trigeminal nerve.

In the 1888 and 1893 editions of his *Manual of the Diseases of the Nervous System*, William Gowers dealt with trigeminal neuralgia as part of the overall topic of neuralgia, rather than considering it as a separate entity. Further, he then went into the manifestations of the neuralgia mainly in relation to particular branches of the nerve in whose distributions the pain appeared to be experienced, so that he tended to deal with trigeminal branch neuralgias, for example infraorbital neuralgia. He indicated that the neuralgia could be due to various pathological processes that caused local damage to trigeminal nerve fibers and made no clear mention that any idiopathic variety existed. In considering neuralgia in general, he made the ingenious suggestion that pressure on a peripheral nerve might disturb the function of the neurons that innervated the sheath of the nerve more than that of the fibers of the main nerve trunk itself. This effect on the neurons that innervated the nerve sheath might explain why neuralgic pain tended to follow the line of the involved nerve rather than being perceived as arising in the skin innervated by that nerve.

Harris (1926), in his detailed account of chronic paroxysmal trigeminal neuralgia, stated that there had been many assertions that the disorder was due to chronic degenerative change in the Gasserian ganglion, for example fibrosis and arteriosclerosis. However, there were also many reports that the ganglion on the affected side was normal. He seemed aware that attempted surgical treatments of the neuralgia might themselves cause structural abnormalities in the ganglion. He was able to describe the outcome of an autopsy in one of his own trigeminal neuralgia patients who had died untreated. The Gasserian ganglia had identical microscopic appearances on the affected and the unaffected sides. He had often seen the neuralgia begin after severe dental operations, or be associated with long-standing bad teeth or maxillary antrum abscesses. Harris therefore proposed that trigeminal neuralgia was the manifestation of a septic infection of dental nerve filaments. His idea explained why the neuralgia so much more often involved the second and third divisions of the nerve than the first.

Frazier et al. (1937) carried out a number of operative procedures on a woman with a thalamic syndrome who also suffered from trigeminal neuralgia. Based on their observations of the outcomes in relation to her trigeminal pain, they suggested the following:

> Trigeminal neuralgia, and eventually other forms of typical neuralgia, seem to represent special forms of the thalamic syndrome in which the lesions are confined either to the end places of the trigeminal system or to the thalamic sensory arrangement of an extremity, &c. (p. 51)

Kinnier Wilson, in explaining the pathogenesis of the disorder, wrote, "It is simpler to conceive of neuralgic paroxysms as sensory 'epileptiform' discharges. . . . If lesions exist, they should be sought rather in some *efferent* sensory inhibitory mechanisms" (1940, p. 386).Thus an idea had begun to appear that central nervous system events might play a role, at least at times, in the pathogenesis of trigeminal neuralgia.

Since those mid-20th-century days, more material from affected trigeminal nerves, ganglia, and roots has become available, including tissue from the relevant neural structures obtained during surgical procedures. Love and Coakham summarized the situation thus:

> There is now persuasive evidence that trigeminal neuralgia is usually caused by demyelination of trigeminal nerve fibres within either the nerve root or, less commonly, the brainstem. In most cases, the trigeminal nerve root demyelination involves the proximal, CNS part of the root and results from compression by an overlying artery or vein. (2001, p. 124)

The demyelination might be expected to affect the functional properties of the myelinated afferent nerve fibers that convey somatic sensation rather than the unmyelinated pain fibers in the nerve root. However, enthalpic conduction (cross-talk) between the denuded, relatively uninsulated hyperexcitable large fibers and the small diameter unmyelinated pain fibers could occur and account for the production of the neuralgic pain. Devor et al. (2002), in what they term their "ignition hypothesis," proposed that it is the combination of hyperexcitability and after-discharging that explains the pain. In all the various explanations of the pathogenesis of the disorder, attention has been focused on the pathogenesis of the neuralgic pain. The basis of the involuntary facial movements that often accompany the pain episodes has tended to be ignored, though it is easy to assume that neural communications exist between the brain stem pathway mediating facial pain and the neurons of the facial nucleus.

Treatment

Leaving aside dental procedures, particularly tooth extraction, which have undoubtedly been carried out on the basis of mistaken diagnoses, the history of attempts to relieve and, if possible, cure trigeminal neuralgia seems to have gone through several overlapping stages. The earliest attempts aimed at providing pain relief with drugs, or attempted to cure the disorder by correcting its presumed pathogenesis. There was a long period, going back almost to the earliest accounts, in which various operative procedures were carried out on trigeminal nerve branches, the sites of the surgery moving progressively closer to the brain stem, as mentioned in the previous section of this chapter. Then came the injection of the intracranial portions of the trigeminal with chemicals, mainly alcohol, intended to interfere with trigeminal nerve function. Onto this scene in the 1950s and 1960s burst the possibility of using antiepileptic drugs to afford relief. The latter approach, and more refined operative procedures, subsequently achieved the status of standard medical practice.

Locke in 1677, before he sought advice, treated the Countess of Northumberland with oil of turpentine applied locally to the site of the earlier tooth extraction that had been carried out, unsuccessfully, to relieve her facial pain. When his attempt increased her pain, he resorted to the almost inevitable remedies of his day, the emptying of the bowels and the use of blistering plasters, suggesting that he subscribed to the concepts of humoral pathology as being capable of explaining the pain. Indeed, he had suggested that a sharp humor might be irritating a nerve at the site of the earlier tooth extraction. However, he also applied laudanum to the area of the gums where the pain seemed to originate, and this afforded some relief (whether through local effects or as result of absorption into the systemic circulation is a matter for speculation). As mentioned earlier in this chapter, Locke sought advice from several physicians in England. The countess may have had reason to be thankful for the slower communications of those days because, by the time Locke had received the advice, her problem either was settling or had already settled. Most of the four physicians consulted advised purging (with various different prescriptions suggested). Application of various vesicatories behind the ear was proposed, as was cupping, and also the application of laudanum or opiates to the apparently affected area of gum during the paroxysms. Sydenham and Scarburgh tended to take more vigorous lines than the others. The former was in favor of bleeding, though the others saw no need for this, and Scarburgh advocated applying leeches to the apparently affected gum and cauterization of the area where the tooth had been removed previously. According to Dewhurst (1957), Micklethwaite made what now seems the eminently sensible suggestion that she be given "opiates inwardly."

Wepfer (1727) treated his patient with vesicatories applied to the sinciput, fontanel region and vertex, embrocations, repeated arteriotomies, and footbaths with a cephalic decoction. André in 1756, according to Brown et al.,

> begins his discussion by summarizing contemporary efforts at treatment. These include
> jaw bandage; antivenereal, antiepileptic, and antispasmodic agents; ointments; a milk
> diet; anodynes, cauteries, and vesicatories; peripheral neurectomy; and even insertion
> of the diseased portion of the face into the cavity of a recently slaughtered animal.
> (1999, p. 978)

This reads as if André may have been aware of the contents of the correspondence between Locke and the London medical authorities of the day. After such conventional measures failed in his first patient, André arranged for an infraorbital neurectomy to be carried out. This provided no pain relief, and bleeding occurred into the surgical wound. André then inserted a cauterizing stone into the wound and later scraped away the dead tissue, and had the wound irrigated with mercury water. Pain relief ensued. He subsequently applied a similar approach in two other patients in whom the inferior dental nerve seemed the site of origin of the painful episodes.

Fothergill (1773/1883, pp. 183–184) mentioned treatment only incidentally in his account of the disorder. In his initial case, "opium in considerable doses" was the only substance that afforded relief. He recorded of the pain in this woman that "it seemed to decline by the use of extract of hemlock, together with her strength." Hemlock contains various conium alkaloids that have nicotine-like actions on the central nervous system. It is long remembered as the substance that poisoned Socrates. Despite possibly hastening the dispatch of his patient, whose condition declined further before she expired, Fothergill continued to employ hemlock in cautiously increasing dosage in his other cases of painful facial neuralgia. He obtained what he considered to be generally favorable results. Understandably enough, there seems to have been little further reported use of the substance as a medication for trigeminal neuralgia.

As described by Govoni et al. (1996), Ragazzi's trigeminal neuralgia was treated at various times with purgatives, enemas, vesicants, and making a fonticulus (a wound kept open with caustic), musk and opium in large dosage taken by mouth, tartar emetic, mercury liniment, ammonium, cuprous, belladonna, hyoscyamus, and zinc oxide pills, as well as various local applications and electricity. Additional measures are recorded in the Govoni et al. (1996) paper. Poor Ragazzi considered undergoing André's procedure that was described above, and also surgical section of the infraorbital nerve, but decided against them, and finally resigned himself to the knowledge that no effective treatment existed for him.

Méglin (1816), in his review of trigeminal neuralgia, attempted to set down the principles of treating the disorder. In the belief that its basis was a disturbance of the body's humors, previous authors had recommended attempts to get rid of the abnormal humoral materials, for example gouty, scorbutic, and catarrhal ones in the case of Pujol's (1787) writings, using the various methods then in vogue. Various drugs were used to calm nerves. Méglin seemed satisfied by the benefits conferred by pills containing jusquiame (henbane—various solanaceous alkaloids) and zinc oxide, though he sometimes also employed valerian. If medical therapy failed, surgery could be tried. He referred to the operation Maréchal had carried out on the infraorbital nerve of André's first patient as the initial surgical attempt to treat the disorder, and cited a few subsequent ones.

Clearly at this stage, by virtue of the very variety of substances recommended, no effective drug treatment of trigeminal neuralgia had been found, with the exception of the prescription of sufficient dosages of opiates, if these could be tolerated. That remained the situation at the time when Trousseau (1868) stated the following, in relation to his experience of the response of trigeminal neuralgia to drug treatment, including belladonna (citing from Bazire's translation):

These are not excellent results, it is true; but they are favourable upon the whole. Of all the therapeutic agents which I have used—and I have tried a good many with extreme perseverance—opium, then, is the drug which has least disappointed me. (p. 115)

When there was failure of medical therapy, Trousseau considered surgical approaches, commenting that

> division of the affected nerves in the points where they can be reached without danger almost certainly gives immediate relief, . . . yet I do not expect a lasting good result. Even if I were to see a patient remain better for a pretty lengthened period, I should always dread a recurrence of the disease. I formerly believed, like many others, in the complete efficacy of this measure, but as I grew older, I unfortunately lost all my illusions on that score. (p. 110)

Anstie (1869) preferred the use of injected rather than oral morphia, which Trousseau had recommended, and claimed that the daily application of direct electrical current from a battery of 5 to 15 Daniell cells could be of benefit.

As already mentioned, Gowers (1888) chose to deal with the subject of neuralgia in an overall manner, though material relevant to trigeminal neuralgia may be extracted from his text. He began by pointing out that there were two aspects to the treatment—relieving the pain, and removing its cause—and that these aims were to be achieved by means of hygiene, by drugs applied internally or externally, and by certain surgical operations. Because neuralgia tended to be accompanied by states of debility, various dietary measures were advocated, as well as "nervine" tonics such as strychnine and ammoniosulphate of copper. At the beginning of attacks of trigeminal neuralgia, nervine stimulants such as alcohol, sulfuric ether, and valerian might occasionally cut the attack short. The most satisfactory anodynes were opium or morphia, particularly when injected—their oral use had gone out of fashion (for valid, though then not understood, pharmacokinetic reasons). Aconite and gelsemium were reputed to have "a special action on the fifth nerve." In addition, Gowers wrote, "I have found, for instance, in neuralgia of the fifth, the combination of arsenic, quinine, and Indian hemp of great value." In trigeminal neuralgia, he suggested the application of a blister beneath the occiput or behind the ear, and mentioned the recent use of local injections of carbolic acid or osmic acid, said to give immediate pain relief. Gowers commented that the procedure "does not appear entirely free from danger." He remarked that acupuncture had been introduced from China and Japan, but its value was not great. Aquapuncture, an injection of pure water into or beneath the skin, resulted in much pain and did little good. He described various skin applications that could be used for neuralgia in general, but did not specify trigeminal neuralgia in this connection, possibly because the eye was close to where the materials would have to be applied. In like fashion, he mentioned the use of electricity for treating neuralgia, without specific reference to the trigeminal variety.

He did not mention the application of the magnet, which Blundell (1833) for instance had reported produced transfer of the pain from the head to the extremity of the little finger of the same side over a period of some five weeks. The variety of treatments suggested for trigeminal neuralgia was extremely wide, and authors had to exercise some discrimination in the selections that they recommended.

Until this time, the surgical treatment of trigeminal neuralgia, apart from removing any causative lesion, comprised division, excision, and stretching of trigeminal nerve branches, and ligation of arteries. Gowers commented that it was a very large subject, and it remained so.

> Neurotomy has been frequently adopted in cases of severe, old-standing neuralgia, especially in the branches of the fifth nerve. Sometimes it is successful, more often it fails. Temporary relief may be given, and may continue for some months, but is too often succeeded by a return of the pain in all its old severity. . . . In cases of neuralgia of the second division of the fifth, the excision of Meckel's ganglion has sometimes given better results than simple division of the nerve. It is probable, however, that the transient relief is often due to the influence of the surgical irritation on the centre, which soon passes off. (1888, p. 770)

In those words, Gowers summarized the story of the surgical endeavors to his day. They yielded temporary benefit only, and the preferred site of nerve traumatizing moved progressively toward the neuraxis as time passed. Gowers's skeptical view of the mechanism whereby surgery achieved its ends may well have been valid, and may remain so in relation to the other surgical and other physical approaches that were subsequently described. He mentioned that stretching the lingual nerve had been reported to relieve trigeminal neuralgia and that, when all else had failed, the carotid had been ligated. Clearly he was not enthusiastic about this: "All that can be said to justify so dangerous an operation is that it has sometimes, but very rarely, been successful."

However, as Tubbs et al. (2010) pointed out, in 1858, the American surgeon John Murray Carnochan had relieved the pain of trigeminal neuralgia by operating through the maxillary sinus to remove the whole second division of the trigeminal nerve.

Within a few years of Gowers's writing the above, William Rose, professor of surgery at King's College in London, gave the Lettsomian lectures on the surgical treatment of trigeminal neuralgia (Rose 1892-a, 1892-b). He provided a comprehensive account of the history of previous surgical endeavors to relieve the disorder, acknowledged their limitations, and described how the more-or-less favorable outcome of operations removing Meckel's sphenopalatine ganglion had led him to move the site of his operative procedure even more centrally along trigeminal nerve branches and to enter the skull itself. He attempted to achieve surgical isolation of the Gasserian ganglion, or its actual removal. Horsley was also carrying out similar procedures, though by means of a different route of intracranial approach. The anatomical and procedural niceties of Rose's operations are for others to appreciate, but, at the time of his lectures, the durations of pain relief achieved in his five cases ranged from 22 months to 16 days. The site of surgical onslaughts on the fifth nerve had moved to the Gasserian ganglion within the skull by 1893. All that remained was for the site to move fractionally more centrally to the trigeminal nerve root beside the brain stem itself, as described in the material quoted earlier in the present chapter from Dandy's (1934) paper, which dealt with the mechanism of the disorder. Of course, surgical techniques and technologies have advanced since those pioneering days, and a very considerable amount of relevant material and historical detail has since appeared in the neurosurgical literature, but conceptually the usual target of the surgical approach to trigeminal neuralgia appears to have reached its present preferred site some eight decades ago. However, some more adventurous surgeons have operated on pain pathways within the brain stem itself (medullary and mesencephalic selective tractomy of pain fibers). As mentioned earlier, a history of the surgical endeavors to the mid-20th century was provided by Wilfred Harris (1951).

The increasing success of surgery for the neuralgic pain, despite the hazards in those relatively early days of intracranial operating, the failure of medical treatment to provide an answer better than that provided by the provision of narcotics, and perhaps Gowers's insight that the surgery was no more than a way of injuring a strategic part of the trigeminal afferent system, may have been responsible for an attempt to produce local injury of the nerve by some less drastic measure. By 1931, the choice of treatment for the condition was seen to lie between intracranial surgery and percutaneous injection of alcohol into parts of the trigeminal nerve (Harris 1931).

Wilfred Harris achieved what seems to have been very considerable mastery of the technique of injuring selectively the intracranial branches of the trigeminal nerve and the Gasserian ganglion itself by injecting alcohol via a long needle inserted through the appropriate nerve exit foramina in the base of the skull. Harris (1951) traced the origin of the idea of this method to Abadie and Verger in 1902, and to Sclöesser in 1903. Harris himself first injected the Gasserian ganglion in November 1910, and by 1940 was in the position of being able to analyze the outcome of 1433 such injections. He also injected alcohol into more peripheral trigeminal branches when he judged that appropriate, always acknowledging that the benefits were likely to be temporary. However, he thought that about 25 percent of his subjects who had undergone peripheral trigeminal nerve injections remained pain-free for as long as three years. Further, it was possible to repeat the peripheral procedure. The injected alcohol was intended to produce tissue destruction. It probably acted relatively selectively by damaging unmyelinated pain fibers in preference to the larger myelin-coated fibers responsible for conveying other types of sensation.

As time passed, in principle, similar, minimally surgical, percutaneous approaches to the intracranial portion of the trigeminal nervous structures came to be used with reasonable success in producing brief extrinsic compression of the relevant trigeminal nerve structures while avoiding the risk of alcohol diffusing too far from where its action was intended. For several decades, such methods became the treatment of choice for the disorder. However, the situation changed with the advent of drug therapy that had genuine efficacy in trigeminal neuralgia, and with refinements of neurosurgical technology—for example, the operating microscope, microsurgical decompression of the nerve, the significantly enhanced safety of intracranial operations, and the advent of stereotaxic radiosurgery.

Probably on a trial-and-error basis, the antiepileptic agent phenytoin came to be used for trigeminal neuralgia soon after it first became available on the market. It seemed to yield results that were satisfactory enough to warrant persevering with its use (Pennybacker 1961). Possibly on the basis of this experience, the newer antiepileptic agent carbamazepine appears to have been tried in the treatment of trigeminal neuralgia relatively early in the course of the drug's clinical development (Blom 1962). It achieved such success that it rapidly became the treatment of first choice for the disorder, a situation that prevailed at the end of the 20th century. As other antiepileptic agents came on the market, several have also appeared to prove efficacious: for example clonazepam (Court and Kase 1976), valproate (Peiris et al. 1980), gabapentin (Khan 1998), and lamotrigine (Canavero et al. 1995), as well as the antispasticity agent baclofen (Fromm 1989). Other possible drug therapies were discussed by Cheshire (1999) and Sindrup and Jensen (2002). With this plethora of pharmacological alternatives, it might have been expected that little place would remain for surgery. Trigeminal injection procedures seem to have largely disappeared from contemporary practice, but some intracranial procedures continue to be carried out, possibly because of either a failure of drug therapy in tolerated dosage or an unwillingness on the part of some neuralgia sufferers to take medication for prolonged periods of time.

GLOSSOPHARYNGEAL NEURALGIA

In November 1921, Wilfred Harris mentioned the existence of glossopharyngeal neuralgia in a paper on the topic of persistent pain in peripheral and central nervous system lesions that he presented to the Royal Society of Medicine in London (Harris 1922). There he recorded the features of the two instances of the disorder that he had seen by that time, and mentioned a further instance in which the local effects of a carcinoma of the tonsillar region may have been responsible for similar pain. In his monograph, he was in a position to write the following:

> In addition to chronic paroxysmal neuralgia affecting the trigeminal and geniculate systems there is a still rarer form of intense tic douloureux attributable to the glossopharyngeal nerve. I have met with three well-marked examples of this chronic tic, two lasting for many years, which in the suddenness of onset of the paroxysms closely resemble trigeminal neuralgia. (Harris 1926, p. 327)

The three instances he mentioned had no discernable cause, but he had also seen four other cases with similar symptoms, three with known and one with suspected malignancy in the tonsillar region on the side of the pain. In his cases, the pain appeared in the tonsil region and spread to the ear and neck on the same side. Attacks were precipitated by yawning and swallowing. In two of his cases, Harris injected the third division of the trigeminal at the foramen ovale, producing anesthesia in the appropriate territory but without relieving the pain; in the third, he injected the glossopharyngeal itself near the jugular foramen, with pain relief, but he cautioned against others attempting the procedure unless they had considerable experience of such injection work.

Pearce (2008) managed to trace earlier reports of this type of neuralgia in the literature, though the initial one, that of Wiesenberg (1910), was associated with the presence of local structural pathology situated where the nerve could have been involved. There were other early reports, from Sicard and Robineau (1920) and from Doyle (1923), in which no associated pathology was detected on clinical examination.

In almost every respect, clinical pattern, etiology, and therapeutic response, such paroxysmal glossopharyngeal neuralgia appears analogous to trigeminal neuralgia, but it is arguable whether it would be appropriate to devote further space to a pain that, because of its site of occurrence, can hardly be regarded a headache in the usual sense in which that word is employed.

CHAPTER 10

Some Thoughts from the History of Headache

When historical material concerning the understanding of a disorder has been presented in an overall chronological fashion, as has been attempted in this book in relation to headache, the reader may be left with an overall impression that knowledge has moved forward toward its current state in a reasonably smooth, orderly, and almost preordained progression. Admittedly, the tempo of the progress may have been uneven and there may have been long fallow periods. Yet, in reality, chance may have played parts that have escaped recording or notice, and testimony to false directions in thought and action, particularly in the more distant past, may have been less likely to be preserved in memory than those that led to what were perceived to be useful outcomes.

What seems to have often happened in relation to the growing understanding of headache, at least in more recent centuries, is that someone has collected an appreciable number of instances of the disorder and then thought about their characteristics. Sometimes the occurrence of a particular set of features has then been noticed to be present in part of the whole group. This realization has then permitted the demarcation of a hitherto unrecognized headache entity. Once the reality of this new headache entity has been accepted, and its diagnostic criteria have been agreed, knowledge has begun to move forward in developing an understanding of the new disorder and in finding treatments for it. In addition, those with knowledge may have then sometimes looked backward in time and been able to detect instances of the recently recognized headache disorder, or probable instances of it, recorded in the earlier literature. Such a set of processes probably happened in ancient times to allow the traditional headache triad of *cephalalgia*, *cephalaea*, and *hemicrania* to emerge in stages from the generality of headache that seems to have been all that was known prior to the second century A.D. It also happened in relation to cluster headache centuries afterward, once that disorder had emerged out of the general collection of headaches embraced by the idea of migraine and became a possible new entity in the writings of Harris and Horton. The features of the disorder were then firmly defined by writers such as Symonds and Kunkle. After this, probable examples of the condition could be traced in the literature up to three centuries earlier. On a lesser scale, a similar set of events may currently be occurring in relation to other trigeminal autonomic cephalalgias. It probably also occurred in relation to migraine with aura, where Tissot's (1780) account, and, more so, that of Piorry (1831), were followed by the identification of occasional much earlier descriptions of the aura phenomena. A disorder cannot be recognized until it has achieved the status of an accepted entity and its essential features have been defined and agreed. As well, if observations made on a disorder as it is currently known cannot all be accounted for by a hypothesis that seeks to explain it, it may be that the disorder category actually contains one or more currently unrecognized entities. It may be worth keeping this latter possibility in mind when thinking about present-day migraine and tension-type headaches.

Possibly it would have been more convenient, and may have been easier for the generalist reader, if the present history of headache had ended a little less than half a century ago. There would then have been no risk of the account transgressing from the past into the province of the present, that ever-shifting boundary where past abuts on future. As well, the story probably would then have appeared as if it was close to having come to a reasonably satisfactory finality after many centuries of intellectual endeavor. Medicine would have appeared to have achieved an understanding of the mechanisms of all of the important types of nonsymptomatic—in other words, primary—headache and to have acquired reasonably satisfactory treatments for them that merely needed further refinement to become totally efficacious. In earlier times also, individuals and groups of those concerned with headache may well have also reached stages in which they thought their understandings of the disorder had achieved a satisfactory approximation to what would prove to be the ultimate one. That may have been the state in the Greco-Roman world of later antiquity, after which the intellectual situation concerning headache became virtually frozen for a millennium, and also perhaps in the later 17th-century times of Willis and Wepfer. However, on each occasion, further events and advances in knowledge dispelled such illusory hopes. That was to happen again in the later decades of the 20th century. Therefore, while the apparent tidiness of a headache history ending at the mid-20th century might satisfy the professional historian, it might also leave the modern clinician who is interested in headache with a sense that the account was quaintly old-fashioned, indeed dated, and somewhat irrelevant to the present-day world of headache understanding.

Much has changed in the second half of the 20th century, and is still in the process of changing. This is the result of a very considerable awakening of interest in headache and its mechanisms, and the increased capacity and availability of technologies that permit the ethically acceptable investigation of headache mechanisms in humans, as well as in animal models. The whole mid-20th-century interpretation of the mechanism of the main types of headache, centered on the belief that they were primarily matters of cranial artery misbehavior or excessive extracranial muscle contraction, appears to have been overturned, for the most part. The mechanisms underlying the initiation of the most common forms of primary headache are coming to be seen as situated within the brain itself. If the intracranial and extracranial arteries are involved, this involvement occurs as a secondary event mediated via their trigeminal nerve supply. In the case of migraine, ideas have become available suggesting that the cortical spreading depression that seems to be responsible for the migraine aura may also be able to activate peripheral elements of the trigeminal system.

It may appear that, at the present time, a new and plausible interpretation of at least the migraine mechanism, or set of mechanisms, is in the process of becoming accepted. If that happens, and the interpretation holds, it may open new therapeutic possibilities as molecular tools are devised to counter the underlying and associated biochemical disturbances that are being recognized. Yet reading the history of interpretations of headache mechanisms over some hundreds of years, particularly those of migraine, shows that they have alternated between those primarily based on neural malfunction at various levels of the central and peripheral nervous systems, and those that have regarded the primary event as vascular. The present-day statement that migraine is a neurovascular or trigeminovascular headache acknowledges this changing interpretation of headache mechanisms. It also provide a neat verbal device that may permit the currently favored understanding of headache mechanisms to partly escape criticism if further events bring its deficiencies to light and the dominant direction of the headache mechanism interpretation changes yet again.

Does the history of headache up to the time of writing suggest that particular deficiencies in understanding do exist? To use a military analogy for a moment, recent change in the interpretation of headache has moved in rather a blitzkrieg-like fashion, tending to overwhelm its main opponents but leaving behind, unaccounted for, pockets of facts that may have the potential of coalescing into sources of opposition sufficient to undermine and perhaps alter the direction of the forefront of the advance. For instance, although the concept of cortical spreading depression seems to account adequately for the migraine visual aura, can such a relatively brief event explain those occasional recorded instances in which the neurological deficit of the aura persists for many hours or days, or even, as it rarely does, remains permanently? Can it explain those very infrequent instances of auras associated with the presence of fatal brain infarction in which no obstruction of the relevant brain arteries has been found at postmortem? Is it adequate to explain migraine auras restricted to the vision of one eye, or the reversible individual cranial nerve palsies that occur during some migraine attacks, or the phenomenon of migrainous vertigo? If the spreading depression alters the molecular environment around trigeminal nerve endings in the meninges to activate the trigeminovascular system and thus produce the headache of migraine, how are those unusual instances to be explained in which the onset of migraine headache precedes the aura?

Then there is the question of the whole set of observations made some years ago in relation to altered platelet function and abnormal circulating serotonin concentrations during, and in some instances before, migraine attacks. Considerable attention was being paid to these matters half a century ago, but once it was decided that they did not provide an adequately explanation for all aspects of the migraine mechanism, they seem to have been discreetly swept under an intellectual carpet. There they still lurk, out of sight, never proved to be incorrect but simply deemed insufficient. They can be left to remain there, unaccounted for, only to constitute a potential peril to the validity of any hypothesis of migraine pathophysiology that currently exists or is developed. And there is an older question from headache history—how Gowers's mixture, containing an agent that provokes migraine, glyceryl trinitrate, could survive as a recommended migraine preventative for more than 50 years. And there may be another example of a similar situation in that reserpine, a now superseded antihypertensive agent claimed to activate migraine, was also reported to prevent migraine if its use was continued beyond the stage when it might cause the disorder to worsen (Genefke et al. 1975).

Further, present-day genetics has so far not provided anything like an adequate accounting for the long-known tendency for migraine to run in families, let alone how the genetic undesirabilities (can one write of abnormalities in a disorder that has such a high prevalence?) interdigitate with other aspects of the pathophysiology of the condition. Could it be that the record of so many failures to explain fully the mechanisms of migraine over so long a time is due to there existing more than one headache type within the category of migraine, rather than there being a single entity of migraine? After all, John Hughlings Jackson in the 1870s introduced the concept of "the many epilepsies" when he tried to escape the limitations of the idea of epilepsy as it was then favored. Has medicine been searching for an explanation for a single entity when several entities exist within a named headache category, and when more than one of these entities may afflict the individual migraine sufferer at the same, or at different, stages of life?

The affinities of cluster headache to migraine are obvious, and become very apparent when one reads Wilfred Harris's (1926) accounts of ciliary and migrainous neuralgia and relates them to knowledge of migraine phenomenology. The recent demonstration of the activation of the suprachiasmatic nucleus region of the hypothalamus prior to the onset of cluster headache attacks suggests the presence of a mechanism that explains the peculiar time pattern of this disorder. There seems to be a tacit, still being developed but not unreasonable, assumption that a migraine-type trigeminovascular mechanism is responsible for the headache in the disorder. There seems to be no answer yet as to whether the customary explanation still holds, namely that carotid arterial dilatation in the cavernous sinus during the attacks explains the ocular sympathetic paresis that may occur in the attacks, and sometimes persist afterward, or whether sympathetic and parasympathetic function are altered as result of some temporary change in the central nervous system itself. How alcohol intake activates the headache attacks during clusters, but not at other times, also awaits explanation.

If one turns to tension-type headache, the history of events can again raise questions. Half a century ago, under the guise of *contraction headache*, the mechanism of production of tension-type headache appeared to be satisfactorily accounted for. The pain was believed to be due to excessive contraction of parts of the musculature of the head with resulting traction on the epicranial aponeurosis. Now this mechanism no longer seems sufficient to account for all instances of the headache, and various items of knowledge appear to be blurring the boundary between this type of headache and migraine. Once it became obvious from the 19th century onward that all headache could not be accounted for as consequences of structural pathology or systemic illness and the lingering concepts of rheumatic, fibrotic nodular and gouty headache failed to convince, tension headache seems to have made its appearance as an entity. In clinical practice, it has at times been used for something like a diagnostic dumping ground for otherwise uncategorizable, but usually not particularly severe or dangerous, headache. Perhaps tension-type headache also comprises more than one nosological entity, and there may be more than one pain-producing mechanism involved in its origin.

Awareness of the history of headache, even if it may provide intellectual pleasure for some, may also cause others to raise questions that arise out of knowledge gained in the past, questions whose answers ultimately may enhance the understanding of this disorder in its various manifestations.

The awareness of existing deficiencies in knowledge may also leave a keener sense that medicine is some very considerable distance from being able to prevent, or immediately alleviate, situations such as that depicted in the words of Shakespeare's *Romeo and Juliet*, when Juliet's old nurse, amid the hustle of the preparations on the day of her mistress's wedding, gave way to the anguished utterance:

> Lord, how my head aches! What a head have I!
>   It beats as it would fall in twenty pieces.

REFERENCES

Abercrombie J (1828) *Pathological and practical researches on diseases of the brain and the spinal cord.* Waugh & Innes. Edinburgh.

Abernethy (1826) Mr Abernethy's physiological, pathological, and surgical observations delivered as the anatomical course of lectures at St Bartholomew's Hospital. *Lancet* 7:65–68.

Adams F (1856) *The extant works of Aretaeus, the Cappadocian.* New Sydenham Society. London.

Adams F (1849) *The genuine works of Hippocrates.* Williams and Wilkins. Baltimore.

Adams F (1844) *The seven books of Paulus Aegineta.* Sydenham Society. London.

Ad Hoc Committee on Classification of Headache (1962) Classification of headache. *Archives of Neurology* 6:172–176.

Airy G B (1865) The Astronomer Royal on hemianopsy. *Philosophical Magazine* 30:19–21.

Airy H (1870) On a distinct form of transient hemiopsia. *Philosophical Transactions* 159: 247–264.

Albucasis (1861) *La chirurgie d'Albucasis.* Ballière. Paris.

Allbutt T C (1883) Case of epileptiform migraine. *Brain* 6:246–249.

Allory A-L (1859) *De la migraine.* Thesis. Paris.

Ambrosini A, Vandenheede M, Rossi P, Aloj F, Sauli E, Pierelli F, Schoenen J (2005) Suboccipital injection with a mixture of rapid- and long-acting steroids in cluster headache: A double-blind placebo-controlled study. *Pain* 118:92–96.

Ameli N O (1965) Avicenna and trigeminal neuralgia. *Journal of the Neurological Sciences* 2:105–107.

André N (1756) *Observations pratiques sur les maladies de l'urèthre et sur plusiers faits convulsifs, & la guérison de plusiers maladies chirurgicales, avec la décomposition d'un remède propre à réprimer la dissolution gangréneuse & cancéreuse, & à la réparer; avec des principes qui pourront servir à employer les différens caustiques.* Paris: Delaguette. Cited by Brown et al. (1999) *loc. cit.*

Anonymous (1745) Cephalalgia. In: James R (ed.) *A medical dictionary.* Roberts. London: 205–211.

Anonymous (1999) Radix Valerianae. In: *WHO monograph on selected medicinal plants.* WHO. Geneva: 267–276.

Anstie F E (1866) Lettsomian lectures on certain painful affections of the fifth nerve. *Lancet* 87:653–664; 88:31–33; 199–201.

Anstie F (1869) On the treatment of "epileptiform" neuralgia in its earlier stages. *Lancet* 93: 41–43.

Anstie F E (1873) The pathology of sick-headache. *British Medical Journal* 1:61.

Anstie F E (1880) Neuralgia. In: Reynolds J R, Hartshorne H (eds.) *A system of medicine.* Vol. 1. Lea's Son & Co. Philadelphia: 1026–1048.

Anstie F E (1882) *Neuralgia and the diseases that resemble it*. Bermingham & Co. New York.

Anthony M, Hinterberger H, Lance J W (1967) Plasma serotonin in migraine and stress. *Archives of Neurology* 16:544–552.

Anthony M, Lance J W (1969) Monoamine oxidase inhibition in the treatment of migraine. *Archives of Neurology* 21:263–268.

Anthony M, Lance J W (1971) Histamine and serotonin in cluster headache. *Archives of Neurology* 25:225–231.

Anthony M, Lord G D A, Lance J W (1978) Controlled trials of cimetidine in migraine and cluster headache. *Headache* 18:261–264.

Anzola G P, Magoni M, Guindani M, Rozzini I, Dalla Volta G (1999) Potential source of cerebral embolism in migraine with aura: a transcranial Doppler study. *Neurology* 52:1622–1625.

Arago F (1858) *Oeuvres complètes*. Giles & Baudry. Paris.

Aring C D (1959) Tension headache. In: Friedman A P, Merritt H H (eds.) *Headache: diagnosis and treatment*. Davis. Philadelphia: 401.

Arkink E B, van Buchem M A, Haan J, Ferrari M D, Kruit M S (2010) An early 18th-century case description of cluster headache. *Cephalalgia* 30:1392–1395.

Ashina M, Bendtsen L, Jensen R, Sakai F, Olesen J (1999-a) Muscle hardness in chronic tension-type headache: relation to actual headache state. *Pain* 79:201–205.

Ashina M, Bendtsen L, Jensen R, Lassen L H, Sakai F, Olesen J (1999-b) Possible mechanism of action of nitric oxide synthase inhibitors in chronic tension-type headache. *Brain* 122:1629–1635.

Ashina M, Larsen L H, Bendtsen L, Jensen R, Olesen J (1999-c) Effect of inhibition of nitric oxide synthase on chronic tension-type headache: a randomised cross-over trial. *Lancet* 353:287–289.

Ashina M, Bendtsen L, Jensen R, Sakai F, Olesen J (2000-a) Nitric oxide-induced headache in patients with chronic tension-type headache. *Brain* 123:1830–1837.

Ashina M, Bendtsen L, Jensen R, Schifter S, Jansen-Olesen I, Olesen J (2000-b) Plasma levels of calcitonin gene-related peptide in chronic tension-type headache. *Neurology* 55: 1335–1339.

Ashina M, Stallknecht B, Bendtsen L, Pedersen J F, Galbo H, Dalgaard P, Olesen J (2002) In vivo evidence of altered skeletal muscle blood flow in chronic tension-type headache. *Brain* 125:320–326.

Auerbach S (1913) *Headache: its varieties, their nature, recognition and treatment*. Henry Froude; Hodder & Stoughton. London. (Translated Playfair E).

Aurora S K, Kori S H, Barrodale P, McDonald S A, Haseley D (2006) Gastric stasis in migraine: more than just a paroxysmal abnormality during a migraine attack. *Headache* 46:57–63.

Auzias-Turenne (1849-a) *Théorie ou mécanisme de la migraine*. De Plon Frères. Paris.

Auzias-Turenne (1849-b) Theory on the production of hemicrania. *Lancet* 53:177–179.

Babington B G (1841) Observations on epilepsy. *Guy's Hospital Reports* 6:10.

Babinski J F F (1890) De la migraine ophthalmique hystérique. *Archives de neurologie* 20: 305–335.

Baralt R L (1880) *Contribution à l'étude du scotome scintillant ou amaurose partielle temporaire*. Thesis. Paris.

Barger G (1931) *Ergot and ergotism*. Gurney & Jackson. London.

Barnett C (1974) *The first Churchill: Marlborough, soldier and statesman*. Putnam's Sons. New York.

Barré M (1926) Sur un syndrome sympathetique cervical posterior et sa cause frequente: l'arthrite cervicale. *Revue Neurologique Paris* 33:1246–1248.

Barrough P (1610) *The method of physick: containing the causes, signes and cures of inward diseases in mans bodies, from the head to the foote*. Field. London.

Bärtschi-Rochaix W (1948) Le diagnostic de l'encephalopathi posttraumatique d'original cervicale ("migraine cervicale"). *Praxis* 37:673–677.

Barudel M (1867) De l'hémicrânie causée par l'anémie: de son traitment par le bromure de potassium. *Recuil de mémoires de médecine, de chirurgie et de pharmacie militaires* 35:371–390.

Bendtsen L, Jensen R, Olesen J (1996) A non-selective (amitriptyline) but not a selective (citalopram) serotonin reuptake inhibitor is effective in the prophylactic treatment of chronic tension-type headache. *Journal of Neurology, Neurosurgery and Psychiatry* 61:285–290.

Bendtsen L, Jensen R, Hindberg I, Gammeltoft S, Olesen J (1997) Serotonin metabolism in chronic tension-type headache. *Cephalalgia* 17:843–848.

Bendtsen L, Evers S, Linde M, Mitsakostas D D, Sandrini G, Schoenen J, EFNS (2010) EFNS guideline on the treatment of tension-type headache—report of an EFNS task force. *European Journal of Neurology* 17:1318–1325.

Berde B, Schild H O (1978) *Ergot alkaloids and related compounds.* Springer-Verlag. Berlin.

Berde B, Stürmer E (1978) Introduction to the pharmacology of ergot alkaloids and related compounds as a basis of their therapeutic application. In: Berde B, Schild H O (eds.) *Ergot alkaloids and related compounds.* Springer-Verlag. Berlin: 1–28.

Bickerstaff E (1959) The periodic migrainous neuralgia of Wilfred Harris. *Lancet* 273: 1069–1071.

Bickerstaff E (1961-a) Basilar artery migraine. *Lancet* 277:15–17.

Bickerstaff E R (1961-b) Impairment of consciousness in migraine. *Lancet* 278:1057–1059.

Biggs R S, Milac P A (1979) Timolol in migraine prophylaxis. *Headache* 19:379–381.

Bing R (1952) Histamin-Kopfscmerz oder Erythroprosopalgie. *Journal of Nervous and Mental Diseases* 116:862–873.

Blau J N (1992) Migraine: theories of pathogenesis. *Lancet* 339:1202–1207.

Blom S (1962) Trigeminal neuralgia: its treatment with a new anticonvulsant drug (G-32883). *Lancet* 279:839–840.

Blundell E S (1833) Case of tic douloureux cured by the "mineral magnet." *Lancet* 22:693.

Boes C J, Capobianco D J (2005) Chronic migraine and medication-overuse headache through the ages. *Cephalalgia* 25:378–390.

Boes C J, Capobianco D J, Matharu M S, Goadsby P J (2002) Wilfred Harris' early description of cluster headache. *Cephalalgia* 22:320–326.

Bogousslavsky J, Regli F, Van Melle G, Payot M, Uske A (1988) Migraine stroke. *Neurology* 38:223–227.

Boissier de Sauvages F (1772) *Nosologie méthodique.* Gouvion. Lyon.

Bolay H, Reuter U, Dunn A K, Huang Z, Boas D A, Moskowitz M A (2002) Intrinsic brain activity triggers trigeminal meningeal afferents in a migraine model. *Nature Medicine* 8:136–142.

Bonet T (1700) *Sepulchretum sive anatomia practica.* Cramer & Perachon. Lugundi.

Boquet J, Moore N, Boismare F (1982) Hemicrania and lateralized cervicoscapular muscular hypertonicity. In: Critchley M, Friedman A P, Gorina S, Sicuteri F (eds.) *Advances in Neurology.* Raven Press. New York: 401–405.

Bradshaw P, Parsons M (1964) Hemiplegic migraine, a clinical study. *Quarterly Journal of Medicine* 34:65–85.

Bramwell E (1926) Discussion on migraine. *British Medical Journal* 2:765–769.

Brewster D (1865) On hemiopsy, or half-vision. *Philosophical Magazine* 29:503–507.

Broca P (1861) Remarques sur le siège de la faculté du language articulé; suivies d'une observation d'aphémie (perte de la parole). *Bulletin de la Société anatomique de Paris* 36: 330–357.

Broch A, Horven H, Nornes H, Sjaastad O, Tonjum A (1970) Studies of cerebral and ocular circulation in a patient with cluster headache. *Headache* 10:1–13.

Brock S, O'Sullivan M, Young D (1934) The effect of non-sedative drugs and other measures in migraine, with especial reference to ergotamine tartrate. *American Journal of the Medical Sciences* 188:253–260.

Brown J A, Coursaget C, Preul M C, Sangvai D (1999) Mercury water and cauterizing stones: Nicolas André and tic douloureux. *Journal of Neurosurgery* 90:977–981.

Brown-Séquard C E (1861) Remarques sur le travail précédent. *Journal de la physiologie de l'homme et des animaux* 4:137–139.

Brunton T L (1899) A discussion on headache. *British Medical Journal* 2:1241–1243.

Bruyn G W (1989) Migraine phylakteria: magic treatment of migraine. In: Rose F C (ed.) *Neuroscience across the centuries*. Smith-Gordon. Nishimura: 31–40.

Bryan C P (1930) *Ancient Egyptian medicine: the Papyrus Ebers*. Ares Publishing Co. Chicago.

Buchanan J A (1921) The abdominal crises of migraine. *Journal of Nervous and Mental Diseases* 54:406–412.

Bullokar J (1616) *An English expositor*. Legatt. London.

Buring J E, Peto R, Hennekens C H (1990) Low-dose aspirin for migraine prophylaxis. *Journal of the American Medical Association* 264:1711–1713.

Burstein R, Cutrer M F, Yarnitsky D (2000-a) The development of cutaneous allodynia during a migraine attack. Clinical evidence for the sequential recruitment of spinal nociceptive neurons in migraine. *Brain* 123:1703–1709.

Burstein R, Yarnitsky D, Goor-Aryeh I, Ransil B J, Bajwa Z H (2000-b) An association between migraine and cutaneous allodynia. *Annals of Neurology* 47:614–624.

Bussemaker, Daremberg Ch (1873) *Oeuvres d'Oribase*. Vol. 5. Imprimerie Nationale. Paris.

Bussone G, Leone M, Peccarisi C, Micieli G, Granella F, Magri M, Manzoni G C, Nappi G (1990) Double blind comparison of lithium and verapamil in cluster headache prophylaxis. *Headache* 30:411–417.

Butler S, Thomas W A (1947) Headache: its physiologic causes. *Journal of the American Medical Association* 135:967–971.

Calmeil L-F (1839) Migraine. In: Béclard B (ed.) *Adelon's Dictionnaire de médecine ou répertoire*. Béchet & Labé. Paris: 3–10.

Campbell A W (1933) The treatment of migraine. *Medical Journal of Australia* 1:36–37.

Campbell H (1892) Dyspeptic headache: a historical sketch. *Lancet* 140:933–935.

Campbell H (1893) What constitutes the aching structure in headache? *Lancet* 142:184–188.

Campbell H (1894) *Headache and other morbid cephalic sensations*. Lewis. London.

Canavero S, Bonicalzi V, Ferroli P, Zeme S, Montalenti E, Benna P (1995) Lamotrigine control of idiopathic trigeminal neuralgia. *Journal of Neurology, Neurosurgery and Psychiatry* 59:646.

Castillo J, Martinez F, Leira R, Lema M, Noya M (1994) Plasma monoamines in tension-type headache. *Headache* 34:531–535.

Chadwick J, Mann W N (1978) *Hippocratic writings*. Penguin Books. London.

Charcot J-M (1882) Migraine ophthalmique se manifestant à la periods initiale de la paralysie generale. *Progrés Médicale* 10:593–595.

Charcot J-M (1890) Sur un cas de migraine ophthalmoplégique (Paralysie oculomotorice périodique). *Progrés Médicale* 12:83–86.

Charcot J-M (1897) Contribution à l'étude clinique de la migraine ophthalmoplégique. *Revue Neurologique Paris* 5:217–222.

Chasman D I, Schürks M, Anttila V, de Vries B, Schmink U, Launer L J, Terwindt G M, van den Maagdenberg A M J M, Fendrich K, Völzke H, Ernst F, Griffiths L R, Buring J E, Kallela M, Freilinger T, Kubisch C, Ridker P M, Palotie A, Ferrari M D, Hoffmann W, Zee R U L, Kurth T (2011) Genome-wide association study reveals three susceptibility loci for common migraine in the general population. *Nature Genetics* 43:695–698.

Chaumier E (1878) *Un chapitre de l'histoire des maladies constitutionnelles: la migraine.* Thesis. Paris.

Chazot G, Claustrat B, Brun J, Jordan D, Sassolas G, Schott B (1984) A chronobiological study of melatonin, cortisol, growth hormone and prolactin secretion in cluster headache. *Cephalalgia* 4:213–220.

Cheshire W P (1999) Trigeminal neuralgia. A guide to drug choice. *CNS Drugs* 7:98–110.

Chugani D C, Kiiura K, Chaturvedi S, Muzik O, Fakhouri M, Lee M-S (1999) Increased brain serotonin synthesis in migraine. *Neurology* 53:1473–1479.

Churchill W S (1933) *Marlborough: his life and times.* Vols. 1–4. Harrap & Co. London.

Clarke J M (1910) On recurrent motor paralysis in migraine with report of a family in which recurrent hemiplegia accompanied the attacks. *British Medical Journal* 1: 1534–1538.

Claustrat B, Loisy C, Brun J, Beorchia S, Arnaud J L, Chazot G (1989) Nocturnal plasma melatonin levels in migraine: a preliminary report. *Headache* 29:241–245.

Cohen A, Matharu M S, Goadsby P J (2006) Short-lasting unilateral neuralgiform headache with conjunctival tearing (SUNCT) or cranial autonomic features (SUNA)—a prospective clinical study of SUNCT and SUNA. *Brain* 129:2746–2760.

Cole C D, Liu J K, Apfelbaum R I (2005) Historical perspectives on the diagnosis and treatment of trigeminal neuralgia. *Neurosurgical Focus* 18:E4, 1–10.

Colin L (1873) Céphalalgie, céphalée. In: Dechambre M A (ed.) *Dictionairre encyclopédique des sciences médicale.* Masson, Asselin. Paris: 16–39.

Collier J (1922) Diseases of the nervous system. In: Price F W (ed.) *A textbook of the practice of medicine.* Hodder & Stoughton. London: 1502–1506.

Collier J (1928) Lumleian lectures on epilepsy. *Lancet* 221:587–591; 642–647.

Connor R C R (1962) Complicated migraine: a study of permanent neurological and visual defects caused by migraine. *Lancet* 280:1072–1075.

Cooke L J, Rose M S, Becker W J (2000) Chinook winds and migraine headache. *Neurology* 54:302–307.

Copeman A H (1901) Headache. *Lancet* 158:127–128.

Copland J (1858) Headache. In: Copland J (ed.) *A Dictionary of Practical Medicine.* Vol. 2. Longman, Brown, Green, Longmans, Roberts. London: 141–156.

Corning J L (1888) *A treatise on headache and neuralgia, including spinal irritation and a disquisition on normal and morbid sleep.* Treat. New York.

Couch J R, Ziegler D K, Hassanein R (1976) Amitriptyline in the prophylaxis of migraine. *Neurology* 26:121–127.

Court J E, Kase C S (1976) The treatment of tic douloureux with a new anticonvulsant (clonazepam). *Journal of Neurology, Neurosurgery and Psychiatry* 39:297–299.

Critchley E M R (1996) Migraine. *Journal of Neurology Neurosurgery and Psychiatry* 60:338; 448; 585.

Critchley M (1949) *Sir William Gowers 1845–1915: a biographical appreciation.* Heinemann. London.

Critchley M (1964) *The black hole and other essays.* Pitman. London.

Critchley M (1986) Records of some famous migraineurs. In: Critchley M (ed.) *The citadel of the senses and other essays.* Raven Press. New York: 130–146.

Critchley M, Ferguson F R (1933) Migraine. *Lancet* 221:123–126; 182–187.

Cullen W (1789/1805) *First lines of the practice of physic.* Vols. 1–2. Duyckinck, Swords, Falconer et al. New York.

Culpeper N (1658) *Four books of that learned, and renowned doctor, Lazarus Riverius.* Vol. 1. Cole. London.

Curran D A, Hinterberger H, Lance J W (1965) Total plasma serotonin, 5-hydroxyindoleacetic acid excretion in normal and migrainous subjects. *Brain* 88:997–1010.

Cutrer F M, Limmroth V, Moskowitz M A (1997) Possible mechanisms of valproate in migraine prophylaxis. *Cephalalgia* 17:93–100.

Dalessio D J, Polich J, Ehlers C (1986) Endogenous and psychic determinants of migraine. In: Amery W K, Wauquier A (eds.) *The prelude to the migraine attack*. Ballière-Tindall. London: 3–7.

D'Andrea G, Cananzi A R, Morra M, Martignoni E, Fornasiero S, Zamberian F, Grunfeld S, Welch K M A (1992) Platelet catecholamines in cluster headache. *Journal of Neurology, Neurosurgery and Psychiatry* 55:308–309.

Dandy W E (1934) Concerning the cause of trigeminal neuralgia. *American Journal of Surgery* 24:447–455.

Day W H (1875) On the treatment of different forms of headache. *Lancet* 105:853–855.

Debney L M, Hedge A (1986) Physical trigger factors in migraine—with special reference to weather. In: Amery W K, Wauquier A (eds.) *The prelude to the migraine attack*. Ballière-Tindall. London: 8–24.

de la Pryme A (1702) Extracts of two letters from the Reverend Mr Abraham de la Pryme, F.R.S. to the publisher, concerning subterranean trees, the bitings of mad dogs, & c. *Philosophical Transactions* 23:1073–1077.

Del Sette M, Angeli S, Leandri M, Ferriero G, Bruzzone G L, Finocchi C, Gandolfo C (1998) Migraine with aura and right-to-left shunt on transcranial Doppler: a case-control study. *Cerebrovascular Disease* 8:327–330.

Demeke T, Kidane Y, Wuhib E (1979) Ergotism: a report on an epidemic. *Ethiopian Medical Journal* 17:107–113.

De Villiers (1819) Migraine. In: *Panckoucke's Dictionnaire des sciences médicales*. Société de Médecins et de Chirurgens. Paris: 391–400.

Devor M, Amir R, Rappaport Z H (2002) Pathophysiology of trigeminal neuralgia: the ignition hypothesis. *Clinical Journal of Pain* 18:4–13.

Dewhurst K (1957) A symposium on trigeminal neuralgia, with contributions by Locke, Sydenham, and other eminent seventeenth century physicians. *Journal of the History of Medicine* 12:21–36.

Dewhurst K (1963) *John Locke (1632–1704): physician and philosopher*. Wellcome Historical Medical Library. London.

Dewhurst K (1980) *Thomas Willis' Oxford lectures*. Sandford Publications. Oxford.

Dheur P (1900) *Comment on se défend de la migraine et du mal de tête*. Société d'Editions Scientifiques. Paris.

Diamond S S, Baltes B J (1971) Chronic tension headache—treated with amitriptyline—a double-blind study. *Headache* 11:110–116.

Diamond S, Franklin M A (2005) *Headache through the ages*. Professional Communications. West Islip, N.Y.

Dianoux E (1875) *Du scotome scintillant ou amaurose partielle temporaire*. Thesis. Paris.

Diener H-C (2008) Acupuncture for the treatment of headaches: more than sticking needles into humans. *Cephalalgia* 28:911–913.

Diener H-C, Limmroth V (2004) Medication-overuse headache: a worldwide problem. *Lancet Neurology* 3:475–483.

Diener H-C, Kronfeld K, Boewing G, Lungenhausen M, Maier C, Molsberger A, Tegenthoff M, Trampisch H-J, Zenz M, Meinert R, for the GERAC Migraine Study Group (2006) Efficacy of acupuncture for the prophylaxis of migraine: a multicentre randomised controlled clinical trial. *Lancet Neurology* 5:310–316.

Dodick D W, Mauskop A, Elkind A H, De Gruyse R, Brin M F, Silberstein S D, BOTOX Study Group (2005) Botulinum toxin type a for the prophylaxis of chronic daily headache: subgroup analysis of patients not receiving other prophylactic medications: a randomized double-blind placebo-controlled study. *Headache* 45:315–324.

Doods H, Arndt K, Rudolf K, Just S (2007) CGRP antagonists: unravelling the role of CGRP in migraine. *Trends in Pharmacological Science* 28:580–587.

Doyle JB (1923) A study of four cases of glossopharyngeal neuralgia. *Archives of Neurology and Psychiatry* 9:34–36.

Drabkin I E (1950) *Caelius Aurelianus on acute diseases and on chronic diseases*. University of Chicago Press. Chicago.

Drake F R (1956) Tension headache: a review. *American Journal of the Medical Sciences* 232:105–112.

Du Bois-Reymond E H (1861) De l'hémicrânie ou migraine. *Journal de la physiologie de l'homme et des animaux* 4:130–137.

Ducros A, Tournier-Lasserve E, Bousser M-G (2002) The genetics of migraine. *Lancet Neurology* 1:285–293.

Dudley H W, Moir C (1935) The substance responsible for the traditional clinical effect of ergot. *British Medical Journal* 1:520–523.

Dunlop D M, Davidson L S P, McNee J (1953) *Textbook of medical treatment*. E & S Livingstone. Edinburgh.

Dunning H S (1942) Intracranial and extracranial vascular accidents in migraine. *Archives of Neurology and Psychiatry* 48:396–406.

Dynes J R (1939) Alternating hemiparetic migraine. *British Medical Journal* 2:446–447.

Eadie M J (2001) Clinically significant drug interactions with agents specific for migraine attacks. *CNS Drugs* 15:105–118.

Eadie M J (2004) Could valerian have been the first anticonvulsant? *Epilepsia* 45:1338–1343.

Eadie M J (2009) Hubert Airy, contemporary men of science and the migraine aura. *Journal of the Royal College of Physicians of Edinburgh* 39:263–267.

Eboli P, Stone J L, Aydin S, Slavin K V (2009) Historical characterization of trigeminal neuralgia. *Neurosurgery* 64:1183–1186.

Ekbom K A (1947) Ergotamine tartrate orally in Horton's "histaminic cephalgia" (also called Harris's "ciliary neuralgia"): a new method of treatment. *Acta Psychiatrica et Neurologica Scandinavica* Suppl 46:105–113.

Ekbom K (1977) Lithium in the treatment of chronic cluster headache. *Headache* 17: 39–40.

Ekbom K, Greitz T (1970) Carotid angiography in cluster headache. *Acta Radiologica (Diagn.)* 10:177–186.

Emch-Dériaz A (1992) *Tissot, physician to the enlightenment*. Lang. New York.

Eulenburg A (1877) Vasomotor and trophic neuroses. Hemicrania (migraine). In: van Ziemssen H (ed.) *Cyclopedia of the practice of medicine*. Wood. New York: 3–30.

Eulenburg A (1883) Subcutane injectionen von Ergotin (Tanret) = ergotinium citricum solutm (Gehe). *Deutsche Medizinische Wochenschrift* 44:637–639.

Evers S, Vollmer-Haase J, Schwaag S, Rahmann A, Hussdedt I W, Frese A (2004) Botulinum toxin A in the prophylactic treatment of migraine—a randomized, double-blind, placebo-controlled trial. *Cephalalgia* 24:838–843.

Färkkilä M, Palo J, Saijonmaa O, Fyhrquist F (1992) Raised plasma endothelin during acute migraine attack. *Cephalalgia* 112:383–384.

Féré C (1881) Contribution à l'étude de la migraine ophthalmique. *Revue de médecine* 1: 625–649.

Féré C (1883) Note sur un case de migraine ophthalmique à accès répétés et suivis de mort. *Revue de médizin* 3:194–201.

Féré C (1892) De l'etat de mal migraineux. *Revue de médecine* 12:25–32.

Féré C (1897) Note sur quelques signes physiques de la migraine et en particulier sur un cas de migraine ophthalmospasmodique. *Revue de médecine* 17:954–965.

Féré C (1906) Migraine et épilepsie. *La Belgique médicale* 13:447–451.

Fernandez-de-las-Peñas C, Cuadrado M L, Arendt-Nielsen L, Simons D G, Pareja J A (2007) Myofascial trigger points and sensitization: an updated pain model for tension-type headache. *Cephalalgia* 27:383–393.

Fernel J (1655) *La pathologie ou discours des maladies*. Faret & Guingard. Paris. (Translated Guingard J).

Ferrari M D (1993) Biochemistry of tension-type headache. In: Olesen J, Schoenen J (eds.) *Tension-type headache: classification, mechanisms, and treatment*. Raven Press. New York: 115–126.

Ferrari M D, Odink J, Frölich M, Tapparelli C, Portielje J E (1989) Release of platelet meten-kephalin, but not serotonin, in migraine. *Journal of the Neurological Sciences* 93:51–60.

Ferrari M D, Saxena P R (1993) On serotonin and migraine: a clinical and pharmacological review. *Cephalalgia* 13:151–165.

Ferrier D (1879) Pain in the head in connection with cerebral disease. *Brain* 1:467–483.

Fischer H (1931) *Johann Jakob Wepfer 1620–1696: Ein Beitrag zur Medizingeschichte des 17. Jahrhunderts*. Rudolf. Zurich.

Fogan L (1985) Treatment of cluster headache: a double-blind comparison of oxygen v air inhalation. *Archives of Neurology* 42:362–363.

Fordyce J (1758) *Dissertatio de hemicrania*. Wilson. Durham.

Fothergill J (1773) Of a painful affection of the face. *Medical Observations and Inquiries* 5: 129–142. Reprinted in Lettsom JC (1783) The works of John Fothergill MD. Vol. 2. Dilly. London: 179–189.

Fothergill J (1784) Remarks on that complaint commonly known under the name of the sick headach. *Medical Observations and Inquiries* 6:103–137.

Frank J P (1819) *De curandis hominum morbis epitome, praelectionibus dicata*. Maspero et Buocher. Mediolani.

Franklin W S (1909) The eye as a causative factor in headache with reference to the ear, nose and throat. *California State Medical Journal* 7:405–409.

Frazier C H, Lewy F H, Rowe S N (1937) The origin and mechanism of paroxysmal neuralgic pain and the surgical treatment of central pain. *Brain* 60:44–51.

Fredriksen T A (1989) *Studies on cervicogenic headache*. Dissertation. University of Trondheim.

Friedman A P (1972) The headache in history, literature and legend. *Bulletin of the New York Academy of Medicine* 48:661–681.

Friedman A P, von Storch T (1953) Studies on vascular headache. One thousand cases of migraine and tension headache. *Southern Medical Journal* 46:1127–1132.

Fritsch G, Hitzig E (1870) Ueber die elektrische Erregbarkeit des Grosshirns. *Archiv fur Anatomie und Physiologie* 37:300–332. English translation by von Bonin G (1960) in Von Bonin G (ed.) Some papers on the cerebral cortex. Springfield. Thomas: 73–95.

Fromm G H (1989) The pharmacology of trigeminal neuralgia. *Neuropharmacology* 12: 185–194.

Gabai I J, Spierings E L H (1989) Prophylactic treatment of cluster headache with verapamil. *Headache* 29:167–168.

Gabbai, Lisbonne, Pourquier (1951) Ergot poisoning at Pont St Esprit. *British Medical Journal* 2:650–651.

Galezowski X (1878) Etude sur la migraine ophthalmique. *Archives générales de médecine* June: 669–686; July: 36–56.

Galezowski X (1882) Ophthalmic megrim: an affection of the vaso-motor nerves of the retina and retinal centre which may end in a thrombosis. *Lancet* 116:176–177.

Gallai V, Gaiti A, Sarchielli P, Coata G, Trequattrini A, Peiarone M (1992) Evidence for an altered dopamine beta-hydroxylase activity in migraine and tension-type headache. *Acta Neurologica Scandinavica* 86:403–406.

Gallai V, Sarchelli C, Firenze C, Trequantrini A, Paciaroni M, Usai F, Palumbo R (1994) Endothelin 1 in migraine and tension-type headache. *Acta Neurologica Scandinavica* 89:47–55.

Garcia-Albea Ristol E (1997) Acupunctura y Neurologica. *Revista de neurologica* 25:894–898.

Gardner W J, Stowell A, Dutlinger R (1947) Resection of the greater petrosal nerve in the treatment of unilateral headache. *Journal of Neurosurgery* 4:105–114.

Gee S (1908) *Medical lectures and clinical aphorisms*. Frowde and Hodder & Stoughton. London.

Genefke I K, Dalsgaard-Nielsen T, Bryndum B, Fog-Moller F, Jensen J A P (1975) Concentration of serotonin in blood platelets: effect of reserpine in migraineurs. *Headache* 15: 279–281.

General Chiropractic Council (2004) *Consulting the profession: a survey of UK chiropractors*. http://www.gcc-uk.org/files/link_file/ConsultTheProfession.pdf

Georget E-J, Calmeil L F (1834) Céphalalgie, céphalée. In: Béclard B (ed.) *Adelon's dictionnaire de médecine ou répetoire générales des sciences*. Béchard & Labé. Paris: 117–128.

Gladstone J P (2007) Dopamine and migraine: trigeminovascular nocioception, genetics and migraine. *Cephalalgia* 27:1315–1320.

Goadsby P J (1999) Chronic tension-type headache: where are we? *Brain* 122: 1611–1612.

Goadsby P J (2009) Cervicogenic headache: a pain in the neck for some neurologists? *Lancet Neurology* 8:875–876.

Goadsby P J, Edvinsson L (1994) Human in vivo evidence for trigemino-vascular activation in cluster headache. *Brain* 117:427–434.

Goadsby P J, Edvinsson L, Ekman R (1990) Vasoactive peptide release in the extracerebral circulation of humans during migraine headache. *Annals of Neurology* 28:183–187.

Goadsby P J, Lipton R B (1997) A review of paroxysmal hemicranias, SUNCT syndrome and other short-lasting headaches with autonomic features, including new cases. *Brain* 120:193–209.

Göbel H, Hamouz V, Hansen C, Heininger K, Hirsch S, Linder V, Hauss D, Soyka D (1994) Chronic tension-type headache: amitriptyline reduced clinical headache-duration and experimental pain sensitivity but does not alter pericranial muscle readings. *Pain* 59:241–249.

Göbel H, Isler H, Hasenfratz H-P (1995) Headache classification and the Bible: St Paul's thorn in the flesh. *Cephalalgia* 15:180–181.

Golino P, Piscione F, Willerson J T, Cappelli-Bigazzi M, Foccacio A, Villari B, Indolfi C, Russolillo E, Condorelli M, Chiarello M (1991) Divergent effect of serotonin on coronary-artery dimension and blood flow in patients with coronary atherosclerosis and control patients. *New England Journal of Medicine* 324:641–648.

Gomersall J D, Stuart A (1973) Amitriptyline in migraine prophylaxis. Changes in pattern of attacks during a controlled clinical trial. *Journal of Neurology, Neurosurgery and Psychiatry* 36:684–690.

Gonzáles-Hernández A, Dominguez-Rodriguez M V (2008) Migraine in Gilbertus Anglicus' Compendium medicinae. The cases of MS Sloane 3486 and Wellcome MS537. *Journal of the History of the Neurosciences* 17:147–159.

Goodell H (1967) Thirty years of headache research in the laboratory of the late Dr. Harold G. Wolff. *Headache* 6:158–171.

Gordon N (2004) History of cluster headache. *Current pain and headache reports* 9:132–134.

Gorji A, Ghadiri M K (2002) History of headache in medieval Persian medicine. *Lancet Neurology* 1:510–515.

Govoni V, Ganieri E, Menini C (1996) The history of the tic douloureux: autopathograph of an Italian lawyer who suffered from trigeminal neuralgia from 1803 to 1824. *Journal of the History of the Neurosciences* 5:169–189.

Gowers W R (1888) *A manual of diseases of the nervous system.* Vol. 2. J & A Churchill. London.

Gowers W R (1893) *A manual of diseases of the nervous system.* 2nd ed. Vol. 2. Churchill. London.

Gowers W R (1895) The Bowman lectures on subjective visual sensations. *Lancet* 145: 1562–1566; 1625–1629.

Gowers W R (1907) *The borderland of epilepsy.* Churchill. London.

Gowers W R (1909) An address of the prodromas of migraine. *British Medical Journal* 1: 1400–1403.

Granella F, D'Andrea G (2003) Hemicrania horologica ("clock-like hemicania"). *Neurology* 60:1722–1723.

Grosberg B M, Solomon S, Friedman D I, Lipton R B (2006) Retinal migraine reappraised. *Cephalalgia* 26:1275–1286.

Guest I A, Woolf A L (1964) Fatal infarction of brain in migraine. *British Medical Journal* 1: 225–226.

Gunther R T (1959) *The Greek herbal of Dioscorides. Illustrated by a Byzantine A.D. 512. Englished by John Goodyer AD. 1655.* Hafner. New York.

Haig A (1893) The physics of the cranial circulation and the pathology of headache, epilepsy and mental depression. *Brain* 16:230–258.

Haigler H (1982) Characteristics of extravascular serotonin in the brain. In: Critchley M, Friedman A P, Gorini S, Sicuteri F (eds.) *Headache—Physiopathogenesis and clinical concepts.* Raven Press. New York: 283–289.

Halford H (1833) On the tic douloureux. In: Halford H (ed.) *Essays and addresses.* John Murray. London: 31–45.

Hall M (1833) On the reflex function of the medulla oblongata and medulla spinalis. *Philosophical Transactions* 123:635–665.

Hall M (1836) *Lectures on the nervous system and its diseases.* Sherwood, Gilbert & Piper. London.

Hall M (1849) The neck as a medical region. *Lancet* 53:174–176; 285–287; 394–395; 506–508; 687–688; 54: 66–69; 75–77.

Haller M A (1755) *A dissertation on the sensible and irritable parts of animals.* Nourse. London. (Translated Tissot M).

Handfield-Jones C (1867) *Clinical observations on functional nervous disorders.* Lea. Philadelphia.

Hanington E (1967) Preliminary report on tyramine headache. *British Medical Journal* 2: 550–551.

Hanington E (1978) Migraine: a blood disorder. *Lancet* 312:501–503.

Hardebo J E (1994) How cluster headache is explained as an inflammatory process lesioning sympathetic fibres. *Headache* 34:125–131.

Harris W (1907) The causation and treatment of some headaches. *Lancet* 169:276–278.

Harris W (1922) Persistent pain in lesions of the peripheral and central nervous system. *Brain* 44:557–571.

Harris W (1926) *Neuritis and neuralgia.* Humphrey Milford Oxford University Press. London.

Harris W (1931) Trigeminal neuralgia and its treatment. *Lancet* 217:567–569.

Harris W (1936) Ciliary (migrainous) neuralgia and its treatment. *British Medical Journal* 1:457–460.

Harris W (1940-a) Alcohol injection of the Gasserian ganglion for migrainous neuralgia. *Lancet* 236:481–482.

Harris W (1940-b) An analysis of 1,433 cases of paroxysmal trigeminal neuralgia (trigeminal-tic) and the end-result of Gasserian alcohol injection. *Brain* 63:209–224.

Harris W (1951) A history of the treatment of trigeminal neuralgia. *Postgraduate Medical Journal* 27:18–21.

Headache Classification Committee of the International Headache Society (1988) Classification and diagnostic criteria for headache disorders, cranial neuralgias and facial pain. *Cephalalgia* 8 (Suppl 7): 1–96.

Headache Classification Committee of the International Headache Society (2004) The International Classification of Headache Disorders. *Cephalalgia* 24 (Suppl 1): 1–160.

Heberden W (1802) *Commentaries on the history and cure of diseases.* Payne. London.

Hering-Hanit R (1999) Baclofen for prevention of migraine. *Cephalalgia* 19:589–592.

Heyck H (1972) Varieties of hemiplegic migraine. *Headache* 12:135–142.

Hirsch A (1885) *Handbook of geographical and historical pathology.* New Sydenham Society. London. (Translated Creighton C).

Hoffman A (1978) Historical review on ergot alkaloids. *Pharmacology* 16:1–11.

Horton B T (1941) The use of histamine in specific types of headache. *Journal of the American Medical Association* 116:377–383.

Horton B T (1959) Management of vascular headache. *Angiology* 10:43–56.

Horton B T (1964) Histaminic cephalgia linked with upper respiratory infections. *Headache* 4:228–236.

Horton B T, MacLean A R, Craig W McK (1939) A new syndrome of vascular headache. *Proceedings of the Staff Meetings of the Mayo Clinic* 14:256–260.

Hosack D (1824) Observations on ergot, No 19. In: *Essays on various subjects of medical science.* Seymour. New York: 295–301.

Hotton S (2004) Conway, Anne, Viscountess Conway and Killultagh (1631–1679). In: *Oxford Dictionary of National Biography.* Oxford University Press. Oxford. Online ed., Sept 2010, http://www.oxforddnb.com.ezproxy.library.uq.edu.au/view/article/6119.

Hughes J T (1991) *Thomas Willis 1621–1675. His life and work.* Royal Society of Medicine Services Ltd. London.

Hughson W (1921) A method for the administration of sodium chloride for headaches. *Journal of the American Medical Association* 77:1859–1860.

Humphrey P P A (2007) The discovery of a new drug class for the acute treatment of migraine. *Headache* 47 (Suppl 1): S10–S19.

Hunt T C (1933) Bilious migraine. *Lancet* 222:279–285.

Hurst A F (1924) The Savill Lecture on migraine. *Lancet* 204:1–6.

Hylands P J, Hylands D M, Johnson E S (1987) Feverfew in migraine therapy and research. In: Blau J N (ed.) *Migraine. Clinical and research aspects.* Johns Hopkins University Press. Baltimore: 543–549.

Iadecola C (2002) From CSD to headache: a long and winding road. *Nature Medicine* 8:110–112.

Infeld M (1901) Zur Kenntniss der bleibenden Folke des Migräne-Anfalles. *Weiner Klinische Wochenschrift* 14:673–675.

Isler H (1968) *Thomas Willis 1621–1675. Doctor and scientist.* Hafner. New York.

Isler H (1986) A hidden dimension in headache work: applied history of medicine. *Headache* 26:27–29.

Isler H (1985) Johann Jakob Wepfer (1620–1695): discoveries in headache. *Cephalalgia* 5 (Suppl 3): 423–425.

Isler H (1987-a) Retrospect: the history of thought about migraine from Aretaeus to 1920. In: Blau J N (ed.) *Migraine. Clinical and research aspects.* Johns Hopkins Press. Baltimore: 659–674.

Isler H (1987-b) Independent historical developments of the concepts of cluster headache and trigeminal neuralgia. *Functional Neurology* 2:141–148.

Isler H (1993) Episodic cluster headache from a textbook of 1745: Van Swieten's classic description. *Cephalalgia* 13:172–174.

Isler H, Agarwalla P, Würth G, Agosti R (2005) Migraine in Diderot's Encyclopedia: an historical mainstream text. *Cephalalgia* 25:1173–1178.

Iversen H K, Olesen J (1989) Intravenous nitroglycerine as an experimental model of vascular headache. *Pain* 38:17–24.

Jaccoud S F (1869) Migraine—hémicrânie. In: Jaccoud S F (ed.) *Traité de pathologie interne* Vol. 1, Book 3. Delahaye & Lecrosnier. Paris: 452–456.

Jackson J H (1870) A study of convulsions. *Transactions of the St Andrews Medical Graduates Association* 3:162–204. Reprinted in Taylor, J (ed.) (1931) Selected writings of John Hughlings Jackson. Vol. 1. Staples Press. London: 8–36.

Jackson J H (1873) On the anatomical, physiological, and pathological investigation of epilepsies. *West Riding Lunatic Asylum Medical Reports* 3:315–349. Reprinted in Taylor J (ed.) (1931) Selected writings of John Hughlings Jackson. Vol. 1. Staples Press. London: 90–111.

Jackson J H (1876) On epilepsies and on the after-effects of epileptic discharges (Todd and Robertson's hypothesis). *West Riding Asylum Medical Reports* 6:266–309. Reprinted in Taylor J (ed.) (1931) Selected writings of John Hughlings Jackson. Vol. 1. Staples Press. London: 135–161.

Jelliffe S E, White W A (1923) *Diseases of the nervous system: a textbook of neurology and psychiatry*. Lewis & Co. London.

Jolly P (1830) Céphalalgie. In: Andral (ed.) *Dictionnaire de médicine et de chirugie practique*. Méquigon-Mavais, Ballière. Paris: 150–156.

Jones J M (1999) Great pains: famous people with headaches. *Cephalalgia* 19:627–630.

Jones R J, Wachowicz B, Lush S, Amess J A L (1981) Platelet aggregation studies during the migraine cycle. In: Rose F C, Zilkha K J (eds.) *Progress in migraine research*. Pitman. London: 85–88.

Jowett B (1892) *The dialogues of Plato*. Vol. 1. Oxford University Press. Oxford.

Kallela M, Färkkilä. M, Saijonmaa O, Fyhrquist F (1998) Endothelin in migraine patients. *Cephalalgia* 18:329–332.

Karenberg A, Leitz C (2001) Headache in magical and medical papyri of ancient Egypt. *Cephalalgia* 21:911–916.

Karwautz A, Wöber-Bingöl C, Wöber C (1996) Freud and migraine: the beginnings of a psychodynamically oriented view of headache a hundred years ago. *Cephalalgia* 16: 22–26.

Kelly E C (1971) *Classics of neurology*. Kreiger Publishing. Huntington, N.Y.

Khan O A (1998) Gabapentin relieves trigeminal neuralgia in multiple sclerosis patients. *Neurology* 51:611–614.

Kimball R W, Friedman A P, Vallejo E (1960) Effect of serotonin in migraine patients. *Neurology* 10:107–111.

Kirkpatrick P J, O'Brien M D, Mac Cabe J J (1993) Trigeminal nerve section for chronic migrainous neuralgia. *British Journal of Neurosurgery* 7:483–490.

Klimek A (1982) Plasma testosterone levels in patients with cluster headache. *Headache* 22:162–164.

Koehler P J (1993) Prevalence of headache in Tulp's Observationes Medicae (1641) with a description of cluster headache. *Cephalalgia* 13:318–320.

Koehler P J (1996) Neurology in Tulp's Observationes Medicae. *Journal of the History of the Neurosciences* 5:143–151.

Koehler P J (1997) Etiology and pathophysiology of headache in the early 17th century, as illustrated by the work of Johan van Beverwijck. *Cephalalgia* 17:817–821.

Koehler P P J, Boes C J (2010) A history of non-drug treatment in headache, particularly migraine. *Brain* 133:2489–2500.

Koehler P J, Isler H (2002) The early use of ergotamine in migraine. Edward Woakes' report of 1868, its theoretical and practical background and its international reception. *Cephalalgia* 22:686–691.

Koehler P J, Tfelt-Hansen P C (2008) History of methysergide in migraine. *Cephalalgia* 28:1126–1135.

Kovalesky P (1906) L'épilepsie et la migraine. *Archives de neurologie* 21:356–379.

Kudrow L (1976) Plasma testosterone levels in cluster headache: Preliminary results. *Headache* 16:28–31.

Kudrow L (1977) Lithium prophylaxis for chronic cluster headache. *Headache* 17:14–18.

Kudrow L (1979) Thermographic and Doppler flow asymmetry in cluster headache. *Headache* 19:204–208.

Kudrow L (1981) Response of cluster headache attacks to oxygen inhalation. *Headache* 21:1–4.

Kudrow L (1987) Cluster headache. In: Dalessio D J (ed.) *Wolff's headache and other head pain.* 5th ed. Oxford University Press. New York: 112–130.

Kühn K G E (1821–1833) *Galen's Omnia opera.* Vols. 1–20. Cnoblochii. Leipzig.

Kunkle E C (1959) Mechanism of headache. In: Friedman A P, Merritt H H (eds.) *Headache. Diagnosis and treatment.* Davis. Philadelphia: 3–22.

Kunkle E C, Pfeiffer J B, Wilhoit W W, Hamrick L W (1952) Recurrent brief headache in cluster pattern. *Transactions of the American Neurological Association* 56 (77th meeting): 240–243.

Kunkle P C, Pfeiffer J B, Wilhoit W M (1954) Recurrent brief headaches in cluster pattern. *North Carolina Medical Journal* 15:510–512.

Labarraque H (1837) *Essai sur la céphalalgie et la migraine.* Thesis. Paris.

Labarthe P (1868) *Nos médecins contemporains.* Lebigre-Duquesne. Paris.

Lampl C, Buzath A, Klinger D, Neumann K (1999) Lamotrigine in the prophylactic treatment of migraine aura—a pilot study. *Cephalalgia* 19:58–63.

Lampl C, Katsarava Z, Diener H C, Limmroth V (2005) Lamotrigine reduces migraine aura and migraine attacks in patients with migraine with aura. *Journal of Neurology, Neurosurgery and Psychiatry* 76:1730–1732.

Lampl C, Voelker M, Diener H C (2007) Efficacy and safety of 1000mg effervescent aspirin: individual patient data meta-analysis of three trials in migraine headache and migraine accompanying symptoms. *Journal of Neurology* 254:705–712.

Lance J (2004) Federigo Sicuteri (1920–2003), a headache medicine pioneer. *Cephalalgia* 24:1090–1091.

Lance J W, Anthony M (1971) Thermographic studies in vascular headache. *Medical Journal of Australia* 1:240–243.

Lance J W, Anthony M, Hinterberger H (1967) The control of cranial arteries by humoral mechanisms and its relation to migraine. *Headache* 7:93–102.

Lance J W, Curran D A (1964) Treatment of chronic tension headache. *Lancet* 283: 1236–1239.

Lance J W, Fine R D, Curran D A (1963) An evaluation of methysergide in the prevention of migraine and other vascular headaches. *Medical Journal of Australia* 1:814–818.

Lance J W, Anthony M, Somerville B (1970) Comparative trial of serotonin antagonists in the management of migraine. *British Medical Journal* 2:327–330.

Larner A J (2005) Caleb Hillier Parry (1755–1822): clinician, scientist, friend of Edward Jenner (1749–1823). *Medical Biography* 14:189–194.

Langmead F (1905) On recurrent vomiting of childhood (cyclical vomiting), with the reports of two cases. *British Medical Journal* 1:350–352.

Lashley K S (1941) Patterns of cerebral integration indicated by the scotomas of migraine. *Archives of Neurology and Psychiatry* 49:331–339.

Latham P W (1872) Nervous or sick headache. *British Medical Journal* 1:305–306; 336–337.

Latham P W (1873) *On nervous or sick-headache, its varieties and treatment.* Deighton, Bull & Co. Cambridge.

Leão A A P (1944-a) Pial circulation and spreading depression of activity in the cerebral cortex. *Journal of Neurophysiology* 7:391–396.

Leão A A P (1944-b) Spreading depression of activity in the cerebral cortex. *Journal of Neurophysiology* 7:359–390.

Leão A A P (1947) Further observations on the spreading depression of activity in the cerebral cortex. *Journal of Neurophysiology* 10:409–414.

Leão A A P, Morison R S (1945) Propagation of spreading cortical depression. *Journal of Neurophysiology* 8:33–46.

Lee M R (2009, 2010) The history of ergot of rye. I. from antiquity to 1900. II. 1900–1940. III. 1940–1980. *Journal of the Royal College of Physicians of Edinburgh* 39:179–184; 365–369; 40: 77–80.

Lempert T, Neuhauser H (2009) Epidemiology of vertigo, migraine and vestibular migraine. *Journal of Neurology* 256:333–338.

Lennox W G (1946) *Science and seizures: new light on epilepsy and migraine.* Harper & Bros. New York.

Lennox W G, von Storch T J C (1935) Experience with ergotamine tartrate in 120 patients with migraine. *Journal of the American Medical Association* 105:169–171.

Leone M, D'Amico D, Moschiano F, Fraschini F, Bussone G (1996) Melatonin versus placebo in the prophylaxis of cluster headache: a double-blind pilot study with parallel groups. *Cephalalgia* 16:494–496.

Leone M, D'Amico D, Frediani F, Moschiano F, Grazzi L, Attanasio A, Bussone G (2000) Verapamil in the prophylaxis of episodic cluster headache: a double-blind study versus placebo. *Neurology* 54:1382–1385.

Leone M, Franzini A, Bussone G (2001) Stereotaxic stimulation of posterior hypothalamic grey matter in a patient with intractable cluster headache. *New England Journal of Medicine* 345:1428–1429.

Le Pois C (1618) *Selectiorum observationum et consiliorum de praetervisis hactenus morbis affectibusque praeter naturam.* Carolum Mercatorem. Pont-à-Mausson.

Leslie W, Dunsworth F A (1947) Headache: treatment with histamine. *Canadian Medical Association Journal* 56:509–512.

Lewis W (1783) *A system of the practice of medicine from the Latin of Dr Hoffman.* Vol. 1. Murray & Johnson. London.

Lewy F H (1938) The first authentic case of major trigeminal neuralgia. *Annals of Medical History* 10:247–250.

Leyton N (1954) *Migraine and periodic headaches. A modern approach to successful treatment.* Heinemann. London.

Leyton N (1958) Treatment of migraine. *Pharmacy Journal* 180:470–. Cited by Wolff H G (1963) *loc. cit.*

Li B U K, Murray R D, Heitlinger L A, Robbins J L, Hayes J R (1999) Is cyclic vomiting related to migraine? *Journal of Pediatrics* 134:567–572.

Limmroth V, Katsarava Z, Diener H-C (1999) Acetylsalicylic acid in the treatment of headache. *Cephalalgia* 19:545–551.

Liu Z, Liu L (2009) *Essentials of Chinese medicine.* Vol. 3. Springer. Dordrecht.

Liveing E (1872) Observations on megrim or sick-headache. *British Medical Journal* 1: 364–366.

Liveing E (1873) *On megrim, sick-headache, and some allied disorders: a contribution to the pathology of nerve-storms.* Churchill. London.

Locock C (1857-a) Discussion following Dr Sieveking "Analysis of fifty-two cases of epilepsy observed by the author." *Medical Times and Gazette* 1: 524–526.

Locock C (1857-b) Discussion of paper by E. H. Sieveking. Analysis of fifty-two cases of epilepsy observed by the author. *Lancet* 59:527.

Logan A H, Allen E V (1934) The treatment of migraine with ergotamine tartrate. *Proceedings of the Mayo Clinic* 9:585–588.

Lorry A C (1760) Sur les mouvememts du cerveaux et de la dure-mère. Premier mémoir, sur le mouvement des parties contenues dans le crâne, considerées dans leut état naturel. *Mémoires de Mathématique et de Physique* 3:277–313. Cited by Neuburger M (1897/1981) *loc. cit.*

Love S, Coakham H B (2001) Trigeminal neuralgia. Pathology and pathogenesis. *Brain* 124:2347–2360.

Loveless M (1950) Milk allergy: a survey of its incidence: experiments with a masked ingestion test; allergy for corn and its derivatives: experiments with a masked ingestion test for its diagnosis. *Journal of Allergy* 21:489–499.

MacGregor W A (1996) "Menstrual" migraine: towards a definition. *Cephalalgia* 16:11–21.

MacGregor E A, Wilkinson M, Bancroft K (1993) Domperidone and paracetamol in the treatment of migraine. *Cephalalgia* 13:124–127.

Magnus H (1908) *Superstition in medicine.* Funk & Wagnall. New York, London. (Translated Salinger J L).

Maier H-W (1926) L'ergotamine, inhibiteur du sympathetique étudié en clinique, comme moyen d'exploration et comme agent thérapeutique. *Revue Neurologique Paris* 33:1104–1108.

Manack A, Turkel C, Silberstein D (2009) The evolution of chronic migraine: classification and nomenclature. *Headache* 49:1206–1213.

Marcus D A, Scharff L, Turk D, Gourley L M (1997) A double-blind provocative study of chocolate as a trigger of migraine. *Cephalalgia* 17:855–862.

Marcus Aurelius (1906) *Meditations.* Dent & Sons. London.

Martin P (1829) *Traité de la migraine, et des autres sortes de maux de tête.* Charpentier. Paris.

Martineau L (1867) Céphalgie, céphalée. In: S. Jaccoud (ed.) *Nouveau dictionnaire de médecine et de chirurgie pratique.* Ballière. Paris: 641–665.

Mascia A, Afra J, Schoenen J (1998) Dopamine and migraine: a review of pharmacological, biochemical, neurophysiological, and therapeutic data. *Cephalalgia* 18:174–182.

Masel B E, Chesson A L, Peters B H, Levin H S, Alperin J B (1980) Platelet antagonists in migraine prophylaxis. A clinical trial using aspirin and dipyramidole. *Headache* 20:13–18.

Mathew N T, Reuveni U, Perez F (1987) Transformed or evolutive migraine. *Headache* 27:102–106.

Mathew N T, Rapoport A, Saper J, Magnus L, Kapper J, Ramadan N, Stacey B, Tepper S (2001) Efficacy of gabapentin in migraine prophylaxis. *Headache* 41:119–128.

Matossian M K (1989) *Poisons of the past: molds, epidemics and history.* Yale University Press. New Haven.

May A, Bahra A, Büchel C, Frackowick R S, Goadsby P J (1998) Hypothalamic activation in cluster headache attacks. *Lancet* 352:275–278.

Mazzotta G, Sarchielli P, Gaggioli A, Gallai V (1997) Studies of pressure pain and cellular concentrations of neurotransmitters related to nociception in episodic tension-type headache patients. *Headache* 37:565–571.

Mearse J (1832) *On the causes, cure and prevention of the sick-headache.* Porter. Philadelphia.

Méglin M (1816) *Recherches et observations sur la névralgie faciale ou le tic douloureux de la face.* Levrault. Strasbourg.

Melchart D, Linde K, Fischer P, White A, Allais G, Vickers A, Berman B (1999) Acupuncture for idiopathic headache. *Cephalalgia* 19:779–786.

Melis P M L, Rooimans W, Spierings E L H, Hoogduin A L (1991) Treatment of chronic tension-type headache with hypnotherapy: a single-blind time controlled study. *Headache* 31:686–689.

Mendizabal J E (1999) Cluster headache. *Archives of Neurology* 56:1413–1416.

Mett A, Tfelt-Hansen P (2008) Acute migraine therapy: recent evidence from randomized comparative trials. *Current Opinion in Neurology* 21:331–337.

Milner P M (1958) Note on a possible correspondence between the scotomas of migraine and spreading depression of Leao. *Electroencephalography and Clinical Neurophysiology* 10:705.

Mitchell S W (1874) Headaches from heat-stroke, from fever, after meningitis, from over use of the brain, from eye-strain. *Medical and Surgical Reporter* 31:67–70; 81–84. Reprinted in Knapp B D (1963) *Headache* 3:69–77.

Moebius P J (1894) *Die migräne*. Holder. Wein.

Moench L G (1947) *Headache*. Year Book Publishers. Chicago.

Moffett A M, Swash M, Scott D F (1972) Effect of tyramine in migraine: a double-blind study. *Journal of Neurology, Neurosurgery and Psychiatry* 35:496–499.

Moffett A M, Swash M, Scott D F (1974) Effect of chocolate in migraine: a double-blind study. *Journal of Neurology, Neurosurgery and Psychiatry* 37:445–448.

Möllendorf (1867) Ueber Hemikranie. *Archiv für Pathologie* 47:385–395.

Morgagni G B (1779) *The seat and causes of diseases, investigated by anatomy*. Vol. 1. Miller & Cadell. London. (Translated Alexander B). Reprinted in Kelly E C (1971) *loc. cit.*

Moskowitz M A (2007) Pathophysiology of headache—past and present. *Headache* 47 (Suppl 1): S58–S63.

Moxon W (1875) Clinical lecture on treatment of headache from organic intracranial disease. *Lancet* 105:749–751.

Murphy P J (1854) On headache and its varieties. *Lancet* 63:182–183; 209–210; 300–301.

Nattero G, Savi L, Pisanti G (1980) Doppler blood flow in cluster headache. *International Congress Headache '80*. Cited by Kudrow L (1987), *loc. cit.*

Nattero G, Bulla A, Levi E, Peyretti F (1981) Platelet aggregability and migraine: is their relationship a reality? In: Rose F C, Zilkha K J (eds.) *Progress in migraine research*. Pitman. London: 69–79.

Nelson R F (1978) Testosterone levels in cluster and non-cluster migrainous headache patients. *Headache* 18:265–267.

Neuberger M (1897/1981) *The historical development of experimental brain and spinal cord physiology before Flourens*. Johns Hopkins Press. Baltimore & London. (Translated Clarke E).

Norström G (1885) *Traitment de la migraine par le massage*. Delahaye Lecrosnier. Paris.

Nunn J F (2002) *Ancient Egyptian medicine*. University of Oklahoma Press. Norman.

Olesen J (1986) Chemicals which may trigger migraine attacks. In: Amery W G, Wahlquier A (eds.) *The prelude to the migraine attack*. Ballière-Tindall. London: 25–35.

Olesen J (1991) Clinical and pathophysiological observations in migraine and tension-type headache explained by integration of vascular, supraspinal and myofascial inputs. *Pain* 46:125–132.

Olesen J, Tfelt-Hansen P, Hansen L, Larsen B (1981) The common migraine attack may not be initiated by cerebral ischaemia. *Lancet* 318:438–440.

Olesen J, Thomsen L L, Lassen L H, Olesen I J (1995) The nitric acid hypothesis of migraine and other vascular headache. *Cephalalgia* 15:94–100.

O'Neill B P, Mann J D (1978) Aspirin prophylaxis in migraine. *Lancet* 312:71–76.

Oppenheim H (1904) *Diseases of the nervous system. A textbook for students and practitioners.* Lippincott. Philadelphia. (Translated Mayer E H).

Oppenheim H (1894) *Lehrbuch der Nervenkrankheiten für Ärzte und Studirende*. Karger. Berlin.

Oppenheim H (1911) *Textbook of nervous diseases*. Vol. 2. Schulze. Edinburgh. (Translated Bruce A N).

Oppermann J C V (1747) *Dissertatio medica inauguralis de hemicrania horologica*. Hilligeri. Halle Magdeberg.

Osler W (1892) *The principles and practice of medicine*. Appleton & Co. New York.

Ostergaard S, Russell M B, Bendtsen L, Olesen J (1997) Comparison of first degree relatives and spouses of people with chronic tension-type headache. *British Medical Journal* 314:1092–1093.

Parry C H (1792) On compression of the arteries in various diseases and particularly in those of the head: with hints towards a new mode of treating nervous disorders. *Memoirs of the Medical Society of London* 3:77. Cited by Liveing E (1873) *loc. cit.*

Parry C H (1811) On a case if nervous affection cured by pressure of the carotids; with some physiological remarks. *Philosophical Transactions* 101:89–95.

Parry C H (1825-a) *Elements of pathology and therapeutics.* 2nd. ed. Vol. 1. Cruttwell. London.

Parry C H (1825-b) Scintillating scotoma. In: Parry C H (ed.) *Collections from the unpublished writings of the late Caleb Hillier Parry MD, FRS.* Underwood. London: Vol. 1: 557.

Paterson D R (1890) Recurring ocular palsy. *Lancet* 136:558–559.

Patsioti J G, Rose F C (1995) What did the Greeks mean? *Journal of the History of the Neurosciences* 4:67–76.

Pearce J M S (1999) Edward Liveing's (1831–1919) theory of nerve-storms in migraine. In: Rose F C (ed.) *A short history of neurology. The British contribution 1660–1910.* Butterworth Heinemann. Oxford: 192–203.

Pearce J M S (2003) Freud's migraine, and contributions to neurology. In Pearce J M S, *Fragments of neurological history.* Imperial College Press. London: 615–621.

Pearce J M S (2008) Glossopharyngeal neuralgia. *European Neurology* 55:49–52.

Peikert A, Wilimzig C, Köhne-Volland R (1996) Prophylaxis of migraine with oral magnesium: results from a prospective, multi-centre, placebo-controlled randomized study. *Cephalalgia* 16:257–263.

Peiris J B, Perera G L S, Devendra S V, Lionel N D W (1980) Sodium valproate in trigeminal neuralgia. *Medical Journal of Australia* 2:278.

Pelletan de Kinkelin J P (1832) *Coup d'oeil sur la migraine.* De Deville Cavellin. Paris.

Pennybacker J (1961) Some observations on trigeminal neuralgia. In: Garland H (ed.) *Scientific aspects of neurology.* Livingstone. Edinburgh: 153–167.

Peroutka S J (1997) Dopamine and migraine. *Neurology* 49:650–656.

Peters R (1934) Tödliche Gehirnblutung bei menstruller Migräne. *Beitrage zur pathologischen Anatomie und zur allegemainen Pathologie* 93:209–218.

Peters G A, Horton B T (1951) Headache: with special reference to the excessive use of ergotamine preparations and withdrawal effects. *Proceedings of the Staff Meetings of the Mayo Clinic* 26:153–161.

Peto R, Gray R, Collins R, Wheatly K, Hennekens C, Jamrozik K (1988) Randomized trial of prophylactic daily aspirin in British male doctors. *British Medical Journal* 296:313–316.

Petroz (1817) Hemicrania. In: Pancoucke (ed.) *Dictionnaire des sciences médicale.* Sociétè de Médecins et de Chirurgie. Paris: 260–263.

Pfaffenrath V, Wessely P, Meyer C, Isler H R, Evers S, Grotemeyer K H, Taneri Z, Soyka D, G'bel H, Fischer M (1996) Magnesium in the prophylaxis of migraine—a double-blind, placebo-controlled study. *Cephalalgia* 16:436–440.

Piorry P A (1831) *Mémoire sur la migraine.* Ballière. Paris.

Piorry P A (1835) Quatrième partie. Mémoire. Sur l'une des affections désignées sous le nom de migraine ou hémicranie (Reprint of Piorry 1831, *loc. cit.*). In Piorry P A, *Du procédé opératoire a suivre dans l'exploration des organes par la percussion médicale.* Ballière. Paris: 405–425.

Piorry P A (1875) Mémoire sur le vertige. *Bulletin de l'Academie de médecine* 66:1–12.

Pliny (first cent. a.d.) *Natural history.* Heinemann and Harvard University Press. London and Cambridge, Mass. (Translated Jones W H S).

Pöllmann W, Keidel M, Pfaffenrath V (1997) Headache and the cervical spine: a critical review. *Cephalalgia* 17:801–816.

Posadzki P, Ernst E (2011) Spinal manipulation for the treatment of migraine: a systematic review of randomized clinical trials. *Cephalalgia* 31: 964–970.

Pravaz (1825) Considérations sur quelques anomalies de vision. *Archives Générales de Médecine* Series 1, 8:59–84.

Pujol M (1787) Essai sur la maladie de la face, nammée le tic douloureux avec réflexions sur le captus caninus, de Caelius Aurelianus. *Journal de Médecine, Chirurgie et Pharmacie* 72:287–290.

Puschmann T (1878) *Alexander von Tralles.* Vol. 1. Bräunmuller. Wien.

Quave C L, Pieroni A (2005) Ritual healing in Arbereshe Albanian and Italian communities of Lurania, Southern Italy. *Journal of Folklore Research* 42:57–97.

Raeder J G (1924) "Paratrigeminal" paralysis of oculo-pupillary sympathetic. *Brain* 47: 149–158.

Raskin N H (1988) The hypnic headache syndrome. *Headache* 28:534–536.

Rasmussen B K, Jensen R, Schroll M, Olesen J (1991) Epidemiology of headache in a general population—a prevalence study. *Journal of Clinical Epidemiology* 44:1147–1157.

Remahl I N, Waldenlind E, Bratt J, Ekbon K I (2000) Cluster headache is not associated with signs of a systemic inflammation. *Headache* 40:276–281.

Reynolds J R (1855) *The diagnosis of diseases of the brain, spinal cord, nerves and their appendages.* J. Churchill. London.

Reynolds J R (1874) *Lectures of the clinical uses of electricity.* Lea & Blakiston. Philadelphia.

Reynolds J R (1876) *Lectures on the clinical uses of electricity.* 2nd. ed. Lindsay & Blakiston. Philadelphia.

Reynolds J R (1890) On the therapeutical uses and toxic effects of cannabis indica. *Lancet* 135:637–638.

Riley H A (1932) Migraine. *Bulletin of the Neurological Institute of New York* 2:429–544.

Ringer S (1877) A suggestion concerning the condition of the nervous centres in migraine, epilepsy, and other explosive neuroses. *Lancet* 109:228–229.

Rollnik J D, Tanneberger O, Schubert M, Schneider U, Dengler R (2000) Treatment of tension-type headache with botulinum toxin type A: a double-blind, placebo-controlled study. *Headache* 40:300–305.

Romberg M H (1853) *A manual of the nervous diseases of man.* New Sydenham Society. London. (Translated Sieveking E H).

Rose F C (1999-a) John Fothergill (1712–1780). In: Rose F C (ed.) *A short history of neurology: the British contribution 1660–1910.* Butterworth Heinemann. Oxford: 88–92.

Rose F C (1999-b) Trigeminal neuralgia. *Archives of Neurology* 56:1163–1164.

Rose W (1892-a) Abstract of the Lettsomian lectures on the surgical treatment of trigeminal neuralgia. *Lancet* 139:71–73; 182–184; 295–301.

Rose W (1892-b) *The surgical treatment of neuralgia of the fifth nerve (tic douloureux).* Baillière, Tindall, Cox. London.

Rosner F (1993) Headache in the writings of Moses Maimonides and other Hebrew sages. *Headache* 33:315–319.

Ross J (1885) *Handbook of the diseases of the nervous system.* J & A Churchill and Lea Brothers & Co. London and Philadelphia.

Rothlin E (1955) Historical development of the ergot therapy of migraine. *International Archives of Allergy and Immunology* 7:205–209.

Rowland R (1838) *A treatise on neuralgia.* Higley. London.

Rucker W C (1958) The concept of a semidecussation of the optic nerves. *Archives of Ophthalmology* 59:159–171.

Rudnick G, Bencuya R, Nelson P J, Zito R A J (1981) Inhibition of platelet serotonin transport by propranolol. *Molecular Pharmacology* 20:118–123.

Russell D (1984) Chronic paroxysmal hemicrania: severity, duration and time of occurrence of attacks. *Cephalalgia* 4: 53–56.

Russell M B (1997) Genetic epidemiology of migraine and cluster headache. *Cephalalgia* 17:683–701.

Russell M B, Andersson P G, Thomsen L L (1995) Familial occurrence of cluster headache. *Journal of Neurology, Neurosurgery and Psychiatry* 58:341–343.

Russell M B, Rasmussen B K, Fenger K, Olesen J (1996) Migraine without aura and migraine with aura are distinct clinical entities; a study of four hundred and eighty-four male and female migraineurs from the general population. *Cephalalgia* 16:239–245.

Russell M B, Ulrich V, Gervil M, Olesen J (2002) Migraine without aura and migraine with aura are distinct disorders. A population-based twin study. *Headache* 42:332–336.

Russo E (1998) Cannabis for migraine treatment: the once and future prescription? An historical and scientific review. *Pain* 76:3–8.

Ryan R E S, Ryan R E J (1982) The use of platelet inhibitors in migraine. *Advances in Neurology* 33:247–252.

Sakai F, Ebihara S, Akiyama M, Horikawa M (1995) Pericranial muscle hardness in tension-type headache. A non-invasive measurement method and its clinical application. *Brain* 118:523–531.

Sakula A (1979) Pierre Adolphe Piorry (1794–1879): pioneer of percussion and pleximetry. *Thorax* 34:575–581.

Saundby R (1882) A case of migraine, with paralysis of the third nerve. *Lancet* 120:345–346.

Saxena P R (1992) Historical aspects of 5-hydroxytryptamine: discovery and receptor classification. In: Olesen J, Saxena P R (eds.) *5-Hydroxytryptamine mechanisms in primary headaches*. Raven Press. New York: 3–18.

Schiller F (1962) Prophylactic ergot and other treatments for limited migraine variant. *Headache* 2:90–93.

Schobelt C H (1776) *Tractatio de hemicrania*. Impensis Bibliopol. Scholae Realis. Berolini.

Schoenen J, Jacquy J, Lenaerts M (1998) Effectiveness of high-dose riboflavin in migraine prophylaxis. *Neurology* 50:466–470.

Schrader H, Stovner L J, Helde G, Sand T, Bovim G (2001) Prophylactic treatment of migraine with angiotensin converting enzyme inhibitor (lisinopril): randomised, placebo controlled, crossover study. *British Medical Journal* 1:19–22.

Schumacher D (1878) Ergot in the treatment of angioparalytic megrim. *Lancet* 112:212–213.

Selby G, Fryer J A (1984) Fatal migraine. *Clinical and Experimental Neurology* 20:85–92.

Seller W (1848) On the seat of headache in the sympathetic nerve, and on some of the rules of treatment drawn from its connexion with chronic ill health. *Monthly Journal of Medical Sciences* 9:137–146.

Shiels J W (1909) The medical side of headache. *California State Medical Journal* 7:400–405.

Shimomura T, Takahashi K (1990) Alteration of platelet serotonin in patients with chronic tension-type headache during cold pressor test. *Headache* 30:581–583.

Shuldham E B (1876) *Headaches: their causes and treatment*. Gould & Son. London.

Shulka R, Shanker K, Nag D, Verma M, Bhargava K P (1987) Serotonin in tension headache. *Journal of Neurology, Neurosurgery and Psychiatry* 50:1682–1684.

Sicard R, Robineau J (1920) Algie vélo-pharangyée-essentiellle. *Revue Neurologique* 36: 256–257.

Sicuteri F (1959) Prophylactic and therapeutic properties of 1-methyl-lysergic acid butanolamide in migraine. *International Archives of Allergy and Applied Immunology* 15: 300–307.

Sicuteri F (1972) Headache as a possible expression of deficiency of brain 5-hydroxytryptamine (cental denervation supersensitivity). *Headache* 12:68–71.

Sicuteri F (1976) Hypothesis: migraine, a central biochemical dysnociception. *Headache* 16:145–159.

Sicuteri F (1977) Dopamine, the second putative protagonist in headache. *Headache* 17: 129–131.

Sicuteri F, Testi A, Anselmi B (1961) Biochemical investigations in headache: increase in the hydroxyindoleacetic acid excretion during migraine attacks. *International Archives of Allergy and Applied Immunology* 19:55–58.

Siegel R E (1976) *Galen on the affected parts.* Karger. Basel.

Sieveking E H (1854) On chronic and periodical headaches. *Medical Times and Gazette* 9: 156–168; 181–182; 208–210.

Sieveking E H (1858) *On epilepsy and epileptiform seizures. Their causes, pathology, and treatment.* Churchill. London.

Silberstein S D (1997) Preventive treatment of migraine: an overview. *Cephalalgia* 17:67–72.

Sindrup S H, Jensen T S (2002) Pharmacotherapy of trigeminal neuralgia. *Clinical Journal of Pain* 18:22–27.

Singer C (2005) The visions of Hildegard of Bingen. *Yale Journal of Biology and Medicine* 78: 57–82 (Reprint of 1917 paper).

Singh N N, Misra S (2002) Sertraline on chronic tension-type headache. *Journal of the Association of Physicians of India* 50:873–878.

Sjaastad O (1970) Kinin-OG histaminiunders o kelser ved migrene. *Kiliniske Aspecter i Migrene Forshningen*: pp. 61–69. Norlundes Bogtrykkeri. Copenhagen.

Sjaastad O (1987) Chronic paroxysmal hemicrania (CPH) and similar headaches. In: Dalessio D J (ed.) *Wolff's headache and other head pain.* 5th ed. Oxford University Press. New York: 131–135.

Sjaastad O, Dale I (1974) Evidence for a new (?) treatable headache entity. *Headache* 14: 105–108.

Sjaastad O, Spierings E L H (1984) "Hemicrania continua." Another headache with absolute indomethacin response. *Cephalalgia* 4:65–70.

Sjaastad O, Rootwelt K, Horven I (1974) Cutaneous blood flow in cluster headache. *Headache* 13:173–175.

Sjaastad O, Hovdahl H, Breivik H, Gronback E (1983) "Cervicogenic" headache. An hypothesis. *Cephalalgia* 3:249–256.

Sjaastad O, Saunte C, Salvesen R, Fredriksen T A, Seim A, Roe O D, Fosted K, Lobben O-P, Zhao J-M (1989) Short-lasting unilateral neuralgiform headache attacks with conjunctival injection, tearing, sweating, and rhinorrhoea. *Cephalalgia* 9:147–156.

Sjaastad O, Fredriksen T A, Pfaffenrath V (1990) Cervicogenic headache: diagnostic criteria. *Headache* 30:725–726.

Skwire S E (1999) Women, writers, sufferers: Anne Conway and An Collins. *Literature and Medicine* 18:1–23.

Slater R (1979) Benign recurrent vertigo. *Journal of Neurology, Neurosurgery and Psychiatry* 42:363–367.

Sluder G (1918) *Concerning some headache and eye disorders of nasal origin.* Mosby. St Louis.

Smith W D (1994) *Hippocrates.* Vol. 7. Harvard University Press. Cambridge, Mass.

Sneader W (2000) The discovery of aspirin: a reappraisal. *British Medical Journal* 2:1591–1594.

Somerville B W (1972) The influence of progesterone and estradiol upon migraine. *Headache* 12:93–102.

Sorensen K V (1988) Valproate: a new drug in migraine prevention. *Acta Neurologica Scandinavica* 778:346–348.

Spector J T, Kahn S R, Jones M R, Jayakumar M, Dalai D, Nazarian S (2010) Migraine headache and ischaemic stroke risk: an up-dated meta-analysis. *American Journal of Medicine* 123:612–624.

Speight T M, Avery G S (1972) Pizotifen (BC-105): a review of its pharmacological properties and its therapeutic efficacy in vascular headaches. *Drugs* 3:159–203.

Spencer W G (1938) *Celsus De Medicina.* Harvard University Press. Cambridge, Massachusetts.

Spitzer A (1901) *Uber migraine.* Fischer. Jena.

Spriggs E (1935) A clinical study of headache. *Lancet* 226:1–8; 63–67.

Stahl J S, Daroff R B (2001) Time for more attention to migrainous vertigo? *Neurology* 56: 428–429.

Stearns J (1808) Account of the pulvis parturiens, a remedy for quickening child-birth. *Medical Repository of New York* 5:308–309.

Steiner T J, Findley L J, Yuan A W (1997-a) Lamotrigine versus placebo in the prophylaxis of migraine with and without aura. *Cephalalgia* 17:109–112.

Steiner T J, Hering R, Couturier E G, Davies P T, Whitmarsh T E (1997-b) Double-blind placebo-controlled trial of lithium in episodic cluster headache. *Cephalalgia* 17: 673–675.

Stensrud P, Sjaastad O (1976) Short-term clinical trial of propranolol in racemic form (Inderal) d-propranolol and placebo in migraine. *Acta Neurologica Scandinavica* 53:229–232.

Stensrud P, Sjaastad O (1980) Comparative trial of Tenormin (atenolol) and Inderal (propranolol) in migraine. *Headache* 20:206–207.

Stewart W F, Lipton R B, Chee E, Sawyer J, Silberstein S D (2000) Menstrual cycle and headache in a population sample of migraineurs. *Neurology* 55:1517–1523.

Stoll A (1918) Zur Kenntnis der Mutterkornalkaloide. *Varhandlungen der Schweizerischen Naturforschungsgesellschaft* 101:190–191.

Stookey B, Ransohoff J (1959) *Trigeminal neuralgia: its history and treatment.* Thomas. Springfield.

Storey J R, Calder C S, Hart D E, Potter D L (2001) Topiramate in migraine prevention; a double-blind, placebo-controlled study. *Headache* 41:968–975.

Stowell A (1970) Physiologic mechanisms and treatment of histaminic or petrosal neuralgia. *Headache* 9:187–194.

Sutherland J M, Hooper W D, Eadie M J, Tyrer J H (1974) Buccal absorption of ergotamine. *Journal of Neurology, Neurosurgery and Psychiatry* 37:1116–1120.

Swanson J W, Vick N A (1978) Basilar artery migraine: 12 patients, with an attack recorded electroencephalographically. *Neurology* 28:782–786.

Sydenham T (1848) On the affection called hysteria in women; and hypochondriasis in men. In: *The works of Thomas Sydenham MD.* Sydenham Society. London: 231–235.

Symon D N K, Russell G (1986) Abdominal migraine. A childhood syndrome defined. *Cephalalgia* 6:223–228.

Symonds C P (1956) A particular variety of headache. *Brain* 79:217–232.

Symonds C (1970) Migrainous variants. In: Symonds C (ed.) *Studies in neurology.* Oxford University Press. London: 191–199 (Reprinted from *Transactions of the Medical Society of London* [1951] 67: 237–).

Symonds J A (1858) Gulstonian lectures for 1858. On headache. *Medical Times and Gazette* 37:285–288; 393–396; 419–422.

Takeshima T, Takao Y, Urakami K, Nishakawa S, Takahashi K (1989) Muscle contraction headache and migraine. Platelet activation and plasma norepinephrine during the cold pressor test. *Cephalalgia* 9:7–13.

Tamin O (1860) *Etude et traitment de la péricranalgie.* Thesis. Paris.

Tanret C (1875) Sur la présence d'un nouvel alkaloide, l'ergotinine, dans la seigle ergoté. *Comptes Rendus de Acadamie des Science* 81:896–897.

Teed J L (1876) On migraine. *Journal of Nervous and Mental Diseases* 3:241–252.

Tepper S J, Sheftell F D, Bigal M E (2007) The patent foramen ovale—migraine question. *Neurological Science* 28:S118–S123.

Tflet-Hansen P (2006) A review of evidence-based medicine and meta-analytic reviews in migraine. *Cephalalgia* 26:1265–1274.

Thomas A (1889) *Contribution à l'etude de la migraine.* Thesis. Montpellier.

Thomas J J (1907) Migraine and hemianopsia. *Journal of Nervous and Mental Diseases* 34: 153–155.

Thomas L H (1887) *La migraine.* Delahaye & Lecrosnier. Paris.

Thompson A P (1932) A contribution to the study of intermittent headache. *Lancet* 220: 229–235.

Thompson D W (2007) *Aristotle's The history of animals.* eBooks@Adelaide. Adelaide.

Thompson R (1903) *The devils and evil spirits of Babylonia.* Luzac & Co. London.

Thompson W H (1894) Ergot in the treatment of periodic neuralgias. *Journal of Nervous and Mental Diseases* 21:124–126.

Thouret M (1776) Observation sur les vertus de l'Aimant. *Histoire de la Société Royale de Médecine:* 281–285.

Timme W (1926) General discussion. *British Medical Journal* 2:771–772.

Tissot S (1754) *L'inoculation justifiée.* Bousquet. Lausanne.

Tissot S A (1778–1780) *Traité des nerfs et de leurs maladies.* Vols. 1–4. Didot. Paris.

Todd J (1955) The Alice in Wonderland syndrome. *Canadian Medical Association Journal* 73:701–704.

Tournier-Lasserve E (1999) CACNA1A mutations. Hemiplegic migraine, episodic ataxia type 2, and the others. *Neurology* 53:3–4.

Trompoukis C, Vadikolias K (2007) The "Byzantine classification" of headache disorders. *Headache* 47:1063–1068.

Trousseau A (1868) *Lectures on clinical medicine.* Vol. 1. New Sydenham Society. London. (Translated Bazire P V).

Trovnik E, Stovner L J, Helde G, Sand T, Bovim G (2003) Prophylactic treatment of migraine with an angiotensin II receptor blocker: a randomized clinical trial. *Journal of the American Medical Association* 289:65–69.

Troxler F, Hoffman A (1957) Substitutionem am Ringsystem der Lysergsäure II. Alkylierung. *Helvetica Chimica Acta* 40:1721–1732.

Tubbs R S, Loukas M, Sjoha M M, Cohen-Gadol A A (2010) John Murray Carnochan (1817–1877): the first description of successful surgery for trigeminal neuralgia. *Journal of Neurosurgery* 112:199–201.

Tzanck M A (1928) Le traitment des migraines par le tartrate d'ergotamine. *Bulletin et mémoires de Societie médicale de Hopitaux Paris* 52:1057.

Tzanck M A (1931) Le traitment des migraines par le tartrate d'ergotamine. *Bulletin et mémoires de Societe médicale de Hopitaix Paris* 55:1663.

Ulrich V, Gervil M, Olesen J (2004) The relative influence of environment and genes in episodic tension-type headache. *Neurology* 62:2065–2069.

Van der Linden J A (1666) *De hemicrania menstrua. Historia et consilium.* Elsevirum. Lugundum Batavorum.

van Dongen P W J, de Groot A N J A (1995) History of ergot alkaloids from ergotism to ergometrine. *European Journal of Obstetrics and Gynecology and Reproductive Biology* 60:109–116.

Vane J R (1971) Inhibition of prostaglandin synthesis as a mechanism of action of aspirin-like drugs. *Nature* 231:232–234.

van Swieten G (1745) *Commentaria in Hermanni Boerhaave Aphorismos de cogniscendi et curandis morbis.* Vol. 2. Johannera & Harmanum Verbeek. Lugundi Batavorum.

Vaughan W (1825) *An essay on headachs, and on their cure.* Longman, Hurst, Rees, Orme, Brown & Green. London.

Volans G (1978) Migraine and drug absorption. *Clinical Pharmacokinetics* 3:313–318.

Ware J (1814) On the muscae volitantes of nervous persons. *Proceedings of the London Medico-Chirurgical Society* 5:255–277.

Warner J S (1997) Analgesic rebound as a cause of hemicrania continua. *Neurology* 48: 1540–1541.

Weatherhead G H (1835) *A treatise on headachs, their various causes, prevention, and cure.* Robson, Levey & Franklyn. London.

Weiller C, May A, Limmroth V, Jüptner M, Kaube H, Schayck R V, Coenen H H, Diener H C (1995) Brain stem activation in spontaneous human migraine attacks. *Nature Medicine* 1:658–660.

Weisenberg TH (1910) Cerebello-pontine tumor diagnosis for six years as tic douloureux: the syndrome of irritation of the ninth and twelfth cranial nerves. *Journal of the American Medical Association* 54:1600–1604.

Wepfer J J (1727) *Observationes medico-practicae de affectibus capitis internis et externis.* Ziegler. Schaffenhausen.

Wesley J (1858) *Primitive physic; or, an easy and natural method of curing most diseases.* Cyrus Stone. Boston.

Wessman M, Terwindt G M, Kaunisto M A, Palotie A, Ophoff R A (2007) Migraine: a complex genetic disorder. *Lancet Neurology* 6:521–532.

Whitty C W M (1953) Familial hemiplegic migraine. *Journal of Neurology, Neurosurgery and Psychiatry* 16:172–177

WHO Task Group on Selected Mycotoxins, Ochratoxins, Trichothecenes, and Ergot (1990) Selected mycotoxins: ochratoxins, trichothecenes, and ergot. http://www.inchem.org/documents/ehc/ehc/ehc105.htm

Whytt R (1768) Observations on the nature, causes, and cure of those disorders which are commonly called nervous, hypochondriac, or hysteric. In: Whytt R (ed.) *The works of Robert Whytt, MD.* Becket, DeHondt & Balfour. Edinburgh: 487–762.

Wilkinson J (1992) The medical history of John Calvin. *Journal of the Royal College of Physicians of Edinburgh* 22:368–383.

Wilkinson M, Isler H (1999) The pioneer woman's view of migraine: Elizabeth Garrett Anderson's thesis "Sur la migraine." *Cephalalgia* 19:3–15.

Wilks S (1866) Observations on the pathology of some of the diseases of the nervous system. *Guy's Hospital Reports* 12:157–244.

Wilks S (1869) Lectures on diseases of the nervous system. Hemicrania or sick-headache. *Medical Times and Gazette* 1:1–2.

Wilks S (1872) On sick headache. *British Medical Journal* 1:8–9.

Wilks S (1878) *Lectures on diseases of the nervous system.* Churchill. London.

Wilks S (1911) *Biographical reminisences.* Adlard & Son. London

Willis T (1670) *Pathologiae cerebri et nervosi generis specimen, in quo agitur de morbis convulsivis et de scurbuto studio.* Denielem Elzevirium. Amsterdam. Translated by Pordage S (1684) as Pathology of the brain and nervous stock: on convulsive diseases. In: Pordage S (ed.) *The remaining medical works of that famous and renowned physician Dr Thomas Willis of Christ Church in Oxford, and Sidley Professor of Natural Philosophy in that Famous University.* Dring, Harper, Leigh & Martyn. London: 1–89.

Willis T (1672) *De anima brutorum quae hominis vitalis ac sensitiva est.* (translated by Pordage S [1683] as *Two discourses concerning the soul of brutes*). Oxford. Davis. Translated version: London. Dring, Harper and Leigh.

Wilson S A K (1940) *Neurology.* Vols. 1 and 2. Arnold. London.

Witteridge G (1964) *The anatomical lectures of William Harvey.* Livingstone. Edinburgh. (Translated Witteridge G).

Woakes E (1868) On ergot of rye in the treatment of neuralgia. *British Medical Journal* 2: 350–361.

Wolff H G (1963) *Headache and other head pain.* 2nd ed. Oxford University Press. New York.

Wollaston H (1824) On semi-decussation of the optic nerves. *Philosophical Transactions* 114:222–231.

Woolhouse R (2007) *Locke: a biography.* Cambridge University Press. Cambridge.

Wright H G (1867) *Headaches: their causes and their cure.* Lindsay & Blakiston. Philadelphia.

Zayas V (2007) On headache tablets: headache incantations from Ur III (2113–2038 BC). *Medicine and Health* 90:46–47.

INDEX

Page numbers followed by *t* or *f* indicate tables or figures, respectively.

Haller, Albrecht von
  De partibus corporis humani sensilibus
    et irritabilibus by, 82
  seat of headache and, 24–25
  wine and, 121
Haly Abbas, 8, 56
Handfield-Jones, C., 27
Harris, Wilfred, 138, 186, 205*f*
  ciliary neuralgia of, 205–8, 212, 217, 269
  on cluster headache, 204–8, 211–12,
    216–17, 222
  on glossopharyngeal neuralgia, 263–64
  migrainous neuralgia of, 204–8, 211, 269
  Neuritis and Neuralgia by, 197–98, 204–8
  on trigeminal neuralgia, 245, 252,
    254–56, 262–63
Harvey, William, 114
headache. *See also specific types*
  classification, xiii, 3–17
    by Ad Hoc Committee on the
      Classification of Headache,
      15–16, 16*t*
    American Neurological Association's,
      15–16, 16*t*
    cranial neuralgias, 243
    diagnosis and, 14–15
    First International, 227
    International Headache Society's, 16,
      17*t*, 74, 197–98, 227, 235–36,
      241, 243
    migraine, xiii, 11–12, 12*t*, 14–15, 53,
      60, 73
    Murphy's, 12–13, 12*t*
    Second International, 227
    Sieveking's, 13, 13*t*
    Wolff and, 16
  in *De Anima Brutorum*, vii, 6, 7*f*, 23, 60,
    83, 107–8, 115–16, 159, 199–200
  growing knowledge of, 265–70
  history of, vii–viii, xi–xiv
  pre-1800, 35–56
  psychosomatic origin of, 229,
    232–39, 240
  resources on, viii–ix, xii–xiii
  scientific work on, vii–viii
  seat of
    in ancient world, 19–21
    Aretaeus and, 19–20
    defined, 19
    dura as, 20–21, 25, 29–30
    in early modern times, 22–24, 22*f*, 24*f*

  in 18th century, 24–26
  Galen and, 20–21, 23, 32
  Gowers and, 27–28, 28*f*
  Haller and, 24–25
  in medieval world, 21–22
  migraine, 33
  in 19th century, 26–29, 27*f*–28*f*
  pericranium as, 20–21, 23, 25, 29, 120
  in 20th century, 29–33, 31*f*–32*f*
  Wilks and, 27, 27*f*
  Willis and, 22–24
  Wolff and, 30–33, 31*f*–32*f*
  terminology, 4–11
  trigeminal nerve in, 33, 123–25, 128, 132
  types, xii
Headache and Other Head Pain (Wolff),
  30, 31*f*–32*f*, 140, 187–88
Heberden, William, 10, 26, 71–72, 123, 181
Heinicke, J. Christian, 85
hemicrania
  chronic paroxysmal, 197, 222–24
  continua, 197, 224–25
  crotaphos, 8
  in early modern times, 60, 63, 68–71
  in Greco-Roman medicine, 47–54
  Harvey and, 114
  insultus, 79
  in medieval medicine, 58–59
  menstrua, 154
  migraine and, xiii, 73–74, 78–80, 82,
    113–16, 118–19, 122–23, 132,
    157–60, 164, 168, 197
  origin of, 26
  sympathotonica, 130
  temporal muscle and, 21
  terminology, 4–10, 12–13, 12*t*, 73–74
  treatment of, 177–78
hemiopia, 94
hemiopsia, 94–95
hemlock, 258–59
heterocrania
  Aretaeus defining, 4, 20, 45–46,
    113, 244
  in Greco-Roman medicine, 45–46, 48
  trigeminal neuralgia as, 244
Hildegard of Bingen, 78, 79*f*
Hippocrates, 3, 40–41, 77, 84–85
histamine, 210, 212, 218
The History of Animals (Aristotle), 40
Hoffman, Frederick (Friedrich), 25, 68–69
homonymous hemianopia, 88

Horton, Bayard, 208–12, 209*f*, 218
humoral pathology
    in Greco-Roman medicine, 46–47,
        50–56
    in medieval world, 56–58
    Whytt and, 119
    Willis and, 61, 64–65
Hunt, Thomas, 187
Hunter, John, 251
Hurst, Arthur, 187
hydrocephalus, 42

iatrochemists, 61, 117–18
ignition hypothesis, 257
indomethacin, 223–24
infratentorial structures, 32
L'inoculation justifée (Tissot), 81
International Headache Society
    classification by, 16, 17*t*, 74, 197–98,
        227, 235–36, 241, 243
    cranial neuralgias and, 243
    tension-type headache and, 227,
        235–36, 241
intracranial arteries, 141
irisalgia, 124
irritability, 24–25
ischemic damage, 105–6
Isis, 38
isovaleric acid, 179
Israel, ancient, 39

Jaccoud, Sigismond, 131, 132*f*, 133–34,
    136, 163
Jackson, John Hughlings, 135–36,
    151–52, 268
James, Robert, 3–4, 8–9
Jellife, S. E., 138, 186
Jenyns, Sarah, 75
Julian the Apostate, 50

Labarraque, Henri, 182–83
lamotrigine, 192, 263
Lance, James, 144
Lashley, K. S., 148
Latham, Peter Wallwork, 95, 134–35,
    138, 163
Leão, Aristides, 144, 148–50
Lectures on Diseases of the Nervous System
    (Wilks), 99
Lennox, W. G., 153
Le Pois, Charles, 22, 22*f*, 79, 83

migraine pathophysiology and, 114–15
    on prevention, 178
Le Pois, Nicolas, 120
Lewis, W., 25, 68
Lewy, Frederick, 245
Leyton, Nevil, 193
ligation, of arteries, 195
lisinopril, 194
lithium, 221
Liveing, Edward
    on attack prevention, 184–85
    On Megrim, Sick-Headache and Some
        Allied Disorders by, 95–98, 97*f*, 135,
        163, 184
    migraine and, 95–98, 96*f*–97*f*, 128,
        135–37, 163
Locke, John, 246–50, 257–58
Locock, Charles, 162, 185
long-term continuing management,
    in attack prevention, 157
Lorry, A. C., 26
Lower, Richard, 249
Luther, Martin, 59

magical papyri, 37–38
magnesium dicitrate, 194
Maimonides, Moses, 57–58
A Manual of Diseases of the Nervous System
    (Gowers), 100, 137, 165, 186
    seat of headache in, 27–28, 28*f*
    trigeminal neuralgia in, 255
Mapletoft, Dr., 247–48
Marcus Aurelius, 74
Marduk, 36
Marlborough, Duke of
    (John Churchill), 75–77
Martin, Prosper, 123, 162
Mearse, J., 181
Medical Aphorisms (Maimonides), 57
Medical Dictionary (James), 3–4, 8–9
Medicina (Fernel), 5, 58
medieval world
    Arabian physicians in, 56–59,
        177–78, 245
    cephalea in, 58–59
    Fernel in, 5, 21, 58–59, 178
    hemicrania in, 58–59
    Maimonides in, 57–58
    migraine in, 78, 79*f*, 113–14, 159
    seat of headache in, 21–22
    treatment in, 57, 159

serotonin
    in biochemical studies of
        tension-type headache, 236
    in circulating serotonin hypothesis, 145
    drugs affecting, 188–90, 240
    in migraine pathophysiology, 142,
        144–46, 149
sertraline, 240
serum, 63–64
Seven Books (Paul of Aegina), 5
shaqhiqheh (recurrent unilateral
        headache), 5, 56
Shuldham, E. B., 73
sick headache, 95, 151. *See also* migraine
Sicuteri, Federigo, 144–45
Sieveking, Edward, 13, 13*t*, 73, 151
Sluder, G., 213
Socrates, 39–40, 259
soda (simple nonrecurrent headache), 5
sodium valproate, 192
Soranus of Ephesus, 5, 120
spinal manipulation, 195
sporadic ergotism, 173
status migrainosus, 109
steroids, 220
stilboestrol, 193
Stoll, Arthur, 169
strategically timed preventive
        intervention, 157
substance P, 147
subtypes, of migraine, 103–9
sumatriptan, 174, 219
SUNCT/SUNA syndrome, 197, 224
superior sagittal sinus, 31
supernatural causes
    in ancient Egypt, 38–39
    in ancient Greece, 39–41
    in Babylonia, 36
    Celsus and, 43
    protective charms and, 40, 55–56
supratentorial structures, 30, 32
Sydenham, Thomas, 8, 68, 247, 258
Symonds, Charles, 13, 210, 213
Symonds, J. C., 27
sympathy, 120–21, 123–24, 254
System of Medicine (Reynolds), 128

Talmud, 58
Tanret, C., 190
Teed, J. L., 136
Tefrut (goddess), 38

teichopsia (town-wall vision), 95
temporal muscle, *hemicrania* and, 21
tension
    defined, 228–29, 232–34
    emotional, 232–33
    muscle, 232–39
tension-type headache
    biochemical studies of, 236–38
    cervicogenic headache and, 241–42
    defined, 228–32
    genetic investigations of, 236
    growing knowledge of, 269
    history of, 228–32
    International Headache Society
        and, 227, 235–36, 241
    mechanism, 232–39
    muscle tension aspects, 232–39
    pain pathway studies, 238–39
    physical therapy for, 240
    prevalence of, 227
    psychological aspects, 229, 232–39, 240
    severity of, 228
    subdivision of, 227
    treatment, 239–41
    Wolff and, 230, 233–35
thalamic syndrome, 29
Thomas, Auguste, 186
Thomas, Louis Hyacinthe, 102, 164–65
Thompson, R., 35–36
Thompson, W. H., 169
tic douloureux. *See* trigeminal neuralgia
Tissot, Samuel
    on attack prevention, 179–80
    Avis au peuple sur sa sante by, 81–82
    Caelius Aurelianus and, 120
    L'inoculation justifée by, 81
    migraine and, 10, 11*f*, 25, 72, 80–84,
        90–91, 120–22, 161, 179–80
    L'onanisme by, 82
    Traité des nerfs by, 10, 11*f*, 72, 120
tizanidine, 240
Todd, J., 106–7
Todd, Robert Bentley, 184
topiramate, 192
Traité des nerfs (Tissot), 10, 11*f*, 72, 120
trapezius muscle, 141
treatment
    in ancient world, 39–41, 158–59
    by Aretaeus, 19–20, 158
    Babylonian, 35–36
    by Celsus, 3–4, 41–43

on prevention, 179
treatment recommended by, 160
on trigeminal neuralgia, 252, 258
Wesley, John, 160
White, W. A., 138, 186
Whitty, Charles, 105
*WHO Monographs on Selected
    Medicinal Plants*, 179
Whytt, Robert, 26, 119, 201
Wilks, Samuel
    *Lectures on Diseases of the
        Nervous System* by, 99
    migraine and, 98–99, 98*f*, 133
    seat of headache and, 27, 27*f*
Willis, Thomas. *See also De Anima
        Brutorum*
    on cluster headache, 199–200, 216
    in early modern times, vii, 6–8, 6*f*–7*f*,
        15, 22–24, 60–68
    Galen and, 60–61
    on genetics, 150
    humoral pathology and, 61, 64–65
    as iatrochemist, 61, 117–18
    Locke and, 249–50
    migraine and, 79–80, 113, 115–18,
        159–60

Pathologiae Cerebri by, 61
    on prevention, 178–79
    seat of headache and, 22–24
    traditional thought and, 113
Wilson, Kinnier, 138
wine, 41, 121
Woakes, Edward, 166–70
Wolff, Harold
    classification and, 16
    cluster headache and, 213
    ergot and, 169
    Headache and Other Head Pain by, 30,
        31*f*–32*f*, 140, 187–88
    migraine pathophysiology and, 140–44,
        149, 235, 239
    seat of headache and, 30–33, 31*f*–32*f*
    tension-type headache and, 230,
        233–35
Wollaston, William Hyde, 88
Wriothesley, Elizabeth. *See* Northumberland,
        Countess of

Zeus, 39
zolmitriptan, 219